T0248983

Dyslipidemia Essentials

Dyslipidemia Essentials

Edited by **Donna Thompson**

FOSTER
ACADEMICS

New Jersey

Published by Foster Academics,
61 Van Reypen Street,
Jersey City, NJ 07306, USA
www.fosteracademics.com

Dyslipidemia Essentials
Edited by Donna Thompson

© 2015 Foster Academics

International Standard Book Number: 978-1-63242-120-3 (Hardback)

This book contains information obtained from authentic and highly regarded sources. Copyright for all individual chapters remain with the respective authors as indicated. A wide variety of references are listed. Permission and sources are indicated; for detailed attributions, please refer to the permissions page. Reasonable efforts have been made to publish reliable data and information, but the authors, editors and publisher cannot assume any responsibility for the validity of all materials or the consequences of their use.

The publisher's policy is to use permanent paper from mills that operate a sustainable forestry policy. Furthermore, the publisher ensures that the text paper and cover boards used have met acceptable environmental accreditation standards.

Trademark Notice: Registered trademark of products or corporate names are used only for explanation and identification without intent to infringe.

Printed in the United States of America.

Contents

Preface

Dyslipidemia has intricate physiopathology, often due to genetic, diet and lifestyle factors. It has various adverse impacts, especially in the development of chronic non-communicable diseases. Important ethnic differences exist due to the prevalence and types of lipid ailment, while elevated serum total and LDL-cholesterol are the main concerns in the developed countries, in other countries hypertriglyceridemia and low HDL-cholesterol are more widespread. The growing cases of obesity, changes in lifestyle and environmental factors will make dyslipidemia a global medical and public health peril, not only for adults but also for children. Various experimental and clinical researches are going on related to the basic mechanisms and treatment of dyslipidemia. This book will deliver an overview of dyslipidemia from distinct facets of physiopathology, ethnic differences, genetics and role in metabolic syndrome.

The researches compiled throughout the book are authentic and of high quality, combining several disciplines and from very diverse regions from around the world. Drawing on the contributions of many researchers from diverse countries, the book's objective is to provide the readers with the latest achievements in the area of research. This book will surely be a source of knowledge to all interested and researching the field.

In the end, I would like to express my deep sense of gratitude to all the authors for meeting the set deadlines in completing and submitting their research chapters. I would also like to thank the publisher for the support offered to us throughout the course of the book. Finally, I extend my sincere thanks to my family for being a constant source of inspiration and encouragement.

Editor

Obesity Related Lipid Profile and Altered Insulin Incretion in Adolescent with Policystic Ovary Syndrome

Annamaria Fulghesu and Roberta Magnini
Department of Obstetrics and Gynecology, University of Cagliari, Cagliari, Italy

1. Introduction

Polycystic ovary syndrome (PCOS) is the most common female endocrine disorder, present in 5 – 7% of women of reproductive age. The diagnosis of PCOS was made according to Rotterdam criteria in presence of at least two of the following: 1) oligomenorrhea and/or anovulation; 2) hyperandrogenism (clinical and/or biochemical); 3) polycystic ovaries with the exclusion of other etiologies (1). The disorder is characterized by irregular menstrual cycle, chronic anovulation and hyperandrogenism. Women with PCOS demonstrate marked clinical heterogeneity: the commonly associated features of hirsutism, acne, polycystic-appearing ovaries, obesity and acanthosis nigricans are neither uniform nor universal (2-3). In time the disorder may lead to onset of hyperinsulinemia, insulin resistance, gestational diabetes, early onset of type 2 diabetes mellitus (DM), dyslipidemia and cardiovascular disease (CVD) (4-5).

PCOS is characterized by a complex physiology implicating an interaction with environmental and genetic factors, resulting in a broad spectrum of reproductive and metabolic disorders. (6-7) Adult females with PCOS may be at increased risk for atherosclerotic cardiovascular disease (CVD) due to increased prevalence of obesity and central adiposity as well as to hypertension, hyperinsulinemia, type 2 DM, and dyslipidemia in these patients (8).The prevalence of obesity and consequently the presence of metabolic abnormalities reported in Italian and American published studies differs considerably, underlining the presence of important ethnic differences. (9, 10, 11, 12).

A percentage ranging from 30-75% of women with PCOS are obese, European women generally weighing less than their American counterparts (20,21). Hyperinsulemia and/or insulin resistance (IR) are frequently manifested in obese, and to a lesser extent (50%) in lean, PCOS patients (3, 13, 14). Hyperandrogenaemia, hyperinsulemia and obesity are considered as risk factors for the development of hypertension and dyslipidemia, diabetes mellitus and coronary disease in PCOS (15-16). The causes of metabolic disorders in PCOS remain to be clarified, but include obesity-related IR, an intrinsic abnormality of postreceptor insulin signaling (e.g. excess serine phosphorylation), and abnormal insulin secretion. On the other hand, increased resistance to insulin is a hallmark of the onset of normal pubertal development with natural to pre-pubertal values at the end of puberty in non-obese subjects. Consequently, in early adolescence a physiological resistance to insulin should be taken into account (12).

Dyslipidemia in PCOS is frequently manifested and is characterized by elevated plasma levels of low- density lipoproteins (LDL), very-low-density lipoproteins (VLDL) and triglycerides with concomitantly reduced concentration of high-density lipoproteins (HDL) in obese subjects (17, 18). A decrease in HDL, rise in triglyceride, VLDL, and LDL levels, as well as qualitative disorders of the LDL have all been described in young and adult PCOS (19). Moreover, recent data have shown a higher prevalence of metabolic syndrome in adolescent PCOS compared to controls (20) as well as an early impairment of endothelial structure and function even in non-dyslipidemic subjects with PCOS syndrome (21). Nevertheless, metabolic disorders in PCOS have not been extensively studied in the adolescent population. Several studies have shown how both lean and obese adolescents with PCOS appear to present an increased risk of both metabolic disorders and impaired glucose tolerance and diabetes (22), similar to their adult counterparts. A previous study carried out by our group demonstrated that the Italian young PCOS population is characterized by a high incidence of insulin alterations also in presence of normal weight and normal peripheral insulin resistance (12). Although the prevalence of dyslipidemia differs between PCOS subjects and young healthy girls, it however remains to be clarified whether dissimilarities in dyslipidemia occur in relation only to BMI or also to alterations to the insulinmetabolism and/or hyperandrogenemia.

Carmina recently demonstrated that MBS in women with PCOS is less common in Southern Italy compared to rates reported in the USA, the former reaching only 8.2% compared to a prevalence of 43-46% reported by US authors (23). The prevalence of MBS in the adult Italian PCOS population is higher than in control population matched for BMI, suggesting that body weight may be only in part responsible for this metabolic disorder (24).

Although few studies have investigated the latter condition in adolescents, it could prove to be of considerable importance in view of the health implications involved, requiring medical counseling to implement an adequate change in lifestyle. Likewise, obesity rate in adolescent PCOS subjects differs between Europe and the USA. In Sardinia, the incidence of obesity is lower than throughout the rest of Italy, with only 3-4% of high school female population presenting a BMI >25 (25). A combination of genetic factors, different lifestyle and diet are likely involved. In view therefore of the regional peculiarity, the patient population attending our Clinic was deemed to be of interest.

Therefore it is important to understand the relationship between lipid pattern and BMI, hyperinsulinemia and/or insulin resistance and circulating androgens in adolescent PCOS. In a study carried out in July 2005 to the Adolescent Center for gynecological diseases of the Department of Obstetrics and Gynecology, University of Cagliari, San Giovanni di Dio Hospital seventy-one adolescent (age 13-18) subjects affected by PCOS were recruited for this study. On the basis of the various aspects linking PCOS dyslipidemia and CVD risk, the present study was designed to investigate the influence of BMI and insulin metabolism derangement on lipid levels. All subjects were screened for other causes of hyperandrogenism, such as androgen secreting tumors and congenital adrenal hyperplasia (tested by evaluation of 17- dydroxyprogesterone). All subjects were euthyroid and devoid of hyperprolactinemia, diabetes mellitus and cardiovascular disease. No subjects had taken hormonal contraceptives or other type of medication or been on a diet that may have affected lipid profile, carbohydrate metabolism or insulin levels for at least 3 months preceding the study. No subjects were either smokers or drinkers. No subjects practiced sports on a regular basis (3 or more 20-min sessions of aerobic exercise per week).

These patients were linked with a control group consisting of healthy patients referred to the Adolescent centre for ultrasound screening of ovarian disease.

Control subjects and PCOS were studied 5 to 8 days following menstrual bleeding, which was progestin-induced in amenorrhoic patients. All patients were studied at least 15 days following Medrossi-Progesteron-Acetate administration (MAP 10 mg for 5 days). At the time of admittance to the study the presence of a dominant follicle, recent ovulation, or luteal phase was excluded by ultrasound examination and serum P evaluation. Height and weight were measured on the morning of testing. Waist and hip circumference were measured as previously referred. Blood pressure was measured in the second position and in the right arm (26) after 15 minutes resting.The hormonal study (after 12 hours overnight) included baseline plasma determination of LH, FSH, Estradiol (E2), Androstenedione (A), Testosterone (T), Dehydroepiandrosteronesulphate (DHEAS), 17hydroxyprogesterone (17-OHP) and Sex-hormone-binding globulin (SHBG). Lipid assay was performed to measure total cholesterol level, high-density lipoprotein cholesterol level (HDL), low-density lipoprotein cholesterol level (LDL) and triglyceride level. Homocysteine levels were also determined.

Adolescents meeting three or more of the following criteria were diagnosed with MBS: waist circumference of at least 90th percentile for age and gender; systolic or diastolic blood pressure at least 90th percentile for age, height and gender; fasting TG at least 110mg/dl (90th percentile for age); fasting HDL not exceeding 40mg/dl (10th percentile for age); and fasting glucose at least 110mg/dl.

Subsequently, patients underwent a 75-g oral glucose tolerance test (OGTT). Insulin, C-peptide, and glucose serum concentrations were analyzed prior to (time 0) and 30, 60, 90, 120 and 180 min after oral glucose load. A normal glycemic response to OGTT was defined according to the criteria of the National Diabetes Data Group (27). Insulin, C-peptide and glucose response to glucose load were expressed as area below the curve (AUC), calculated according to the trapezoidal rule. The homeostatic index of IR (HOMA) was calculated as follows: HOMA = [fasting insulin (μU/ml) x fasting glucose (mmol/L/22, 5)]. (28) The body mass index (BMI) was calculated according to the following formula: body weight in kilograms/ height in m2. Normal weight was considered as $18 \leq BMI \geq 25$. The degree of hirsutism was quantified using Ferriman and Gallwey (F-G) score (28).

No differences were observed with regard to the presence of overweight and obese subjects between PCOS and controls (30% vs. 23%); a similar finding was obtained also for waist measurement and WHR, confirming that obesity is not a common finding in young PCOS subjects in the population studied.Moreover, no subjects affected by metabolic Syndrome or diabetes either among PCOS or in the control group were detected. No differences were revealed in lipid levels between PCOS and controls. In addition, no differences were reported for any of the fasting metabolic parameters (i.e. Glucose fasting insulin, HOMA ratio), whilst a higher insulin response under OGTT was obtained for PCOS subjects. On the other hand, statistical correlations clearly demonstrated the influence produced by BMI and waist measurement on HDL, triglyceride and LDL levels. However, dividing the population into tertiles for BMI and waist measurement significant differences were revealed for both HDL and LDL levels in lean overweight and obese subjects and in relation to the presence of visceral fat.The above features have also been reported by several authors carrying out studies on young subjects.

Glueck published a study regarding PCOS and regular cycling adolescents in USA demonstrating a higher prevalence of obesity and dyslipidemia in PCOS.

However, when subjects were matched one-by-one for BMI and age, differences in lipids were no longer significant. In a recent paper on young obese subjects Shroff failed to demonstrate any difference in lipid as well as traditional CV factors in PCOS and control populations, but demonstrated a higher BMI in subjects presenting subclincal coronary atherosclerosis (CAC) (10). In young subjects from southern Italy, Orio demonstrated normal lipid levels in lean PCOS even in the presence of increased dimensions of heart ventricles.The above findings all seem to indicate that rather than being an insulin-correlated factor BMI may well be implicated in lipid alteration. On the other hand, the presence of increased waist measurements in PCOS population suggests that the presence of visceral fat may represent an additional risk factor, independent from BMI in PCOS. The influence of insulin on lipid profile was also determined.

Indeed, to date very few authors have investigated this aspect: Mather found a significant increase in traditional CV risk factors in PCOS women with fasting hyperinsulinemia in respect to their normoinsulinemic counterparts; this difference persisted when BMI was included as covariate. (29) Through reduction of hyperinsulinemia by means of metformin treatment Banazewska obtained a significant increase of HDL and reduction of triglycerides in a group of 43 adult PCOS. Our group recently published a paper on the peculiar insulin derangement observed in a population of normal weight young PCOS demonstrating a low incidence of insulin resistance but high incidence of hyperinsulinemia under OGTT (30). This peculiar metabolic alteration was confirmed in the present sample, thus allowing the separation of hyperinsulinemia from peripheral insulin resistance in data analysis.

Ibanez et al. also demonstrated higher serum insulin levels after OGTT with normal insulin sensitivity in a population of adolescent girls with PCOS. The causes underlying the increased response of β-cells in these subjects are, as yet, unknown. It is not clear whether high levels of insulin necessarily indicate the presence of a disorder although it may be hypothesized that adaptation to the chronic risk of hypoglycemia in hyperinsulinemic subjects could lead to IR after some time. Moreover, our group recently demonstrated that a normal HOMA score is not sufficient to exclude earlymetabolic abnormalities such as hyperinsulinemia in young lean PCOS subjects. Hyperinsulinemia per se could contribute toward onset of hyperandrogenism independently of peripheral IR.(12)

In this study was found a significant negative correlation between HDL and fasting insulin and HOMA, but this correlation was no longer significant when the influence of BMI was excluded, whereas insulin AUC was not related to any lipid parameters.

Furthermore, although the PCOS sample studied here was divided into tertiles on the basis of both insulin resistance and insulin AUC levels, the data obtained clearly indicate the failure to detect any relationship between insulin levels and lipid profile. Nevertheless, surprisingly a positive correlation was observed between A levels and HDL and a negative correlation between A and triglycerides. Reports present in literature did not afford any explanation for this result. A negative effect of A on HDL levels has previously been reported in males to whom A supplements had been administered (31). Moreover, exogenous T is reported to influence negatively HDL via hepatic lipase (HL) (31) an enzyme that increases the clearance of HDL. Less is known about the regulation of HDL by endogenally-derived androgens. A study performed in women with PCOS was not able to demonstrate any correlation between T and HDL. Considerable controversy exists as to the effect of androgens on lipoprotein lipase (LPL) activity.

In obese women LPL activity correlated positively with plasma free testosterone (32), whereas in women with PCOS a correlation with LPL activity was demonstrated.

Other authors have attributed to coexisting (29) insulin resistance the negative effect of androgen observed on lipid profile. In this case, the low incidence of insulin resistant subjects in a population may explain this unexpected result.

In conclusion, no lipid differences were revealed between our population of adolescent PCOS from southern Italy and controls.

Anthropometric characteristics (BMI, waist measurement and WHR) are the main parameters correlated to lipid derangement, confirming the importance of treating obesity at an early age to prevent onset of complex metabolic syndromes in the future. The latter may be of particular importance in PCOS populations in which insulin alterations (hyperinsulinemia and insulin resistance) are well known peculiarities potentially capable of influencing the long-term evolution of this endocrine disorder towards CVD and diabetes mellitus. A targeted support program should be set up for these young patients aimed at altering life style with the specific aim of reducing BMI and preventing onset of dyslipidemia.

	PCOS (n°71)	CONTROLLI (n°94)	P
Age (years) (M±ES) (range 13-19)	18,61 ± 0,4	18,10 ± 0,38	NS
BMI (kg\m²) (M±ES)	23,97 ± 0,72	22,56 ± 0,50	NS
Overweight (BMI 25 - 29) (%)	10%	11%	
Obesity (BMI > 29) (%)	20%	13%	
Waist (cm) (M±ES)	78,60 ± 1,79	75,56 ± 1,18	NS
WHR (M±ES)	0,77 ± 0	0,77 ± 0	NS
Hirsutism (score F&G) (M±ES)	11,24 ± 0,67	6,7 ± 0,45	0,005°
LH (IU/L)(M±ES)	5,21 ± 0,55	4,19 ± 0,36	NS
FSH (IU/L)(M±ES)	6,42 ± 0,63	5,96 ± 0,19	NS
E_2 (pmol/L)(M±ES)	129,30 ± 20,58	136,81 ± 13,25	NS
A (nmol/L)(M±ES)	0,08 ± 0	0,05 ± 0	0,005°
Tot T(nmol/L)(M±ES)	0,02 ± 0	0,01 ± 0	0,005°
17OHP (ng/mL)(M±ES)	1,49 ± 0,18	1,18 ± 0,07	NS
DHEAS (µmol/L)(M±ES)	2,05 ± 0,12	1,6 ± 0,09	NS
SHBG (nmol/L)(M±ES)	65,83 ± 4,54	71,18 ± 3,35	NS

°P < 0,05

Table 1. Shows the clinical and hormonal characteristics of PCOS population vs. Control group. No significant differences were revealed in age, body weight, waist and WHR between PCOS and control group. Likewise, no differences were observed in the incidence of overweight or obesity in the two groups. As expected, the prevalence of hirsutism and circulating androgen levels were higher amongst PCOS.

	PCOS (n° 71)	CONTROLLI (n°94)	P
Fasting Glucose (mmol/L)(M±ES)	81,13 ± 0,65	88,00 ± 3,27	NS
Fasting Insulin (pmol/L)(M±ES)	119,98 ± 6,14	96,68 ± 4,73	NS
HOMA (M±ES)	61,02 ± 3,09	57,81 ± 2,41	NS
I-AUC 180 min (UI/ml)(M±ES)	21069 ± 978,39	16578 ± 729,37	0,05°
Cholesterol (mg/dl)(M±ES)	166,48 ± 3,53	169,51 ± 2,62	NS
HDL-Cholesterol (mg/dl)(M±ES)	54,26 ± 1,44	51,25 ± 0,89	NS
LDL-Cholesterol (mg/dl)(M±ES)	96,78 ± 3,08	104,55 ± 2,34	NS
Cholesterol/ HDL (mg/dl)(M±ES)	3,16 ± 0,09	3,37 ± 0,07	NS
Triglycerides (mg/dl)(M±ES)	73,91 ± 3,75	78,35 ± 3,86	NS
Homocysteine (μmol/L) (M±ES)	8,16 ± 0,20	7,68 ± 0,25	NS
PCR (M±ES)	2,04 ± 0,36	0,89 ± 0,11	NS

° $P < 0,05$

Table 2. Reports the metabolic features of PCOS and control group. Fasting metabolic indexes detected for glucose, insulin and HOMA were similar between the two groups. On the contrary, insulin secretion after glucose load (I-AUC) was significantly higher in PCOS subjects. Total cholesterol, HDL, LDL, triglycerides and homocysteine levels did not differ between PCOS and control groups

	Cholesterol	LDL-Cholesterol	HDL-Cholesterol	Triglycerides
BMI (kg\m²)	R = 0,0727	R = 0,2579 ·	R = - 0,404 ▪	R = 0,1576
WAIST (cm)	R = 0,0869	R = 0,2960 ·	R = - 0,5934 ▪	R = 0,1704
WHR (cm)	R = 0,1645	R = 0,2872 ·	R = - 0,1853	R = 0,1362
A (nmol/L)	R = 0,0136	R = - 0,0523	R = 0,3705 ▪	R = -0,2948 ·
Tot T (nmol/L)	R = - 0,1016	R = - 0,0948	R = 0,0012	R = - 0,0157
FSH (mIU/L)	R = - 0,0134	R = - 0,0143	R = 0,0623	R = - 0,0687
E2(pmol/L)	R = - 0,1011	R = - 0,0895	R = 0,0698	R = - 0,1984
DHEAS (μmol/L)	R = - 0,0498	R = - 0,0022	R = - 0,0447	R = - 0,0441
HOMA	R = 0,0762	R = 0,1770	R = -0,3335	R = - 0,0214
I-AUC 180 min(UI/ml)	R = - 0,0098	R = - 0,0272	R = - 0,0701	R = - 0,0287
SHBG (nmol/L)	R = - 0,0689	R = - 0,1514	R = 0,1102	R = 0,1013
17OHP (nmol/L)	R = 0,0418	R = 0,0582	R = 0,0854	R = - 0,1720
Homocysteine (μmol/L)	R = - 0,0670	R = - 0,0786	R = 0,0463	R = - 0,1108 ▪
Fasting Glucose	R = 0,0049	R = 0,0260	R = -0,0829	R = 0,0643
Fasting Insulin	R = 0,0586	R = 0,1557	R = -0,3314	R = -0,0174

P < 0,05
P < 0,01
P < 0,001

Table 3. Illustrates linear regression relationship featured between lipid and physical, hormonal and metabolic parameters. Total cholesterol levels were significantly related to WHR but not to other antropometric parameters. On analyzing cholesterol fractions LDL levels were found to correlate positively with BMI, Waist, WHR and HOMA but not with I-AUC. HDL results correlated in a markedly negative manner with the same physical parameters as BMI, WHR and waist circumference. Moreover, HDL was negatively correlated with both fasting insulin and HOMA but not I-AUC. Finally, HDL was positively correlated with circulating A and negatively with circulating T levels.
Triglycerides appeared to correlate positively with BMI, Waist and WHR, and negatively with A levels. Homocysteine levels correlated positively with plasma triglyceride content. In view of the potential capacity of BMI to affect insulin sensitivity, conditional regression analysis was performed on HOMA and lipid assays to exclude any possible influence of BMI: HOMA resulted as being no longer correlated with any lipid parameter.To determine whether lipid alterations were primarily caused by increased BMI, lipid assay was repeated stratifying the population into 3 weight categories: normal weight, overweight and obese, and waist measurements were classified (normal and excessive).

BMI (kg\m²)

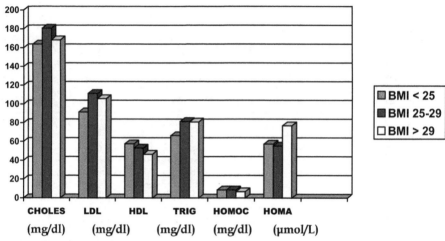

P < 0,05 LDL BMI < 25 VS BMI 25-29
P < 0,05 LDL BMI < 25 VS BMI > 29
P < 0,05 HDL BMI < 25 VS BMI > 29

WAIST (cm)

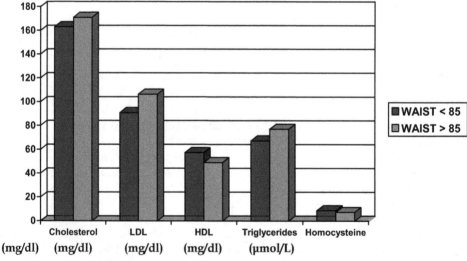

P < 0,05 LDL WAIST < 85 VS LDL WAIST > 85
P < 0,05 HDL WAIST <85 VS HDL WAIST > 85

Fig. 1. Shows the lipid levels in relation to the BMI and the waist of PCOS group.Normal weight and normal waist subjects featured lower LDL and Higher HDL compared to increased waist overweight or obese counterparts. On the other hand, in order to evaluate the influence of metabolic alteration subjects were also stratified on the basis of both HOMA and Insulin AUC values (fig.2).

HOMA

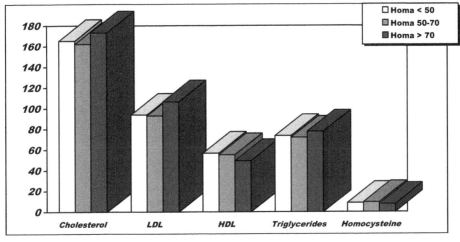

(mg/dl)   (mg/dl)   (mg/dl)   (mg/dl)   (µmol/L)

I-AUC (UI/ml)

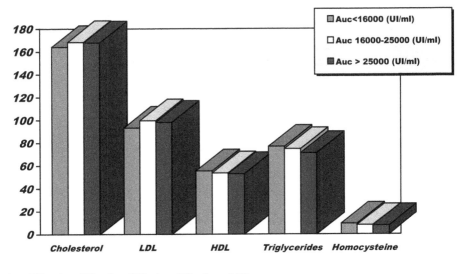

(mg/dl)   (mg/dl)   (mg/dl)   (mg/dl)   (µmol/L)

Fig. 2. Shows lipid levels in subjects divided into tertiles for both HOMA and Insulin AUC levels. Similar lipid values were demonstrated in all subjects.

	Cholesterol	LDL-Cholesterol	HDL-Cholesterol	Triglycerides
BMI (kg\m²)	R = 0,0800	R = - 0,0017	R = - 0,4762▪	R = 0,6962
WAIST (cm)	R = 0,1410	R = 0,0753	R = - 0,4253▪	R = 0,6765
WHR (cm)	R = 0,0326	R = - 0,1535	R = - 0,1878	R = 0,4262
A (nmol/L)	R = - 0,1921	R = - 0,0280	R = - 0,1845	R = 0,0007
Tot T (nmol/L)	R = - 0,3425	R = - 0,4544▪	R = - 0,1377	R = 0,3692
FSH (IU/L)	R = 0,3094	R = 0,3909▪	R = 0,3711▪	R = - 0,1603
E2(pmol/L)	R = 0,0150	R = 0,0124	R = - 0,0264	R = - 0,0876
DHEAS (µmol/L)	R = 0,1230	R = 0,1925	R = - 0,1793	R = 0,2206
SHBG (nmol/L)	R = - 0,2226	R = - 0,2834	R = 0,0655	R = - 0,0942
17OHP (nmol/L)	R = - 0,0925	R = - 0,0586	R = 0,1667	R = - 0,3703▪
HOMA	R = 0,4724	R = 0,5140	R = 0,2293	R = - 0,0123
I-AUC 180 min(UI/ml)	R = - 0,0021	R = 0,0331	R = - 0,3391	R = 0,2882
Homocysteine (µmol/L)	R = 0,2148	R = 0,1214	R = - 0,2604	R = 0,5656▪
Fasting Glucose	R = 0,0440	R = 0,1325	R = - 0,1952	R = - 0,0396
Fasting Insulin	R = 0,1226	R = 0,1315	R = 0,0435	R = 0,0972

P < 0,05
P < 0,01
P < 0,001

Table 4. Linear relationships between lipid assays and phisical endocrine and metabolic parameters in CONTROLS.

	Cholesterol	LDL-Cholesterol	HDL-Cholesterol	Triglycerides
BMI (kg\m²)	R = 0,1058	R = 0,2252	R = - 0,3930	R = 0,2933
WAIST (cm)	R = 0,1298	R = 0,2624	R = -0,3756	R = 0,2856
WHR (cm)	R = 0,2174	R = 0,3039	R = - 0,1924	R = 0,2063
E2(pmol/L)	R = - 0,0912	R = - 0,0912	R = 0,0541	R = - 0,1495
A (nmol/L)	R = - 0,0401	R = - 0,0953	R = 0,2933	R = -0,2400
Tot T (nmol/L)	R = - 0,1848	R = - 0,2191	R = 0,0181	R = 0,0085
SHBG (nmol/L)	R = - 0,1260	R = -0,1973	R = 0,1038	R = 0,0368
Fasting Glucose	R = 0,0107	R = 0.0800	R = - 0,1425	R = -0,0092
Fasting Insulin	R = 0,0773	R = 0,1239	R = - 0,1960	R = 0,0109
HOMA	R = 0,1349	R = 0,2269	R = - 0,2800▪	R = 0,0021
I-AUC 180 min(UI/ml)	R = 0,0324	R = 0,0550	R = - 0,0930	R = 0,0123
Homocysteine (µmol/L)	R = 0,0764	R = 0,0209	R = - 0,0656	R = 0,2863▪

P < 0,05
P < 0,01
P < 0,001

Table 5. Linear relationships between lipid assays and phisical endocrine and metabolic parameters in all patients.

2. References

[1] The Rotterdam ESHRE/ASRM sponsored PCOS consensus workshop group. Revised 2003 consesus on diagnostic criteria and long-term health risks related to polycystic ovary syndrome (PCOS). Human Reproduction 19: 41,47

[2] Hacihanefioglou B. Polycystic ovary syndrome nomenclature: chaos? Fertility and Sterility 2000 73, 1261-1262.2.

[3] Ancien P, Quereda F, Matallin P, Villarroya E, Lopez-Fernandez JA, Ancien M, Mauri M, Alfayate R. Insulin, androgens and obesity in women with and without Policystic ovary syndrome: a heterogeneous group of disorders. Fertility and Sterility 1999 72, 32-40

[4] Franks S. Policystic ovary syndrome. The New England Journal of Medicine 1995 333: 853-861

[5] Ehrmann DA, Barnes RB, Rosenfield RI, Cavaghan MK, Imperial J. Prevalence of impaired glucose tollerance and diabetes in women with Policystic ovary syndrome. Diabetes Care 1999 22: 141-14626.

[6] Diamanti-Kandarakis E, Piperi C. Genetics of polycystic ovary syndrome: searching for the way out of the labyrinth. Human. Reproduction. Update 2005 11, 631-643

[7] Diamanti-Kandarakis E, Piperi C, Spina J, Argyrakopoulou G, Papanastasiou L, Bergiele A, Panidis D. Polycystic ovary syndrome: the influence of environmental and genetics factors. Hormones (Athens) 2006 5, 17-3428.

[8] Conway GS, Agrawal R, Betteridge DJ, Jacobs HS. Risk factors for coronary artery disease in lean and obese women with the polycystic ovary syndrome. Clinical Endocrinology (Oxf) 1992 37: 119-125

[9] Teimuraz Apridonidze, Paulina A. Essah, Maria J. Iuorno and John E. Nestler. Prevalence and Characteristics of the Metabolic Syndrome in Women with Polycystic Ovary Syndrome. Journal of Clinical Endocrinology and metabolism 2005 Apr;90(4):1929-35

[10] Shroff R, Kerchner A, Maifeld M, Van Beek EJ, Jagasia D, Dokras A. Young obese women with polycystic ovary syndrome have evidence of early coronary atherosclerosis. Journal of Clinical Endocrinology and metabolism 2007 Dec;92(12):4609-14

[11] Carmina E, Orio F, Palomba S, Cascella T, Longo RA, Colao AM, Lombardi G, and Lobo RA. Evidence of altered adipocyte function in policystyc ovary sindrome. European Journal of Endocrinology 2005 Mar;152(3):389-94

[12] Fulghesu AM, Angioni S, Portoghese E. Milano F, Batetta B, Paoletti AM, Melis GB. Failure of the homeostatic model assessment calculation score for detecting metabolic deterioration in young patients with polycystic ovary syndrome. Fertility and Sterility. 2006 Aug;86(2):398-404

[13] Chang RJ, Nakamura RM, Judd HL, & Kaplan SA. Insulin resistence in nonobese patients with Policystic ovarian disease. Journal of Clinical Endocrinology and Metabolism 1983 57, 356-359 7.

[14] Morin-Papunen LC, Vauhkonen I, Koivunen RM, Ruokonen A, & Tapanainen JS. Insulin sensitivity, insulin secretion, and metabolic and hormonal parameters in healthy women and women with Policystic ovary syndrome.Human Reproduction 2000 15, 1266-1274

[15] Dunaif A, Graf M, Mandeli J, Laumas V, & Dobrjansky A. Characterization of group of hyperandrogenic women with acanthosis nigricans impaired glucose tolerance, and/or hyperinsulinemia. Journal of Clinical Endocrinology and Metabolism 1987 65, 499-507

[16] Diamanti-Kandarakis E, Kouli CR, Bergiele AT, Filandra FA, Tsianateli TC, Spina GG, Zapanti Ed, & Bartzis MI. A survey of the Policystic ovary syndrome in the greck island of Lesbos: hormonal and metabolic profile. Journal of Clinical Endocrinology and Metabolism 1999 84, 4006-4011

[17] Wild RA, Painter PC, Counlson PB, Carruth KB, Ranney GB. Lipoprotein lipid concentrations and cardiovascular risk in women with Policystic ovary syndrome. Journal of Clinical Endocrinology and Metabolism 1985; 61,946-51 11.

[18] Holte J, Bergh T, Berne C, Lithell H. Serum lipoprotein lipid profile in women with the Policystic ovary syndrome:relation to anthropometric, endocrine and metabolic variables. Clinical Endocrinology 1994; 41: 463-71

[19] Diamanti-Kandarakis E, Papavassiliou AG, Kandarakis SA, Chrousos GP. Patophysiology and types of dylipidemia in PCOS, Trends in Endocrinology and Metabolism 2007 Sep;18(7):280-5

[20] Coviello AD, Richard S, Legro, Dunaif A. Adolescent girls with polycystic ovary syndrome have an increased risk of the metabolic syndrome associated with increasing androgen levels independent of obesity and insulin resistance. Journal of Clinical Endocrinology and metabolism 2006 Feb;91(2):492-7.

[21] Orio F Jr, Palomba S, Cascella T, Tauchmanovà L, Nardo LG, Di Biase S, Labella D, Russo T, Savastano S, Tolino A, Zullo F, Colao A, Lombardi. Is plasminogen activator inhibitor-1 a cardiovascular risk factor in young women with polycystic ovary syndrome? Reprod Biomed Online Journal. 2004 Nov;9(5):505-10

[22] Lewy UD, Danadian K, Witchel SF, Arslanian S. Early metabolic abnormalities in adolescent girl with polycystic ovarian syndrome. Journal of Pediatric 2001 138: 38-44

[23] Carmina E, Legro RS, Stamets K, Lowell J, Lobo RA. Difference in body weight between American and Italian women ith polycystic ovary syndrome: influence of the diet. Hum Reprod 2003 18: 2289-93

[24] Carmina E, Lobo RA. Policystic ovary syndrome (PCOS): arguably the most common endocrinopathy is associated with significant morbidity in women. Journal of Clinical Endocrinology and metabolism 1999 84:1897-1899

[25] Piccione E, Dei M Donna Domani, CIC Edizioni Internazionali

[26] Palmert MR, Gordon CM, Kartashov AI, Legro RS, Emans SJ; Dunaif A. Screening for abnormal glucose tolerance in adolescents with polycistic ovary syndrome. Journal of Clinical Endocrinology and metabolism 2002 87:1017-1023

[27] Matthews DR, Hosker JP, Rudenski AS, Naylor BA, Treacher DF, Turner RC. Homeostasis model assessment: insulin resistence and βcell function from fasting plasma glucose and insulin concentrations in man. Diabetologia 1985 28; 412-419

[28] Ferriman D, Gallwey JD. Clinical Assesmentof body hair growth in women. Journal of Clinical Endocrinology and metabolism 1960 21:1440 – 1447

[29] Mather KJ, Verma S, Corenblum B, Anderson TJ. Normal endothelial function despite insulin resistance in healthy women with the polycystic ovary syndrome. Journal of Clinical Endocrinology and metabolism 2000 May;85(5)

[30] Pasquali R. Obesity and androgens: facts and perspectives; Fertil Steril 2006 May;85(5):1319-40

[31] Brown GA, Vukovich MD, Martini ER, Kohut ML, Franke WD, Jackson DA, King DS. Endocrine responses to chronic androstenedione intake in 30- to 56-year-old men. Journal of Clinical Endocrinology and metabolism 2000 Nov;85(11):4074-80

[32] Tan KC, Shiu SW, Kung AW.Alterations in hepatic lipase and lipoprotein subfractions with transdermal testosterone replacement therapy. Clinical Endocrinology (Oxf) 1999 51, 765-769

2

Nutrigenetics and Dyslipidemia

Maryam Shalileh
Islamic Azad University of Hamedan Branch
Iran

1. Introduction

Dyslipidemia is an abnormal amount of lipids (abnormality in any of the lipoprotein fractions), especially elevated Low Density Lipoprotein (LDLs) and decreased High Density Lipoprotein (HDLs) in the blood (Shalileh et al., 2009). In developed countries, most dyslipidemias are hyperlipidemias; that is, an elevation of lipids in the blood, are often due to diet and lifestyle (Wikipedia., 2011; Shalileh et al., 2009). According to the Katharina studie's, elevated cholesterol levels and dyslipoproteinemia are metabolic abnormalities that are becoming increasingly significant in industrialized countries, but also worldwide (Shalileh et al., 2009).

There is a proportional increase in the risk of Coronary Heart Disease (CHD) with rising serum cholesterol levels (Shalileh et al., 2009). Dyslipidaemia is an important risk factor for Cardiovascular Disease (CVD) (Masson & McNeili., 2005).

CVD is a common killer in both the Western and the developing world and is the leading cause of death globally (Lovegrove & Gitau., 2008).

More people die annually from CVDs than from any other cause. An estimated 17. 1 million people died from CVDs in 2004, representing 29% of all global deaths. Of these deaths, an estimated 7. 2 million were due to CHD and 5. 7 million were due to stroke. By 2030, almost 23. 6 million people will die from CVDs, mainly from heart disease and stroke (WHO. 2011).

Atherosclerosis is the most common cause of CHD and related mortality (Debra., 2008; Shalileh et al., 2009) .Endothelial dysfunction initiates atherosclerosis (Shalileh et al., 2009) . The first observable event in the process of atherosclerosis is the accumulation of plaque (cholesterol from low-density lipoproteins, calcium, and fibrin) in the endothelium in large and medium arteries (Debra., 2008).

One of the factors that causes endothelial dysfunction is dyslipidemia (Shalileh et al., 2009).

2. Treatment

CVD represents the paradigm of multi factorial disorders encompassing multiple genetic and non modifiable risk factors, for example older age and modifiable risk factors such as elevated total and LDL-cholesteroland and triglycerides concentrations, reduced HDL-cholesterol concentrations (Ordovas & Corella., 2004; Ordovas., 2009; Perez-Martinez et al, 2011; Lovegrove & Gitau, 2008). The interactions of those modulate plasma lipid concentrations and potentially CVD risk (Ordovas., 2009; Lovegrove & Gitau., 2008).

The link between serum cholesterol and the development of atherosclerosis was established a few decades ago and is now widely accepted. The National Cholesterol Education Program (NCEP) Adult Treatment Panel (ATP) publishes updated guidelines for treating lipid disorders. The latest version is the ATP III (Ordovas & Corella., 2004; Debra., 2008).

The current recommendations aim to reduce the classical modifiable risk factors, and much emphasis has been placed on controlling high-plasma cholesterol levels (Ordovas & Corella., 004).

Physicians are encouraged to refer patients to Registered Dietitians (RDs) to help patients meet goals for therapy (NCEP) based on LDL cholesterol levels. So the ATP III recommended the therapeutic lifestyle change (TLC) dietary pattern as the cornerstone for primary and secondary prevention of CHD. These guidelines consider dietary modification of treatment with emphasis on reducing the high saturated fat atherogenic diet and increased content of polyunsaturated fatty acid (PUFA) as well as controlling other behavioral factors. These therapies are used primarily to lower elevated blood levels of LDL-C, raise HDL –C and lower triglycerides (TGs) (Rubin & Berglund., 2002; Debra., 2008; Ordovas & Orella., 2004).

3. Response to the diet therapy

Although dietary recommendations have been implemented to improve health and diminish the risk of CVD, type 2 diabetes and obesity, these recommendations have been established based on populations and not the individual. On the other hand the approach has been surprisingly unsuccessful in reducing CVD risk and the drastically different inter individual responses to a diet (Ordovas & Corella., 2004).

So this clearly highlights the limitations of population-based nutritional recommendations and suggests that our understanding of the mechanisms responsible for inter-individual differences are far from being understood (Much et al., 2005).

Recent clinical evidence suggests dramatic inter-individual differences and existence of consistent hypo- and hyperresponders in response of plasma lipids to dietary manipulations, ranging from reduced LDL-C levels and TGs in some, to decreased HDL-C levels to elevated TGs. So in some, a low-fat diet has caused a shift to a lipid pattern that is more atherogenic than the original one. This supports the hypothesis that responsiveness is related to genetic variation and existence of nutrient–gene interactions or person's genotype (defined by the term 'nutrigenetics') (DeBusk, 2008; Perez-Martinez et al., 2011; Masson et al., 2003; Rideout., 2011; Ordovas et al., 2007).

A classic example of this is the large variation in the concentration of serum low-density lipoprotein-cholesterol (LDL-C) in response to fish oil supplementation. The cardio protective effects of the fatty acids in fish oil, Eicosapentaenoic Acid (EPA) and Docosahexaenoic Acid (DHA) are well recognized. However, a potentially deleterious increase in LDL-C (5–10%) has been consistently reported after moderate to high doses of fish oil (>2 g day−1 EPA + DHA) (Lovegrove & Gitau., 2008).

Despite this small, but significant increase in LDL-C, closer examination of the responses revealed a noticeable inter-individual variation. There was a mean increase in LDL-C of 4. 1%, yet the spread of individual responses was substantial, with 33 of the 74 subjects demonstrating a lower serum LDL-C and the remaining 41 demonstrating a higher LDL-C (range −40 to +113%) following fish oil intervention. This heterogeneous response to a change in dietary fat, may be attributed to a number of factors; including age, gender, baseline LDL-C levels, disease status and drug use. However, recent evidence strongly suggests that variations in a number of key genes may also be important (Lovegrove & Gitau., 2008). For example, individuals with specific of genetic variants in a gene may experience different type of lipoprotein changes when placed on a particular diet, whereas individuals with other variants in the gene may be resistant to the effects of the same diet. Although data is sparse in regard to whether such interactions exist, some limited work suggests that interactions may play an important role in determining lipoprotein profiles and may thus be informative for CVD risk prediction. For example, knowledge of a patient's genetic information may allow medical providers and nutritional counselors to predict what lipoprotein changes are likely to occur if the patient starts a particular dietary intervention and, thus, better advise the patient regarding lifestyle changes (Musunuru., 2010; Ordovas & Corella., 2004).

Lipoproteins are macromolecular complexes of lipids and proteins that originate mainly in the liver and intestine and are involved in transporting and redistributing lipids in the body. Lipid homeostasis is achieved by the coordinated action of numerous nuclear factors, enzymes, apolipoproteins, binding proteins, and receptors. Lipid metabolism is also linked with energy metabolism and is subject to many hormonal controls essential for adjusting to environmental and internal conditions. Genetic variability exists in humans for most of these components, and some of these mutations result in abnormal lipid metabolism and plasma lipoprotein profiles that may contribute to the pathogenesis of atherosclerosis. Many of these genes have been explored in terms of gene-diet interactions (Ordovas & Corella., 2004).

So the shift towards personalized nutritional advice is a very attractive proposition, where, in principle, an individual can be given dietary advice specifically tailored to their genotype. However, the evidence-base for the impact of interactions between nutrients and fixed genetic variants on biomarkers of CVD risk is still very limited (Lovegrove & Gitau., 2008; Ordovas., 2006; Masson et al., 2003; Masson & Mc Neil., 2005; Fisler & Warden., 2005).

With the advent of nutritional genomics, it's becoming clear that an individual's genetic makeup (genotype) is an important factor in this response and that dietary interventions must be matched to genotypes to effect the intended lipid-lowering responses (DeBusk., 2008).

A number of such genes have already been identified and include those involved with postprandial lipoprotein and triglyceride responses, homocysteine metabolism, hypertension, blood-clotting, and inflammation (Ordovas & Corella., 2004; DeBusk., 2008).

Genetic polymorphism in human populations is part of the evolutionary process that results from the interaction between the environment and the human genome. Recent changes in diet have upset this equilibrium, potentially influencing the risk of most common morbidities such as cardiovascular diseases, diabetes, and cancer. Reduction of these conditions is a major public health concern, and such a reduction could be achieved by improving our ability to detect disease predisposition early in life and by providing more personalized behavioral recommendations for successful primary prevention. In terms of cardiovascular diseases, polymorphisms at multiple genes have been associated with differential effects in terms of lipid metabolism. The integration of genetic and environmental complexity into current and future research will drive the field toward the implementation of clinical tools aimed at providing dietary advice optimized for the individual's genome (Ordovas., 2009; Engler., 2009).

The recognition that nutrients have the ability to interact and modulate molecular mechanisms underlying an organism's physiological functions has prompted a revolution in the field of nutrition (Much et al., 2005).

For the field of nutrition, this would encompass the ongoing efforts to understand the relationships between the genome and diet, currently termed nutrigenomics and nutrigenetics (Much et al., 2005; Ommen., 2004)

4. Nutritional genomics

Nutrigenetics and nutrigenomics are promising multidisciplinary fields that focus on studying the interactions between nutritional factors, genetic factors and health outcomes. Their goal is to achieve more efficient individual dietary intervention strategies aimed at preventing disease, improving quality of life and achieving healthy aging (Ordovas., 2004).

In contrast to most single gene disorders, chronic disorders (e. g., cardiovascular disease, cancer, diabetes) are far more complex. First, they involve multiple genes, each of which comes in more than one variation, that likely contribute in small ways to the overall condition rather than have the dramatic impact that is more typical with single gene disorders. Second, the genes are more likely to be influenced by environmental factors, which make the resulting phenotype murkier than with single-gene disorders. An individual might have gene variants that predispose to a particular chronic disorder but, depending on that individual's nutritional and other lifestyle choices, the disorder may or may not develop (DeBusk., 2008).

Nutritional genomics or nutrigenomics is the newly developing field of science that focuses on the complex interaction among genes and environmental factors, specifically bioactive components in food and how a person's diet interacts with his or her genotype to influence the balance between health and disease (DeBusk., 2009; Much et al., 2005; Fisler & Warden., 2005).

Nutritional genomics is the umbrella term (Ryan-Harshman., 2008). There are two major subcategories of nutritional genomics: nutrigenetics and nutrigenomics (Much et al., 2005).

The creation of nutrigenomics and nutrigenetics, two fields with distinct approaches to elucidate the interaction between diet and genes but with a common ultimate goal to optimize health through the personalization of diet, provide powerful approaches to unravel the complex relationship between nutritional molecules, genetic polymorphisms, and the biological system as a whole (Much et al., 2005).

Thus, nutrition in the 21st century is poised to be an exciting and highly relevant field of research, as each new day is accompanied by advances in our understanding of how the interactions between lifestyle and genotype contribute to health and disease, taking us one step closer to achieving the highly desirable goal of personalized nutrition (Much et al., 2005).

4.1 Nutrigenetics

Nutrigenetics term was used first time by Dr R. O Brennan in 1975 (Farhud et al., 2010). Nutrigenetics is concerned with the effect of gene variations or gene variant or individual's genetic make-up on the organism's functional ability, specifically its ability to digest, absorb, and use food (DeBusk., 2009; Ordovas & Corella., 2004; Lovegrove & Gitau., 2008). Nutrigenetics embodies the science of identifying and characterizing gene variants associated with differential responses to nutrients or dietary pattern, functional food or supplement on a specific health outcome, and relating this variation to disease states (Much et al., 2005; Michael., 2008). The particular gene variants a person has to determine the nutritional requirements for that person and the gene-based differences in response to dietary components and developing nutraceuticals that are most compatible with health based on individual genetic makeup (DeBusk., 2009; Subbiah., 2007). Nutrigenetics will assist clinicians in identifying the optimal diet for a given individual, i. e., personalized nutrition (Much et al., 2005; Svacina., 2007; Zak & Slaby., 2007; Gillies., 2003).

Furthermore, the concept is that if an individual is genotyped at various genes for disease-associated risk alleles, a genotype-based diet or nutritional supplement regimen may be useful to overcome the genetic variation and reduce risk or prevent the disease altogether (Wood., 2008; Xacur-GarcAa et al., 2008; Kussmann & Fay., 2008).

4.2 Nutrigenomics

Nutrigenomics, is concerned with how bioactive components within food affect genes. The field of nutritional genomics is still evolving, and it is common to see "nutrigenomics" used as a shorthand version of "nutritional genomics ". However, keeping the concepts separate can be helpful when sorting out the underlying mechanisms involved (DeBusk., 2009). Nutrigenomics will unravel the optimal diet from within a series of nutritional alternatives, whereas nutrigenetics will help clinicians in identifying the optimal diet for a given individual, i. e., personalized nutrition (Much et al., 2005).

Although these two concepts are intimately associated, they take a fundamentally different approach to understanding the relationship between genes and diet. Despite the immediate goals differing, the long-term goal of improving health and preventing disease with nutrition requires the amalgamation of both disciplines (Much et al., 2005)

Nutrigenetics is the more familiar of the two subtypes of nutritional genomics (DeBusk., 2009) At one end of the spectrum of nutritional genomics are the highly penetrant monogenic disorders that give rise to inborn errors of metabolism such as phenylketonuria (DeBusk., 2009). More recently less penetrant, more subtle variations have been identified that also affect the gene-encoded protein's function. However, such variations do not in themselves cause disease. Instead, they alter a person's susceptibility for developing a disease. Depending on the specific gene variant, the person's likelihood of developing a disorder may be increased or reduced. These genes are the primary focus of nutritional genomics, because they are common within the global population, they affect dietary recommendations about the types and amounts of food that best fit a person, and practical interventions are possible. These interventions can potentially improve the health potential of individual people and, by extrapolation, the populations in which they live (DeBusk., 2009).

Current nutrition recommendations, directed towards populations, are based on estimated average nutrient requirements for a target population and intend to meet the needs of most individuals within that population. They also aim at preventing common diseases such as obesity, diabetes and cardiovascular disease. So diet has been reported as a major contributor to alarming prevalence of obesity (Shalileh et al, 2010). For infants with specific genetic polymorphisms, e. g. some inborn errors of metabolism such as phenylketonuria, adherence to current recommendations will cause disease symptoms and they need personalized nutrition recommendations (Hernell & West., 2008; Farhud & Shalileh., 2008).

Some other monogenic polymorphisms, e. g. adult hypolactasia, are common but with varying prevalence between ethnic groups and within populations. Ages at onset as well as the degree of the resulting lactose intolerance also vary, making population-based as well as personalized recommendations difficult. The tolerable intake is best set by each individual based on symptoms. For polygenetic diseases such as celiac disease, and allergic disease, current knowledge is insufficient to suggest personalized recommendations aiming at primary prevention for all high-risk infants, although it may be justified to provide such recommendations on an individual level should the parents ask for them.

New technologies such as nutrigenetics and nutrigenomics are promising tools with which current nutrition recommendations can possibly be refined and the potential of individualized nutrition be explored. It seems likely that in the future it will be possible to offer more subgroups within a population personalized recommendations (hernell & West., 2008).

The possibility of offering personalized nutritional advice to the individual is an attractive option for dietitians and nutrition scientists and is becoming practicable with the emergence of nutritional genomics. This developing field promises to revolutionize dietetic practice, with dietary advice prescribed according to an individual's genetic makeup to prevent, mitigate or cure chronic disease (Lovegrove & Gitau., 2008). It has been also termed "personalized nutrition" or "individualized nutrition" (Ordovas & Corella., 2004; Perez-Martinez et al., 2011). The practical applications of this research include a new set of tools that nutrition professionals can use to identify disease susceptibilities and a growing body of knowledge that will form the basis for developing strategies for disease prevention and intervention that are specifically targeted to the underlying genetic mechanisms (DeBusk., 2008).

Nutrigenetics and personalized nutrition are components of the concept that in the future genotyping will be used as a means of defining dietary recommendations to suit the individual. Over the last two decades there has been an explosion of research in this area, with often conflicting findings reported in the literature (Rimbach & Minihane., 2009).

According to WHO reports, diet factors influence occurrence of more than 2/3 of diseases. Most of these factors belong to the categories of nutrigenetics and nutrigenomics. In the future both, nutrigenetics and nutrigenomics, will induce many changes in preventive medicine and also in clinical medicine (Svacina., 2007).

Nutrients interact with the human genome to modulate molecular pathways that may become disrupted, resulting in an increased risk of developing various chronic diseases. Understanding how genetic variations influence nutrient digestion, absorption, transport, biotransformation, uptake and elimination will provide a more accurate measure of exposure to the bioactive food ingredients ingested. Furthermore, genetic polymorphisms in the targets of nutrient action such as receptors, enzymes or transporters could alter molecular pathways that influence the physiological response to dietary interventions. Knowledge of the genetic basis for the variability in response to these dietary factors should result in a more accurate measure of exposure of target tissues of interest to these compounds and their metabolites. Examples of how 'slow' and 'fast' metabolizers respond differently to the same dietary exposures will be discussed. Identifying relevant diet-gene interactions will benefit individuals seeking personalized dietary advice as well as improve public health recommendations by providing sound scientific evidence linking diet and health (EL-Sohemy, 2007; Amouyel., 2000).

A really personalized diet will be a diet considering the nutritional status, the nutritional needs based on age, body composition, work and physical activities, but also considering the genotype. That is, define the "nutritional phenotype (Perez-Martinez et al., 2011; Miggiano & De Sanctis., 2006). It is clear that integrating knowledge of gene variants into dietary recommendations for populations and individuals will increasingly play a role in nutrition counseling and policy making (DeBusk., 2008).

Nutrigenetics will provide the basis for personalized dietary recommendations based on the individual's genetic makeup. This approach has been used for decades for certain single gene diseases; such as phenylketonuria, however, the challenge is to implement a similar concept for common multi factorial disorders and to develop tools to detect genetic predisposition and to prevent common disorders decades before their manifestation. The preliminary results involving gene-diet interactions for cardiovascular diseases and cancer are promising, but mostly inconclusive. Success in this area will require the integration of different disciplines and investigators working on large population studies designed to adequately investigate gene-environment interactions (Ordovas & Corella., 2004; Ordovas & Mooser., 2004).

4.3 Nutritional genomics and lipid metabolism

From a health perspective, the major concerns regarding genes and lipid metabolism center on susceptibility to vascular disease. Genes involved with cholesterol homeostasis offer examples of how genetic variations affect lipid metabolism and, thereby, disease risk (DeBusk., 2009).

The blood lipid response to diet is influenced by polymorphisms within genes for the apolipoproteins as well as within those for enzymes, such as hepatic lipase, that are involved in lipid metabolism (fisler & Warden., 2005).

The major focus of nutritional genomics research is on identifying (1) gene-disease associations, (2) the dietary components that influence these associations, (3) the mechanisms by which dietary components exert their effects, and (4) the genotypes that benefit most from particular dietary choices (DeBusk., 2008).

The following section takes a brief look at some of the key diet-related genes and their known variants and how these variants affect the person's response to diet. Keep in mind that chronic diseases involve complex interactions among genes and bioactive food components, and unraveling the details will require population and intervention studies large enough to have the statistical power needed to draw meaningful conclusions. Although what is known today is but the tip of the iceberg compared to what will come in the years ahead (DeBusk., 2008).

Over the last two decades there has been an explosion of research in this area, with often conflicting findings reported in the literature (Rimbach & Minihan., 2009).

5. Candidate gene approach

The candidate gene approach involves the selection and study of biologically relevant genes. Genetic polymorphisms in these genes, known as Single-Nucleotide Polymorphism (SNPs), can alter susceptibility to a disease. Candidate or "susceptibility" genes should meet one or more of the following conditions: genes that are chronically activated during a disease state and have been previously demonstrated to be sensitive to dietary intervention; genes with functionally important variations; genes that have an important hierarchical role in biological cascades; polymorphisms that are highly prevalent in the population (usually >10% for public health relevance); and/or genes with associated biomarkers, rendering clinical trials useful (Lovegrove & Gitau., 2008).

Many studies have investigated this possibility and have largely focused on genes whose products affect lipoprotein metabolism, eg, apolipoproteins, enzymes, and receptors. Although there have been several reviews of such studies, many of them may have led to articles being omitted and introduced bias toward positive findings (Ordovas., 2006).

5.1 Apolipoprotein A-I (Apo AI)

The Apo AI gene, codes for apolipoprotein A-I, is a major structural and functional component of HDL constituting about 70% to 80% of HDL protein mass, and is the main activator of the enzyme lecithin cholesterol acyl transferase (LCAT) (Ordovas & Corella., 2004; Lovegrove & Gitau., 2008; Much et al., 2005; DeBusk., 2008).

Plasma HDL-cholesterol plays a protective role for CVD (Lovegrove & Gitau., 2008; Much et al., 2005). Its gene product Apo A-I plays a central role in lipid metabolism and CVD risk. Pedigree studies have reported associations between genetic variation at the Apo A1 locus and plasma lipid and lipoprotein levels (Ordovas & Corella., 2004). One of the variants that has been identified to be diet-related is -75G>A, in which the typical guanine has been replaced with an adenine at position 75 within the regulatory region of the Apo *A-I* gene (DeBusk., 2008).

It was reported that this polymorphism was associated with Apo A-I and HDL-C concentrations, and individuals carrying the A-allele presented with the highest levels, compared with subjects homozygotes for the G allele (G/G) but many studies have had contradictory results (Lovegrove & Gitau., 2008; Ordovas & Corella., 2004).

In the context of the Framingham Heart Study, individuals with a polymorphism in the Apo A1 gene promoter region (–75 G/A) were found to respond differently to dietary PUFA (Much et al., 2005; Lovegrove & Gitau., 2008).

The inconsistencies in reported studies outcomes are not necessarily a result of inherent differences, but are a result of a nutrient–gene interaction, i. e. a classic example of where individualized dietary advice could be important in relation to exerting a positive influence on HDL-C levels and CVD risk (Lovegrove & Gitau., 2008; Much et al., 2005). In brief, that individuals with the A allele showed an increase in HDL levels following an increased consumption of PUFA. In contrast, those with the more common G allele showed an inverse relationship between HDL levels and PUFA consumption. This study revealed that differences in sex also mediate the response. Indeed, men did not show a relationship between HDL and PUFA consumption, irrespective of their Apo A1 polymorphism (Lovegrove & Gitau., 2008; Much et al., 2005).

A common practice in treating dyslipidemia is to reduce the saturated fat content of the diet and increase the polyunsaturated fat content. Typically, HDL levels fall in women with the more common G allele as the polyunsaturated content of the diet increases, an effect counter to the desired one. These women would benefit from a fat modified diet that keeps amounts of both saturated and polyunsaturated fat low and increases amounts of monounsaturated fat. Women with the A allele, increasing polyunsaturated dietary fat leads to increased HDL levels, and the effect is "dose-dependent; so in women with the more common G allele, increasing dietary Polyunsaturated Fat (PUFA) levels from less than 4% of total energy to 4% to 8% to greater than 8% resulted in a corresponding decline in HDL levels as PUFA levels increase. However, in women with the A allele, increasing PUFA concentrations (>8% of energy derived from PUFA) increased HDL levels and the increase is more dramatic in the presence of two copies of the A alleles than it is with just one. For these women, a diet low in saturated fat, moderate in polyunsaturated fat (8% or greater of total calories), and supplying the rest in monounsaturated fat has the greatest benefit in raising HDL levels. Clearly, whether a person has the -75G>A Apo AI variant, and how many copies are present, will affect any therapeutic intervention developed to correct dyslipidemia (DeBusk., 2009; Much et al., 2005; Debra., 2008).

Juo et al (Hank Juo., 1999) used a meta analysis approach to show the lack of consistency between the less common A-allele and higher HDL-cholesterol concentrations. In view of the significant gene-diet interaction observed for those intervention studies, they examined whether these results could be extrapolated to a free living population, consisting of about 1600 Framingham Offspring Study participants (Ordovas et al., 2002). The results from the straightforward association between genotype and phenotype were disappointing and suggested that the G/A polymorphism was not associated with HDL-cholesterol, Apo A-I concentrations, nor with any other anthropometrical or plasma lipid variable examined. To examine the potential modifying effect of dietary fat on these associations, they fitted multivariate linear regression models, including interaction terms for fat intake [total, Saturated Fatty Acid (SFA), Monounsaturated Fat (MUFA), and PUFA fat]. No significant interactions were observed between the G/A polymorphism, total, SFA, and MUFA fat intakes. However, in women, HDL-cholesterol concentrations were associated with a significant interaction between PUFA intake and Apo A1 genotype $(p = 0. 005)$. Using PUFA as a dichotomous variable, their data show that G/G women consuming <6% PUFA/day had higher HDL-cholesterol (1. 48 ± 0. 40 m mol/L) than A-carriers (1. 43 ± 0. 40 m mol/L). Conversely, when consuming ≥6% PUFA/day, G/G had lower HDL-cholesterol concentrations (1. 44 ± 0. 39 m mol/L) than A-carriers (1. 49 ± 0. 39 m mol/L). In men, the situation was more complex because the effects were observed using three-way interactions, including smoking and alcohol consumption, in the analyzes (Ordovas & Corella., 2004).

The most evident application of these results may be to help us make more efficacious dietary recommendations based on genetic profile. It is clear that subjects with the A-allele at this Apo A1–75 (G/A) polymorphism will benefit from diets containing a high percentage (it is important to underscore that we are talking about percent in the diet and not about total amounts) of PUFA (i. e., vegetable oils, fish, nuts, and so on). According to their data, this should result in higher HDL-cholesterol concentrations, which in turn should lower CVD risk. These findings suggest that the expression of the Apo A1 gene may be regulated by PUFA (Ordovas & Corella., 2004).

On the other hand, of 13 reports, 5 found that the presence of the Apo A-I–75 (G/A) A allele instead of the common G allele resulted in greater LDL-cholesterol responses to changes in dietary. In addition, significant interactions between the G/A genotype and diet were found for changes in total and LDL cholesterol when subjects changed from a low-fat diet to a diet high in MUFAs. No significant interactions between diet and other polymorphisms in the Apo A-I gene were shown (Ordovas & Corella., 2004).

5.2 Apolipoprotein A-IV (APOA4)

Apo A-IV is a 46-Kd plasma glycoprotein that is synthesized by intestinal enterocytes during lipid absorption and is incorporated into nascent chylomicrons. Apo A-IV enters circulation on lymph chylomicrons, but then dissociates from their surface and circulates primarily as a lipid-free protein. Several genetically determined isoforms of Apo A-IV have been detected; amino acid positions 360 and 347 of the mature protein are the most common. The polymorphism at position 360 is due to a CAG → CAT substitution at codon 360 in the Apo A4 gene and encodes a Q360H (Gln → His) substitution in the carboxyl terminus, and produces an isoform, originally known as Apo A-IV-2, one charge unit more basic than the common isoform, Apo A-IV-. In some population studies the Apo A-IV-2 allele is associated with higher levels of HDL-cholesterol and or Apo A-I and/or lower triglyceride (TG) levels, as well as lower LDL-cholesterol, lower Lp (a), and higher fasting glucose and insulin levels, but no associations have been observed in other studies (Ordovas & Corella., 2004).

The other common mutation (Thr347→Ser) is due to an ACT→TCT substitution at codon 347 in the human Apo A-IV gene, it is found within subjects with the apoA-IV-1 isoform. Several population studies note that carriers of the 347S allele have lower plasma, total, LDL-cholesterol, Apo B levels, and Lp (a) levels, than 347T/T homozygotes. The results of many reports showing that male carriers of the less common allele at the Gln360His polymorphism were less responsive to changes in dietary fat and cholesterol or cholesterol alone (Ordovas & Corella., 2004).

Several studies have focused on the interaction between the Apo A4 locus and dietary factors, both in the fasting and postprandial states. Similar to the findings for other genes, the data are conflicting when it comes to the effect of Apo A-IV polymorphisms on the LDL response to dietary cholesterol. However, according to Weinberg (Weinberg., 2002), the results from different studies can be partially reconciled if one assumes that the dietary fatty acid effects dominate over the allele effects. Therefore, if dietary cholesterol intake is the principal variable, and total fat intake is moderate and constant, Q/H subjects display an attenuated response of LDL-cholesterol. However, when dietary cholesterol intake is changed in the setting of a higher baseline dietary fat intake or with a change in fat saturation, the fatty acid effects on LDL levels predominate and overrule the allele effect. The impact of the Q360H polymorphism on cholesterol absorption may be greater on a high PUFAs intake. However, dietary PUFA counteract the effect of dietary cholesterol on the expression of hepatic LDL receptors. Thus, the final effect of Apo AIV alleles on the LDL response to dietary cholesterol may be determined by the relative amounts of cholesterol, saturated fatty acids (SAFAs), and PUFAs in the diet (winberg et al., 2000; Weggemans., 2000; Lopez-Miranda., 1998; Ordovas & Corella., 2004; Hockey., 2001).

There is more consistency and probably less complexity regarding the impact of Apo A-IV polymorphisms on HDL-cholesterol: When total fat intake is raised or lowered, Q/H subjects have an exaggerated, and Threonine /Serine (T/S) subjects an attenuated, response in plasma HDL levels. It has been suggested, and Weinberg demonstrated, that a high-PUFA intake may amplify this effect (Ordovas & Corella., 2004; Winberg et al., 2000).

Given the relationships between plasma TG and plasma HDL-cholesterol levels, it is possible that the response of plasma HDL-cholesterol levels to changes in dietary fat is mediated by Apo A-IV allele effects on postprandial triglyceride-rich lipoprotein metabolism. These studies clearly illustrate the extreme complexity associated with the interpretation of results from studies involving gene-diet interactions (Ordovas & Corella., 2004).

The presence of serine instead of threonine at position 347 in the Apo A-IV gene was associated with increased total and LDL-cholesterol responsiveness when subjects switched from a high-SFA diet to a National Cholesterol Education Program Step I diet. When the same subjects changed from the National Cholesterol Education Program Step I diet to a high-MUFA diet, subjects with the *Thr /Thr* genotype had a 1% decrease in total cholesterol concentrations, whereas subjects with the *Ser* allele had a 5% increase in total cholesterol concentrations. When the Thr347Ser and the Apo A-I-75 (*G/A*) genotypes were combined, carriers of the *A* and *Ser* alleles showed greater LDL-cholesterol responses to changes in dietary fat. However, Carmena-Ramon et al (Carmena-Ramon et al., 1998) investigated both the Gln360His and Thr347Ser polymorphisms and found no gene-diet or haplotype-diet interactions (Masson et al., 2003). The evidence that exists for an interaction between diet and the Apo A-IV glutamine-histidine mutation at position 360 (Gln360His) suggests that *Gln / Gln* subjects show significantly greater total and LDL-cholesterol responses and that *Gln /His* subjects show greater HDL-cholesterol responses to changes in dietary fat, cholesterol, or both. Although Wallace et al found no significant differences in LDL-cholesterol responses between genotypes, dense LDL cholesterol decreased more in subjects carrying the *His* allele when polyunsaturated fatty acids (PUFAs) replaced SFAs in the diet (Wallace et al, 2000). In the same study, there was a significant difference in HDL-cholesterol responses between genotype groups such that concentrations decreased in *Gln /Gln* subjects and increased in *Gln /His* subjects (Masson et al., 2003).

5.3 Apolipoprotein B (Apo B)

Apolipoprotein B is the main protein component of low-density-lipoprotein (LDL) and contains several domains. The human Apo B is 43 kb in length with 81 bp signal sequence. Numerous polymorphisms have been identified on this gene (Heilbronn et al., 2000).

The evidence for an interaction between the *Xba*I polymorphism and diet is inconsistent. In 2 studies, X-X- subjects showed greater LDL-cholesterol responses, whereas Tikkanen et al, found that subjects carrying the *X+* allele had greater total, LDL-, and HDL-cholesterol responses. However in, analysis of these data, the *Xba*I polymorphism only explained a significant proportion of variance of the change in HDL cholesterol (Tikkanen et al., 1995). In one research they found no significant effect on LDL-cholesterol responsiveness, although X-X-subjects showed the greatest HDL$_2$- and VLDL-cholesterol responses. Finally, in another study researchers studied the effect of the *Xba*I polymorphism in subjects with the common Apo *E3/3* genotype and found that X-X- subjects showed the greatest triacylglycerol response. Rantala et al conducted a meta-analysis of all published dietary trials. In their analysis of 8 studies, X-X+ subjects had greater LDL responses than did X+X+ subjects and no significant differences in the responses of total or HDL cholesterol or triacylglycerol were found between genotypes (Masson et al., 2003; Rantala., 2000). Two of 7 intervention studies found that the *Eco*RI R- allele was associated with significantly greater total and LDL-cholesterol responses to changes in dietary fat and cholesterol. Only one study found an interaction between the *Msp*I polymorphism and response to diet. Ten intervention studies found no significant effects of the Apo B signal peptide insertion/deletion (*I/D*) polymorphism on dietary responsiveness; however, 2 studies reported a significantly greater responsiveness in subjects homozygous for the *I* allele. In a study, 43 men and women were observed to compare the effects of insoluble and soluble fiber on plasma lipids. Their statistical model identified gene-diet interactions. However, they did not look specifically at differences between genotype groups. It was found that D/D subjects had similar decreases in HDL cholesterol after consumption of the insoluble- and soluble-fiber diets. However, I/I subjects had larger HDL-cholesterol decreases with the soluble-fiber diet, whereas I/D subjects had larger HDL-cholesterol decreases with the insoluble-fiber diet. The gene-diet interaction was significant ($P = 0. 021$) (Masson et al., 2003; Rantala., 2000).

In response, low-fat, low-cholesterol diet, I/I subjects showed the greatest decrease in HDL_2. In addition, I/I and I/D subjects showed increased VLDL-cholesterol and decreased LDL-cholesterol concentrations, whereas D/D subjects showed decreased VLDL-cholesterol and increased LDL-cholesterol concentrations. The I/D polymorphism showed no significant effect on the responsiveness of total, LDL, or HDL cholesterol or triacylglycerol in a meta-analysis of 7 studies (Masson et al., 2003).

5.4 Apolipoprotein E (APO E)

Apo E gene variants have implications for nutrition therapy related to preventing and treating CVD and the responses to dietary fat, soluble fiber, and alcohol. The impact of Apo E genotype on individual variability in its LDL cholesterol response to diet interventions and CVD risk has been extensively investigated over the past 30 years. Apo E contains 299 amino acids, considering Apo E's key role in lipoprotein metabolism, being involved in chylomicron metabolism, very low-density lipoprotein synthesis and secretion, and in the cellular removal of lipoprotein remnants from the circulation. Apo E serves as a ligand for multiple lipoprotein receptors. This gene locus is polymorphic, with 84 gene variants being characterized to date. The prevalence of this SNP varies in different populations (Lovegrove & Gitau., 2008; Rubin & Berglund., 2002; Ordovas & Corella., 2004; DeBusk., 2009).

Apo E is present in a subfraction of lipoprotein (a). The receptor-binding properties reside in the N-terminal part of Apo E, whereas the lipid-binding domain resides in the C-terminal portion. It was recognized that Apo E was present as three different Apo E isoforms (E2, E3, and E4), coded by three different alleles (e2, e3, and e4), resulting in six homo and heterozygous genotypes (e2/e2, e2/e3, e2/e4, e3/e3, e3/e4, e4/e4). Apo E2 differs from the wild type, Apo E3, by a substitution of arginine for cysteine at amino acid 158, and Apo E4 differs from Apo E3 by a substitution of cysteine for arginine at amino acid 112. In addition, several other genetic variants have been described at the Apo E locus (Rubin & Berglund., 2002; Lovegrove & Gitau., 2008; Masson et al., 2003; Farhud et al., 2010).

Persons with E4 variant respond to a high-fat diet negatively with an increased risk for coronary heart disease (CHD). In these individuals, low-fat diet should be useful (Farhud et al., 2010; Sheweta et al., 2011).

Population studies show that plasma cholesterol, LDL cholesterol, and Apo B levels are highest in subjects carrying the Apo E4, intermediate in those with the Apo E3, and lowest in those with the Apo E2 isoform. An initial observation was that the association of the Apo E4 isoform with elevated serum cholesterol levels was greater in populations consuming diets rich in saturated fat and cholesterol than in other populations (Ordovas & Corella., 2004).

Corella and Ordovas reviewed the numerous studies that have investigated the diet-gene interaction for Apo E variants. People with at least one E4 allele have the highest basal levels of various lipids and show the greatest lipid-lowering response to a low-fat diet. Taking into account which Apo E alleles a person has is helpful in developing diet and lifestyle interventions for improving serum lipid levels (DeBusk., 2009).

In 46 studies that examined the Apo E locus and alterations in dietary fat content, significantly different responses in total and LDL cholesterol by Apo E genotype were reported in 8 and 11 studies, respectively, with the Apo E4 individuals generally being the most responsive (Lovegrove & Gitau., 2008; Masson et al., 2003).

Note that despite the numerous studies examining the relation between Apo E genetic variability and LDL-cholesterol response to diet intervention, there is considerable inconsistency regarding the magnitude and significance of the reported associations, and this locus continues to be the subject of intense research (Ordovas & Corella., 2004).

In a study, there are 29 intervention studies that examine Apo E-diet interactions. A total of 3224 subjects participated in these studies, ranging from 16 to 420 subjects per study. Of the 29 studies, 12 demonstrated no significant Apo E-diet interactions, 15 reported significant interactions (E4 was usually associated with increased dietary response), and 2 were undefined. Using the same available literature, but different selection criteria, Masson, reviewed 62 dietary intervention periods, including 3223 subject-by-diet interventions (Masson et al., 2003). Again, the range of the studies varied between 8 and 210 subjects per dietary intervention. According to this review, 42 of the diet interventions did not demonstrate significant Apo E-diet interactions, and only 19 provided evidence for significant interactions, clearly demonstrating the diversity of the results presented in the original papers as well as those obtained from review papers (Ordovas & Corella., 2004; Masson et al., 2003).

The heterogeneous response to changes in dietary fat may be attributed to a number of factors including age, gender, baseline LDL-C levels, disease status and drug use (Lovegrove & Gitau., 2008).

One difference between the negative studies and those reporting significant Apo E gene–diet interactions relates to the baseline lipid levels of the subjects. Studies reporting significant associations often included subjects who were moderately hypercholesterolemic and/or had significant differences in base total cholesterol and LDL-cholesterol among the Apo E genotype groups. This suggests that the significant gene-diet interaction is apparent only in subjects susceptible to hypercholesterolemia. Concerning differences in dietary interventions, there were significant interactions in studies in which total dietary fat and cholesterol were modified. Several mechanisms are proposed to explain these Apo E-related differences in individual response to dietary therapy. Some studies show that intestinal cholesterol absorption is related to Apo E phenotype, with Apo E4 carriers absorbing more cholesterol than non-Apo E4 carriers. Other mechanisms such as different distribution of Apo E on the lipoprotein fractions, LDL Apo B production, bile acid, and cholesterol synthesis, and postprandial lipoprotein clearance may also be involved (Ordovas & Corella., 2004).

On the other hand although the obvious dietary factors implicated in gene-diet interactions affecting plasma lipid levels are dietary fats and cholesterol, other dietary components have revealed significant interactions. This is the case for alcohol intake.

Although the raising effect of alcohol consumption on high-density lipoprotein (HDL)-cholesterol levels is well established, the effect on LDL-cholesterol is still unclear. It is possible that the reported variability will be due to interactions between genetic factors and alcohol consumption. Using cross-sectional analysis, researcher examined whether variation at the Apo E locus modulates the association between alcohol consumption and LDL-cholesterol levels in a healthy population based sample of 1014 male and 1133 female participants in the Framingham Offspring Study (Corella et al., 2001). In male nondrinkers, LDL-cholesterol levels were not different across Apo E groups; however, in male drinkers, there were differences in LDL-cholesterol, with Apo E2 subjects displaying the lowest levels. When LDL cholesterol levels were compared among the Apo E subgroups by drinking status, LDL-cholesterol levels in Apo E2 male drinkers were lower than in Apo E2 non drinkers. Conversely, in Apo E4 males, LDL-cholesterol was higher in drinkers than in nondrinkers. This Apo E-alcohol interaction remained significant after controlling for age, BMI, smoking, fat, and energy intake. In women, the expected effect of Apo E alleles on LDL-cholesterol levels was present in both drinkers and nondrinkers. Multiple linear regression models showed a negative association between alcohol and LDL-cholesterol levels in Apo E2 men, with alcohol intake a continuous variable. Conversely, in Apo E4 men, this association was positive. There were no statistically significant associations in either Apo E3 men or in women. These data suggest that in men, variability at the Apo E locus partially modulates the effects of consuming alcoholic beverages on LDL-cholesterol levels (Ordovas & Corella., 2004).

The effect of alcohol was also investigated in the Copenhagen City Heart Study (Frikke-Schmidt., 2000). In that study, there was an interaction between alcohol and Apo E among women, in which higher triglyceride levels were associated with both the E2 and E4 alleles among women who regularly consumed alcohol. For men, increased triglyceride levels among E2 and E4 carriers were seen across the entire alcohol distribution spectrum, perhaps because of some degree of alcohol consumption among all men. Overall, the results suggested that metabolic stresses, such as the postprandial situation or alcohol consumption, might contribute to uncover underlying differences between Apo E genotypes in cholesterol, triglyceride or lipoprotein metabolism (Frikke-Schmidt., 2000).

The effect of the Apo E gene on lipoproteins may differ with age. In elderly individuals as well as in children, there is less difference in LDL cholesterol levels in individuals carrying the E4 allele versus non-E4 carriers. Interestingly, in both of these age groups, the presence of the Apo E2 allele was associated with lower LDL cholesterol levels. An age-dependent variation between Apo E and plasma lipids was also seen by Jarvik et al (Jarvik et al, 1997). By longitudinally following male Caucasian twins, the authors demonstrated that whereas E4 carriers initially had higher triglyceride and cholesterol levels compared with E3 homozygotes, this difference disappeared over an 18-year period (Rubin & Berglund., 2002).

A sex-specific association between Apo E2 and HDL cholesterol levels has been described in Turkish individuals. In Turkish women, but not men, the frequency of the Apo E2 allele increased almost six fold from the lowest to the highest HDL cholesterol tertiary (Rubin & Berglund., 2002). The available information show, significant diet–Apo E gene interactions occurred in male-only studies. In studies including men and women, significant effects were noted only in men, suggesting a significant gene-sex interaction (Ordovas & Corella., 2004).

As pointed out above, in studies in which an Apo E gene nutrient interaction was found, it was generally more common among men than women, suggesting a modulation by sex. Interestingly, in the study by Mahley et al, on HDL levels in Turkish individuals, the authors suggested that the association of Apo E2 with higher HDL cholesterol levels found in women but not in men may be caused by a sex difference in hepatic lipase. Among women, a lower hepatic lipase activity might allow the detection of the modulating effect of Apo E genotypes, whereas this effect might be overwhelmed by a higher enzyme activity in men (Mahley et al., 2000). This is an analogous situation to the suggestion above that differences in susceptibility might be uncovered by a metabolic challenge (Rubin & Berglund., 2002).

Other causes for the observed differences between studies may be the presence of confounders, the type of dietary intervention used, the population studied and, importantly, the number of subjects in the respective studies. A small number of subjects limits the possibility of detecting differences, or could alternatively lead to spurious associations. Although the number of studies addressing the gene nutrient interaction for Apo E is growing, in most studies so far this has been a secondary endpoint, usually analyzed post hoc. Perhaps the most likely possibility is that a number of dietary interventions will elicit variable responses across Apo E genotypes, but that the ability to detect such differences will depend on the strength and type of intervention as well as on specific recipient factors (type of population, presence of hyperlipidemia, etc.). In the end, however, our ability to confirm or refute the presence of Apo E gene nutrient interactions as well as to understand their metabolic basis fully will require larger and more detailed studies (Rubin & Berglund., 2002).

Inconsistency in nutrient–gene interactions in relation to Apo E polymorphisms may be a result, in part, of retrospective genotyping of small study cohorts, for which the genotype-diet–LDL-C interactions were not the primary outcome. This factor has resulted in the under-representation of the less-frequent genotypes and, although trends may have been evident, many of the studies were clearly under-powered to detect significant genotype–treatment effects. The prospective genotyping of larger study cohorts has been used as an alternative approach to increase statistical power (Lovegrove & Gitau., 2008).

However, recent evidence strongly suggests that variations in a number of key genes may also be important, including common variants of the Apo E gene. The most convincing evidence to date for genotypic effects on dietary response comes from the extensively studied Apo E gene variant (Lovegrove & Gitau., 2008).

A metaanalysis has been published recently that summarizes the overall findings from studies using a variety of end-point measures. A mean 40–50% increase in CHD risk was observed in E4 carriers (overall OR 1. 42) relative to the wild-type E3/E3 genotype, with no apparent differences for either the E2 and E3 subgroups (OR 0. 98). Although a causal mechanism to link E4 with increased CHD risk has not been fully elucidated, the association has been ascribed to a higher concentration of LDL-C. This higher LDL-C is believed to arise from the Apo E4 isoform having a relatively higher affinity for its membrane (LDL/chylomicron remnant) receptor and feedback inhibition of receptor activity in E4 carriers Other mechanisms relating to reduced antioxidant status may also be operative (Lovegrove & Gitau., 2008).

There is the large variation that is observed in the concentration of serum LDL-cholesterol (LDL-C) in response to fish oil supplementation. The cardioprotective effects of the fatty acids in fish oil include eicosapantanoiec acid (EPA) and docosahesanoiec acid (DHA) are well recognized. However, a potentially deleterious increase in LDL-C (5–10%) has been consistently reported after moderate to high doses of fish oil (>2 g EPA+ DHA/d). These data showed the DHA rather than the EPA in fish oils that is responsible for the LDL-C raising effects in E4 individuals (Lovegrove & Gitau., 2008).

In contrast, those with one or more E4 alleles have the highest serum total cholesterol, LDL-, and Apo B levels, the lowest HDL-C levels, and have elevated fasting and postprandial triglyceride levels. They respond best to a low-fat diet but are the least responsive to soluble fiber for lowering serum lipids or to exercise for increasing HDL levels. Fish oil supplementation in these people increases total cholesterol and reduces HDL. Whether a person has the U allele or the E4 allele appears to make a difference in the diet and lifestyle recommendations that would be appropriate for improving vascular health (DeBusk., 2009).

Two prospectively genotyped studies designed to test the hypothesis that Apo E polymorphism has a significant effect on the LDL-C response to EPA and DHA have recently been completed (Lovegrove & Gitau., 2008).

Overall, the triglyceride response to the fat load was lower during fish oil supplementation, and interestingly the decrease in the incremental area under the curve for triglyceride levels was significantly higher for E2 carriers compared with E3 homozygotes and E4 carriers (Rubin & Berglund., 2002).

Although a number of previous studies have observed effects of Apo E genotype in response to dietary total fat and saturated fatty acid (SFA) manipulation, only one study to date has examined the Apo E genotype–dietary fat-LDL-C association using prospective recruitment by genotype. A study reported a significant effect of Apo E genotype on the plasma lipid response to a low fat diet, with a 5%, 13% and 16% reduction in LDL-C in E3/E3, E3/E4 and E4/E4 males, respectively. Other studies have examined the association between Apo E genotype and fish oil (EPA/DHA) on LDL-C responses. In a retrospectively genotyped study it was observed that a mean increase of 7. 1% in LDL-C for the group as a whole was solely attributable to a 16% rise in LDL-C in the Apo E4 participants, and it was speculated that Apo E genotype may, in part, predict the blood lipid response to fish oil intervention. Variable effects of EPA and DHA on LDL-C have been reported previously (Kobayashi et al., 2001; Lovegrove & Gitau., 2008).

The ApoE gene locus accounts for approximately 7% of the population variance in total and LDL cholesterol levels; in general, E4 carriers have higher and E2 carriers have lower LDL cholesterol levels. It has also been suggested that Apo E variations impact triglyceride levels, as higher triglyceride levels have been reported for both E4 and E2 carriers compared with E3 homozygotes (Rubin & Berglund, 2002).

In a recent study of more than 9000 individuals from the Copenhagen City Heart Study, Frikke-Schmidt and colleagues demonstrated that the association between the Apo E locus and cholesterol or plasma Apo B levels was invariant, i. e. present in most contexts (e. g. present in both men and women), whereas associations between Apo E and other lipoproteins such as triglycerides, Apo A-I, HDL cholesterol and lipoprotein (a) were found to be context dependent (Frikke-Schmidt., 2000). As the associations of Apo E with Apo B remained significant when adjusting for cholesterol but not the other way around, this suggested that Apo B is the factor primarily associated with Apo E genotype. It should be pointed out, however, that in their study triglyceride levels represented nonfasting conditions, and LDL cholesterol was not included in the analysis (Rubin & Berglund., 2002).

Furthermore, the Apo E2 allele was more common in individuals with high LpA-I levels, i. e. HDL with Apo AI but not Apo A-II. This HDL subfraction generally corresponds to the larger HDL2 subpopulation, which interestingly, in a study by Isasi et al, was associated with Apo E2 in children (Isasi et al., 2000). In view of their results, Mahley et al, suggest that HDL containing Apo E2 might be a poorer substrate for hepatic lipase compared with HDL with Apo E3 or E4, leading to an accumulation of HDL in plasma. In addition, there might be a difference in the clearing mechanisms between HDL containing Apo E2 compared with Apo E3 or E4 (Mahley et al., 2000).

This mixed pattern was recently addressed by Weggemans et al, who performed a meta-analysis of 26 controlled clinical diet trials conducted. The effect of Apo E genotypes on response to dietary change in 395 healthy subjects, well balanced for sex, was evaluated. The authors pooled data in the response of LDL and HDL cholesterol from four types of trials; replacement of cis-unsaturated fat for saturated fat (n = 7 studies), replacement of cis-unsaturated fat for trans unsaturated fat (n = 2), changes in dietary cholesterol (n = 8) and changes in coffee diterpenes (n = 9). Overall, there were small, non-significant differences between Apo E genotypes in the response of LDL cholesterol, and results were unchanged after adjusting for age, sex and body mass index. For HDL cholesterol, a sex difference was noted, as the response to trans fat and cholesterol differed across Apo E genotypes in men but not in women (Weggemans et al., 2001).

Appropriately, the authors caution against the over interpretation of this result because of chance associations (Rubin & Berglund., 2002).

Friedlander et al, compared plasma levels across Apo E genotypes in response to two diets, a high saturated fat/high cholesterol and a low saturated fat/low cholesterol diet, in 214 free-living individuals in two kibbutz settlements in Israel. Although the baseline total and LDL cholesterol levels were higher among E4 carriers and lower among E2 carriers compared with E3 homozygotes, the plasma lipid response to the diet intervention did not differ across Apo E genotypes (Friedlander et al., 2000).

Loktionov et al, investigated 132 free-living healthy individuals participating in the European Prospective Investigation of Cancer study, a cohort study with approximately 25 000 subjects. The reported subgroup was part of a quality control study on the dietary methods used. In the 132 subjects, serum cholesterol levels correlated with the intake of total and saturated fat. For LDL cholesterol, a significant correlation with relative saturated fat intake was seen only for Apo E 4/3, and not for Apo E3/3 or 3/2 (Loktionov et al., 2000).

In another recent study, researchers analyzed lipid levels in relation to Apo E genotypes in 420 randomly selected free-living Costa Rican individuals consuming a low fat intake (53% of energy). In accordance with most previous studies, E2 carriers had lower, and E4 carriers higher LDL cholesterol and Apo B levels compared with E3 homozygotes. The population was dichotomized in two groups depending on the intake of saturated fat. High saturated fat intake (mean intake 13. 5% of energy) was associated with increased VLDL cholesterol, decreased HDL cholesterol and smaller LDL sizes in Apo E2 carriers, whereas the opposite was found for Apo E4 carriers. Effects on LDL size had previously been noted by Dreon et al, in which a more pronounced decrease in large, buoyant LDL particles during reduced fat intake was seen for Apo E4 carriers (Dreon et al, 1995). The findings of Campos et al suggested, as pointed out by the authors, that in E2 carriers, a high saturated fat intake may result in increased VLDL production and delayed clearance. Such a metabolic challenge might thus unmask a relative susceptibility in E2 carriers (Campos et al, 2001).

Finally, the study on plasma lipid response to dietary fat and carbohydrate in men and women with coronary heart disease provided further support for the association of triglyceride metabolism with Apo E2. Overall, E2 carriers had lower LDL cholesterol as well as a tendency to higher triglyceride levels than E3 and E4 carriers. In addition, there was a positive association between dietary sucrose (6±7% of the total energy intake) and plasma triglyceride levels among E2 carriers (Rubin & Berglund., 2002).

Postprandial studies as Apo E have important functions in chylomicron remnant metabolism, there has been substantial interest in the role of Apo E genotypes in the postprandial setting. Furthermore, a postprandial challenge could serve as a tool to uncover more precisely the differences between different Apo E alleles (Rubin & Berglund., 2002).

In a study of normolipidemic adults by Rubin & Berglund, the Apo E2 allele was associated with an increased postprandial triglyceride response. A similar response has also been demonstrated in other studies. Regarding the Apo E4 allele, more controversial results have been obtained (Rubin & Berglund., 2002).

However, although such studies are compatible with a faster clearance of VLDL and chylomicron remnants in E4 compared with E3 carriers, the meta-analysis showed higher triglyceride and lower HDL cholesterol levels among E4/3 individuals compared with E3 homozygotes. This would perhaps suggest an impaired postprandial clearance among E4 carriers (Rubin & Berglund., 2002). In support of this, another study found an impaired clearance of chylomicron and VLDL remnants in normolipidemic male E4 carriers compared with E3/3. Furthermore, several recent studies have also reported an increased postprandial triglyceride excursion in E4 carriers. In children, they did not observe any difference in triglyceride or retinyl palmitate response between E3/3 and E4 carriers, although a non-significant trend towards higher baseline triglyceride levels as well as higher triglyceride and retinyl palmitate levels 3 h postprandially among E4 carriers was seen (Couch et al., 2000). Another research found no significant effects of the Apo E4 allele on the postprandial triglyceride response after adjusting for baseline triglyceride levels, although a delayed retinyl palmitate clearance in E2 carriers was observed (Rubin & Berglund., 2002). In a recent study by Kobayashi et al, individuals with the E3/3 and E3/4 genotypes were matched for intra-abdominal visceral fat accumulation. Postprandial triglyceride levels did not differ between the two genotypes when adjusting for baseline levels, whereas retinyl palmitate levels among lipoproteins with Sf 5400 were higher among male E3/4 subjects, indicating a slower remnant clearance. As pointed out by the authors, there were fewer women in the study, which might contribute to the non-significant finding in this sex group (Kobayashi et al., 2001).

In a study, the researchers investigated postprandial fat load tolerance in 55 healthy volunteers with an atherogenic lipid profile, defined as triglyceride levels of 1. 5±4 m M, cholesterol 5±8 m M and HDL cholesterol less than 1. 1 m M, as part of a double-blind placebo-controlled crossover study with the consumption of either 6 g of fish oil or 6 g of olive oil supplements for 6 weeks. At the end of each period, a postprandial study was carried out. The difference in LDL cholesterol levels among Apo E genotypes is associated with differences in LDL receptor activity, with Apo E2 carriers having higher and Apo E4 carriers lower activity compared with Apo E3 homozygotes. Conditions with increased stress of this system, such as the increased intake of cholesterol and saturated fat, could therefore result in a variable response in LDL cholesterol levels across Apo E genotypes. In addition, E2 carriers may have decreased lipolytic function with an inhibition of the conversion of VLDL to LDL, as well as a compromised clearance system for triglyceride-rich lipoproteins. Therefore, even a modestly increased VLDL production in response to increased precursor availability might result in differences in plasma triglyceride levels across Apo E genotypes (Rubin & Berglund., 2002).

Although the results from postprandial studies are generally in agreement with the established metabolic differences between Apo E2 and E3, it is currently more difficult to explain the reduced postprandial clearance in E4 carriers. However, it is possible that a differential distribution of the varying Apo E isoforms over different lipoprotein fractions, as well as variations in Apo E levels, could play a role. In addition, a lower LDL receptor activity in E4 carriers may contribute to a decreased postprandial clearance (Rubin & Berglund., 2002).

How could we reconcile these varying results? Even if most studies have established associations between Apo E and baseline lipoprotein levels, the absolute differences between the Apo E genotypes are relatively modest. It might thus be expected that inter-genotype differences in response to nutrient variations may generally be even smaller in magnitude, and thus more difficult to detect, although they might be enhanced by metabolic challenges affecting the synthetic or clearance systems in lipoprotein metabolism described above. Examples of such metabolic stresses in which Apo E gene nutrient interactions may be more readily detectable may be hyperlipidemia, an increased intake of saturated fat or cholesterol, the postprandial state, or alcohol intake. In agreement with this, studies indicating Apo E gene nutrient interactions have been more common in hyperlipidemic settings, whereas it has been more difficult to detect differences across Apo E genotypes in normolipidemic individuals or populations. However, Apo E gene± nutrient interaction has not been seen in all hyperlipidemic states. In familial heperlipidemia heterozygotes, no difference in plasma lipid response to a step 1 diet was seen across Apo E genotypes, indicating that the modulating effects of Apo E may be overwhelmed by other genetic defects, such as LDL receptor deficiency (Rubin & Berglund., 2002).

In conclusion, Apo E has important functions in lipoprotein metabolism and the Apo E polymorphism is associated with plasma lipoprotein levels. Although a large number of studies have addressed whether there is an interaction between Apo E genotypes and diet in affecting plasma lipid levels, this issue is presently unresolved. Most studies to date have involved a small number of subjects, analyzed the Apo E polymorphism post hoc, or included populations in which the effects might be modest, making discrepancies difficult to detect. Studies conducted with conditions representing a metabolic challenge have generally been more successful in finding differential effects across Apo E genotypes, and such studies may be helpful in the future to clarify Apo E gene nutrient relationships. The mixed results obtained indicate that, at present, it is premature to suggest the use of genotyping of Apo E in the design of therapeutic diet interventions (Rubin & Berglund., 2002).

All studies have demonstrated a strong association between plasma cholesterol and Apo E phenotypes in the following order: E4/E4 > E4/E3 > E3/E3 > E3/E2. It has been thought possible that the Apo E gene might be involved in the modulation of dietary plasma cholesterol responses, perhaps explaining the differences in cholesterol concentrations. Some dietary intervention studies have suggested that Apo E4 individuals react to dietary change with exaggerated cholesterol responses. In one study, Apo E4/E4 individuals responded by increased cholesterol reductions during low fat intake, and by increased cholesterol elevations during a switchback to high fat diet. Plausible mechanisms have been postulated which could explain such differences. However, other studies have reported no differences in plasma lipid responses among Apo E phenotypes. The studies cannot be directly compared because of different designs and study populations with differing Apo E allele frequencies (Tikkanen., 1995).

Although Tikkanen et al, found that subjects with the E4/4 phenotype showed the greatest total and LDL-cholesterol responses to dietary change (Tikkanen et al., 1995) Xu et al analyzed the same data and concluded that the Apo E polymorphism did not explain a significant proportion of the variation of the response (Xu et al., 1990). In a meta-analysis of 9 studies involving 612 subjects and found that the presence of the E4 allele was associated with a significantly greater LDL response to dietary intervention (Masson et al, 2003).

Four studies found significantly different HDL-cholesterol responses between genotype groups: one study found that carriers of the E4 allele had the smallest HDL-cholesterol response, whereas the other 3 studies found that carriers of the E4 allele had the largest response (Masson et al., 2003).

However, recent evidence strongly suggests that variations in a number of key genes may also be important, including common variants of the Apo E gene. The most convincing evidence to date for genotypic effects on dietary response comes from the extensively studied Apo E gene variant (Lovegrove & Gitau., 2008).

5.5 Cholesteryl ester transfer protein (CETP)

Another gene that affects HDL levels is CETP, encoding for the cholesteryl ester transfer protein that exchanges cholesteryl esters and triglycerids from HDL to other lipoproteins. This protein is also called the "lipid transfer protein:' People with two copies of a common allele at position 279 of this gene tend to have low HDL levels and elevated levels of LDL and VLDL. A variation (279G>A) that decreases plasma levels of CETP is associated with increased HDL levels, decreased LDL and VLDL levels, and a lower risk of cardiovascular disease than the more common (GG) form (DeBusk, 2009; Musunuru., 2010).

A recent meta-analysis which confirms that the I405V and TaqIB variants are indeed associated with lower CETP activity and higher high-density lipoprotein-cholesterol levels (Boekholdt., 2004).

The currently available evidence suggests that several genetic variants in the CETP gene are associated with altered CETP plasma levels and activity, high-density lipoprotein-cholesterol plasma levels, low-density lipoprotein and high-density lipoprotein particle size, and perhaps the risk of coronary heart disease (Boekholdt., 2004).

5.6 Hepatic lipase (LIPC)

Hepatic lipase (HL) is a lipolytic enzyme involved in the hydrolysis of triacylglycerols present in circulating chylomicrons providing nonesterified fatty acids and 2-monoacylglycerol for tissue utilization and phospholipids from plasma lipoproteins that participates in metabolizing intermediate-density lipoprotein and large LDL into smaller, denser LDL particles, and in converting HDL2 to HDL3 during reverse cholesterol transport (Ordovas & Corella., 2004; Fisler, Warden, 2005; Ordovas., 2006; Much et al., 2005). It may suggest a role to play as a ligand for cell-surface proteoglycans in the uptake of lipoproteins by cell-surface receptors (Fisler & Warden., 2005; Ordovas & Corella., 2004).

Given the wide spectrum of effects that HL exerts on lipoprotein metabolism, and the significance of the promoter variant (s), it is reasonable to hypothesize that genetic variation at this locus may also be involved in variability in the response to dietary therapy (Ordovas & Corella., 2004). HL deficiency is characterized by mildly elevated concentrations of triglyceride-rich LDL and HDL particles, as well as impaired metabolism of postprandial triglyceride-rich lipoproteins, which may result in premature atherosclerosis. Conversely, increased HL activity is associated with increased small, dense LDL particles and decreased HDL2 concentrations, which may also result in increased CAD risk. Four common single nucleotide polymorphisms (SNPs) on the 5_-flanking region of the HL gene (*LIPC*) [−763 (A/G), −710 (T/C), −514 (C/T), and –250 (G/A)] are in total linkage disequilibrium and define a unique haplotype that is associated with variation in HL activity and HDL-cholesterol levels (Fisler & Warden., 2005; Ordovas & Corella., 2004).

The less common A-allele of the SNP at position−250 is associated with lower HL activity and buoyant LDL particles. Normal and CAD subjects heterozygous for the A-allele have lower HL activity and significantly more buoyant LDL particles. Homozygosity for this allele (AA) is associated with an even lower HL activity. The A-allele is associated with higher HDL2-cholesterol (Ordovas & Corella., 2004).

An early intervention study with a low-saturated-fat, low-cholesterol diet found that, although significant improvements in fasting lipids occurred, there was no difference in response between genotypes at the hepatic lipase gene (LIPC) polymorphism measured. However, the study of 83 subjects may not have had adequate power to detect a modest effect of genotype (Fisler & Warden., 2005; Masson & McNeill., 2005; Ordovas., 2006).

Dietary information collected from Framingham Heart Study participants shows that subjects carrying the CC genotype react to higher contents of fat in their diets by increasing the concentrations of HDL-cholesterol, which could be interpreted as a "defense mechanism" to maintain the homeostasis of lipoprotein metabolism. Conversely, carriers of the TT genotype cannot compensate, and experience decreases on the HDL-cholesterol levels. These data could identify a segment of the population especially susceptible to diet-induced atherosclerosis. Considering the higher frequency of the T allele among certain ethnic groups (i. e., African-Americans), these data could shed some light on the impaired ability of certain ethnic groups to adapt to new nutritional environments, as clearly seen for Native Americans and Asian Indians. In this regard, they replicated the significant gene-diet interaction demonstrated in the Caucasian population of Framingham in another multiethnic cohort that consisted of Chinese, Malays, and Indians representing the population of Singapore. In addition to the significant gene-diet interactions reported in these papers, these data provides clues about the reasons why genotype-phenotype association studies fail to show consistent results. In theory, this polymorphism at the hepatic lipase gene will show dramatically different outcomes in association studies depending on the dietary environment of the population studies. The impact of these interactions will be magnified in populations with a high prevalence of the T-allele, as it is with Asians and African-Americans (Ordovas & Corella., 2004).

Three larger observational studies on the effect of a common polymorphism in the LIPC promoter gene –514C→T on the response of HDL cholesterol to dietary fat intake have been published. In examining the effects of the –514C→T LIPC polymorphism x dietary fat interaction on HDL in 2130 men and women participating in the Framingham Study, Ordovas et al found that the rarer *TT* genotype was associated with significantly higher HDL-cholesterol concentrations only in subjects consuming <30% of energy from fat. This same interaction was found for saturated and monounsaturated fats but not for polyunsaturated fat. A second association study, in an Asian population of 2170 subjects, found that Asian Indian subjects with a total fat intake of <30% of energy and with *TT* genotype at the –514C→T polymorphism had the highest HDL-cholesterol concentrations. This interaction, however, did not apply to the Chinese or Malay subjects in that study, and the significant interactions found for saturated or monounsaturated fats found by Ordovas et al were not found in the study by Tai et al. However, these 2 studies are consistent with other studies showing that the *TT* genotype at –514C→T is associated with higher HDL concentrations, although, in 1 of those studies, this effect was attenuated by visceral obesity (Fisler & Warden., 2005).

The third association study of the interaction between dietary fat and the –514C→T polymorphism, by Zhang et al that, from a study population of 18159 men, Zhang et al selected 780 men with confirmed type 2 diabetes. After adjustment for age, smoking, alcohol intake, exercise, and BMI, higher HDL-cholesterol concentrations were found in men with the *CT* or *TT* genotype, which is consistent with previous studies. However, they found significantly higher HDL-cholesterol concentrations in men with the *CT/TT* genotype who consumed large amounts of dietary fat (≥32% of energy), saturated fat, and monounsaturated fat, a result that is apparently opposite to the findings of the other 2 association studies. Thus, the interaction effect of dietary fat with the –514C→T polymorphism was not replicated (Zhang et al., 2005).

Two researcher discussed causes of nonreplication of genetic association studies in obesity and diabetes research that should apply to studies of dyslipidemias as well. An important cause of nonreplication is a lack of statistical power. For any polygenic model, such as models with complex phenotypes (eg, obesity, dyslipidemia, or type 2 diabetes), the effect size for any marker will be small to moderate. Thus, larger sample sizes are needed to ensure adequate power to observe an effect. In the study of Zhang et al, the problem of small sample size (despite the fact that >18000 men were screened to identify ≈800 men with type 2 diabetes) is compounded by the fact that the *TT* genotype is rare, especially in a white population. Thus, only 30 subjects in that study had homozygous *TT* genotype at –514C→T LIPC, and subjects with either the *CT* or *TT* genotype were pooled for analysis. Examination of the data of Ordovas et al and Tai et al found that the slope of predicted values for HDL cholesterol versus total fat intake as a percentage of energy is steeply negative in persons with the *TT* genotype, whereas it is positive for persons with the *CT* genotype (Ordovas, et al, 2002; Tai et al, 2003). Assuming that the data of Zhang et al followed the same pattern, combining the smaller number (n = 30) of persons with the *TT* genotype with the larger number (n = 247) of persons with the *CT* genotype would mask the effects of percentage of dietary fat and the *TT* genotype on HDL-cholesterol concentrations. An additional complexity is that BMI and obesity phenotypes may also interact with dietary fat and LIPC genotype to modulate HDL-cholesterol concentrations (Tai et al., 2003; Zhang., 2005). Thus, the nonreplication in the study by Zhang et al of the findings of Ordovas et al and Tai et al is likely due to the small number of persons with the *TT* genotype who were available in the study of Zhang et al (Fisler & Warden., 2005).

5.7 Lipoprotein lipase (LPL)

LPL, encoding lipoprotein lipase, which hydrolyzes triglycerides in chylomicrons and VLDL particles, converting the latter to LDL particles, as well facilitating cellular lipoprotein uptake (Musunuru, 2010).

Several polymorphisms have been described that disrupt normal LPL function and contribute to the premature development of CHD, primarily through the increased levels of circulating TGs (Much et al., 2005).

Indeed, several of the common LPL polymorphisms described by Merkel et al have recently been established to influence circulating lipid levels in pregnant women, whom are often characterized with high levels of circulating TGs and increased total cholesterol (Merkel et al., 2011). Although TG levels were unaffected, certain LPL SNPs modulated HDL levels and may alter the susceptibility of pregnant women to developing CHD. However, further studies are required to definitively define a relationship between lipid levels, CHD, and pregnant women. Therefore, the importance of LPL in the whole-body regulation of lipid metabolism has been avidly demonstrated and merits further exploration.

One common LPL polymorphism, known as T495G *Hind* III, has been extensively examined and demonstrates the complexity of disease prediction associated with a single SNP. Indeed, preliminary indications suggest that this polymorphism may play a role in the onset of several important diseases, such as CHD, diabetes and obesity. This SNP has been associated with the higher plasma TG and lower HDL levels characteristic with the early onset of diabetes. Preliminary results have also suggested a positive association between the *Hind* III polymorphism and a predisposition to developing obesity. Finally, this polymorphism has been associated with variations in lipid levels and heart disease, and that these alterations were attenuated by such environmental factors as physical exercise and low calorie diets, reiterating the important interactions arising between lifestyle, nutrition, and disease. Although these associations are not conclusive, they do suggest that LPL variants play a critically important role in the regulation of whole-body lipid metabolism that may predispose an individual to the onset of several metabolic diseases.

A relationship was established between a low calorie diet and the circulating lipid profile in obese individuals with the *Hind* III polymorphism. Homozygotes (H2H2) were found to have significantly higher levels of plasma VLDL-TG and Apo B than heterozygotes. Caloric restriction reduced lipid levels in both H2H2 and H1 individuals to a point where no difference was observed between the groups. Although H2H2 individuals responded more strongly (larger decreases in plasma lipids) to the low calorie diet, these preliminary results identify an important relationship between LPL polymorphisms, function, and diet (Much et al., 2005).

As such, it is difficult to draw any firm conclusions from any one gene-diet study in the absence of replication by another study that examined the same question using similar methodologies. For example, one study demonstrated that a Mediterranean-style, MUFA-rich diet compared to a high-carbohydrate diet increased LDL size in individuals with certain Apo E gene variants but decreased LDL size in those with other Apo E variants; this is potentially a clinically important observation, but no confirmatory study has yet emerged, calling this observation into doubt. As pointed out by others, the field would greatly benefit from increased collaboration and coordination of studies among international nutrition researchers (Musunuru., 2010).

6. Magnitude of the response

Because of the heterogeneity in the type and duration of the interventions described the magnitude of the lipid response to dietary interventions varied widely: in one study the change in LDL cholesterol in the Apo B *Eco*RI R-R- genotype group was as large as 59% of the baseline concentration. In the studies that showed a significant difference in response between genotype groups, the results also varied widely: in some studies, the difference in response between 2 genotype groups was ≈20% of the baseline lipid concentration (Rantala et al., 2000; Clitfon., 1997). However, the magnitude of these differences cannot be estimated with any accuracy, largely because most studies had only a small number of subjects in the rare genotype group (Masson et al, 2003). The proportion of variance in the lipid response attributable to a single polymorphism is not likely to be > 10% (Xu et sal., 1990). Therefore, individual genes contribute only a small part to the variation in the lipid response; however, when several genes are considered, the proportion of variance explained could be larger (Masson et al, 2003).

7. Evidence for a gene-diet interaction

Evidence suggests that variation in the genes for apolipoproteins A-I, A-IV, B, and E may contribute to the heterogeneity in the lipid response to dietary intervention. Many studies were unable to show significantly different responses between these genotype groups, and the genotypes showing the greatest response are not necessarily consistent between studies. There was insufficient evidence to assess whether lipid responsiveness is affected by variation in the genes for Apo C-III, lipoprotein lipase, hepatic lipase, the cholesteryl ester transfer protein. Although each of these gene products is essential in lipid metabolism, only a handful of studies have investigated variation in these genes, and most of these studies were unable to show significant gene-diet interactions (Masson et al, 2003).

8. Publication bias

Publication bias is a problem with any review because "studies with results that are significant, interesting, from large well-funded studies, or of higher quality are more likely to be submitted, published, or published more rapidly than work without such characteristics" (Sutton, 2000). Therefore, it is possible that other relevant dietary intervention studies with genotype information exist but were not included in this review because they have not been published. It is possible that the literature strategy for this review missed studies because the genotype analyses were not mentioned in their title, abstract, or subject headings (Masson et al, 2003).

In the search for explanations for the heterogeneity in lipid responses, reviewers may tend to highlight studies showing significant effects of genetic variation while ignoring a large proportion of studies that found no such results. Studies showing nonsignificant or conflicting results cannot be ignored, especially because they outnumber the studies showing significant effects, notwithstanding the unpublished studies that could have nonsignificant and uninteresting results. Therefore, one has to ask the question "If genetic variability plays a role in the heterogeneity of lipid and lipoprotein responses to dietary change, why have so many studies been unable to demonstrate this with statistical significance?" (Masson et al, 2003).

9. Possible reasons for conflicting results

There are many possible reasons why studies have been unable to show statistically significant gene-diet interactions. First, it is highly probable that lipid responses to dietary change are under polygenic control, with each gene contributing a relatively small effect. However, most studies have attempted to find only single-gene effects (Masson et al, 2003). Most of the studies summarized in this review lacked sufficient statistical power to detect any but a very strong effect because the sample sizes were too small, particularly for genotypes with low frequencies of the rare allele. However, many of the studies were retrospective and were not designed to examine gene-diet interactions, but data were reexamined after the availability of new information from genotype analyses. Therefore, it is perhaps not surprising that significant effects were not found in many studies because the numbers of individuals in each genotype group were so small. In many studies there were too few subjects homozygous for the rare allele to allow an analysis that would take into account differences in the response between heterozygote's and homozygote's. For Apo E, where there are 6 possible genotypes, differences in the grouping of these could also lead to differences in results between studies. This illustrates that meta-analyses are important because they can detect effects with greater power and greater precision because of their inflated sample size (Rantala et al., 2000; Lopez-Miranda et al., 1994). In addition, in studies with small sample sizes, genotype misclassification of one individual may significantly affect the interpretation and validity of the results. Conflicting results may also occur because of the different dietary protocols that were followed. The studies reviewed varied widely in the composition and length of the baseline and experimental diets. The dietary factors responsible for the changes seen in each genotype group are not clear because many studies modified several dietary factors, and so the dietary content in future studies should be tightly controlled and compliance must be strictly measured not only for cholesterol and the amount and type of fatty acids but also for other influential dietary components such as fiber and plant sterols. In addition, these studies investigated fasting lipid and lipoprotein concentrations; however, the effect of genetic variation may be more evident in the postprandial state than in the less-common fasting state). Differences in the age, sex, body mass index, menopausal status, dietary backgrounds, and baseline lipid values of the participants could also have contributed to the discrepancies between the results. For instance, subjects with the E4 allele tend to have higher baseline total and LDL-cholesterol concentrations, and so greater responses in these subjects could reflect the regression to the mean phenomenon. It is also possible that weight change could account for differences in lipid and lipoprotein changes. In addition, a significant effect may not reflect a causal relation but the allele may be in linkage disequilibrium with another one that does. For example, the base change that results in the *Xba* I site in the gene for Apo B does not alter the amino acid, and so it may be in linkage disequilibrium with another functional mutation (Masson et al., 2003).

The studies varied widely in terms of the number and type of study participants, the composition and duration of the dietary interventions, the nutrients studied and dietary assessment methods used in the observational studies, and the polymorphisms analyzed - some of which had not been studied before with regard to the lipid response to diet (Masson et al., 2005).

10. Conclusion

Evidence suggests that genetic variation may contribute to the heterogeneity in lipid responsiveness. At present, the evidence is limited but suggestive and justifies the need for future studies with much larger sample sizes based on power calculations, with carefully controlled dietary interventions, and that investigate the effects of polymorphisms in multiple genes rather than in single genes. Investigating gene-diet interactions will increase our knowledge of the mechanisms involved in lipid metabolism and improve our understanding of the role of diet in reducing cardiovascular disease risk (Masson et al., 2003).

Future studies will have to be large in order to assess the effects of multiple polymorphisms, and will have to control for many factors other than diet. At present, it is premature to recommend the use of genotyping in the design of therapeutic diets. However, such studies may be useful in identifying the mechanisms by which dietary components influence lipid levels (Masson & McNeill., 2005).

However, current knowledge is still very limited and so is the potential benefit of its application to clinical practice. Thinking needs to evolve from simple scenarios (e. g., one single dietary component, a single nucleotide polymorphism and risk factor) to more realistic situations involving multiple interactions. One of the first situations where personalized nutrition is likely to be beneficial is in patients with dyslipidemia who require special intervention with dietary treatment. This process could be more efficient if the recommendations were carried out based on genetic and molecular knowledge. Moreover, adherence to dietary advice may increase when it is supported with information based on nutritional genomics, and a patient believes the advice is personalized. However, a number of important changes in the provision of health care are needed to achieve the potential benefits associated with this concept, including a teamwork
approach with greater integration among physicians, food and nutrition professionals, and genetic counselors (Ordovas., 2006).

The ultimate goal of nutritional genomics is to provide sufficient knowledge to allow diagnosis and nutritional treatment recommendations based on an individual's genotype. Defining the interaction effects of nutrients and genes on complex phenotypes will be the challenge of this field of nutrition research for some time to come (Fisler & Warden, 2005; Gregori et al, 2011; Ordovas & Corella., 2004).

11. Ethic

Although an increased understanding of how these and other genes influence response to nutrients should facilitate the progression of personalized nutrition, the ethical issues surrounding its routine use need careful consideration (Lovegrove & Gitau., 2008).

The study of nutrigenetics is in its infancy. Many studies published in this area have only considered one SNP in a single gene, with little consideration being given to multiple nutrient–gene–environmental interactions. Although this is scientifically valid, and invaluable for the elucidation of causative mechanisms in disease, multiple gene–nutrient–environment–gender interactions will be required for developing specific personalized nutritional advice. The collation of data in haplotype databases and biobanks is expensive and difficult to establish, but is a necessity if nutrigenetic research is to progress (Lovegrove & Gitau., 2008).

Standardized protocols in nutrigenetics are not yet established, the comparison of studies is challenging and conclusions are often difficult to draw. As discussed previously, studies are often retrospective in design and thus of insufficient power to detect nutrient–gene associations. Prospective genotyping increases the power to resolve these associations and should be used whenever possible. With any research, publication bias results in positive associations being reported more often than negative associations. This has applied to nutrigentic studies and created a false impression of the level of significance of many nutrient–gene interactions (Lovegrove & Gitau., 2008).

There are numerous ethical issues and unavoidable assumptions that need to be considered before personalized nutritional can become routine practice. First, it is important to consider whether the genetic tests and personalized food products would be affordable, cost-effective and socially acceptable. It is also of concern that only the well educated and affluent would benefit. The open accessibility of genetic information to third parties has major implications for the availability of health insurance and increased premiums (Lovegrove, Gitau, 2008).

Moreover, it is still unknown whether people will want to undertake genetic tests or even understand the concept of such technology. A survey was conducted by Cogent Research in 2003 on 1000 Americans in which 62% of respondents reported they had never heard of 'nutrigenomics'. However, if specific products did arise from nutrigenomic research, those interviewed did express interest in an in-depth well-being assessment and also a strong interest in vitamins, fortified foods and natural foods. More research is required to determine whether individuals would want to undergo such tests, and for understanding the value to the individual of an increased awareness of personalized nutrition regimens. There is already a large gap between the existing dietary guidelines and what people actually eat. Knowledge of being at higher than average risk of CVD may motivate people to actually make positive changes to their diets. However, genetic testing could undermine current healthy eating messages, by implying that only those with the 'risky gene' need to eat a healthy diet. These are important unanswered questions that must be addressed if personalized nutritional advice is ever to become part of mainstream disease prevention and treatment. It may be that the interactions between genotype–phenotype and the environment are just too complex to be properly understood from human dietary intervention studies (Lovegrove, Gitau, 2008).

There is resistance to the use and perceived effectiveness of personalized nutrition that is based on genomics, and whether this can offer a solution to diseases caused by a diet that is inappropriate for health (Canon & Leitzmann, 2005). It has been suggested that it may be more beneficial to use current risk factors as a basis for population screening and the management of CVD (McCluskey et al., 2007). There has also been dialogue on the social, economic and environmental causes of CVD, shifting the emphasis away from dietary intake to food manufacturing as being more effective in disease management (Canon & Leitzmann, 2005; Lovegrove & Gitau., 2008).

Progression of knowledge in the fields of nutrient–gene interactions promises a future revolution in preventative health care. However, although there is increasing evidence for interactions between diets/nutrients, genes and environmental factors, there are inconsistencies in the evidence that will limit the application of nutrigenetics in diet-related disease in the immediate future. In addition to the need for adequately powered intervention studies, greater attention should be given to ethical issues, such as the public's acceptance of genetic testing and the economics of this relatively new science (Lovegrove & Gitau., 2008).

Ethical issues fall into a number of categories: (1) why nutrigenomics? Will it have important public health benefits? (2) questions about research, e. g. concerning the acquisition of information about individual genetic variation; (3) questions about who has access to this information, and its possible misuse; (4) the applications of this information in terms of public health policy, and the negotiation of the potential tension between the interests of the individual in relation to, for example, prevention of conditions such as obesity and allergy; (5) the appropriate ethical approach to the issues, e. g. the moral difference, if any, between therapy and enhancement in relation to individualised diets; whether the 'technological fix' is always appropriate, especially in the wider context of the purported lack of public confidence in science, which has special resonance in the sphere of nutrition (Chadwick., 2004).

12. References

Amouyel, P. (2000). Genomics and cardiovascular diseases. *Bull Acad Natl Med.* 184 (7):1431-8.

Boekholdt, SM. & Kuivenhoven, JA. & Hovingh, GK. & Jukema, JW. & Kastelein, JJ. & van, Tol A. (2004). CETP gene variation: relation to lipid parameters and cardiovascular risk. *Curr Opin Lipidol.* 15 (4):393-8.

Campos, H. & D'Agostino, M. & Ordovas, JM. (2001). Gene±diet interactions and plasma lipoproteins: role of apolipoprotein E and habitual saturated fat intake. *Genet Epidemiol;* 20:117±128.

Canon, G. & Leitzmann, C. (2005). The new nutrition science Progect. *Public Health Nutr.* : 8 (6A):673-694.

Carmena-Ramon, R. & Ascaso, J F. & Real, J T. & Ordovas, J M. (1998). Genetic Variation at the ApoA-IV Gene Locus and Response to Diet in Familial Hypercholesterolemia. *Arteriosclerosis, Thrombosis, and Vascular Biology.* 18:1266- 1274.

Chadwick, R. (2004). Nutrigenomics, individualism and public health. *Proc Nutr Soc.* 63 (1):161-6.

Clifton, P. & Kind, K. & Jones, C. & , Noakes, M. (1997). Response to dietary fat and cholesterol and genetic polymorphisms. *Clin Exp Pharmacol Physiol;*24:A21–5.

Corella, D. & Tucker, K. & Lahoz, C. & Coltell, O. & Cupples, L A. & Wilson, P WF. & Schaefer, E J. & Ordovas, J M. (2001). Alcohol drinking determines the effect of the *APOE* locus on LDL-cholesterol concentrations in men: the Framingham Offspring Study. *American Journal of Clinical Nutrition.* 73 (4): 736-745.

Couch, SC. & Isasi, CR. & Karmally. W, et al. (2000). Predictors of postprandial triacylglycerol response in children: the Columbia University Biomarkers Study. *Am J Clin Nutr.* 72:1119±1127.

Debra A. K. (2008). Medical Nutrition Therapy For Cardiovascular Disease. In Mahan KL, Escoott- Stump S (eds). *Krause's Food Nutrition and Diet Therapy.* Suanders. 12th ed. Philadelphia. 833-864. DeBusk, R. . (2008). Nutritional genomic. In Mahan KL, Escoott-Stump S (eds). *Krause's Food Nutrition and Diet Therapy.* 12th ed. Suanders. Philadelphia. Pp: 364- 382.

DeBusk, R M. (2009). Nutritional Genomics: The Foundation for Personalized Nutrition, What Is Nutritional Genomicsl. *In Advanced nutrition and human metabolism.* Sareen S. G, Jack L. Smith, James L. G. FIFTH EDITION. *WADSWORTH-CENGAGE Learning".* USA. pp 29-32.

Dreon, DM. & Fernstrom, HA. & Miller, B. & , Krauss, RM. (1995). Apolipoprotein E isoform phenotype and LDL subclass response to a reduced-fat diet. *Arterioscler Thromb Vasc Biol;* 15:105±111.

El-Sohemy, A. (2007). Nutrigenetics. *Forum Nutr.* 60:25-30.

Engler, M B. (2009). Nutrigenomics in Cardiovascular Disease: Implications for the Future. *Progress in Cardiovascular Nursing.* 24 (4): 190–195.

Farhud, D. & Shalileh, M. (2008). Phenylketonuria and its Dietary Therapy in Children. Iran J Pediatr. 18 (Suppl 1):88-98.

Farhud, DD. & Zarif Yeganeh, M. & Zarif Yeganeh, M. *(2010).* Nutrigenomics and Nutrigenetics. *Iranian J Public Health.* 39 (4) :1-14.

Fenech, M. (2008). Genome health nutrigenomics and nutrigenetics-dignosis and nutritional treatment of genome damage on an individual basis. *FdChem Tox*. 46 (4):1365-70.

Fisler, J S. & Warden, C H. (2005). Dietary fat and genotype: toward individualized prescriptions for lifestyle changes *American Journal of Clinical Nutrition*. 81 (6): 1255-1256.

Friedlander, Y. & Leitersdorf, E. & Vecsler, R. et al. (2000). The contribution of candidate genes to the response of plasma lipids and lipoproteins to dietary challenge. *Atherosclerosis*. 152:239±248.

Frikke-Schmidt R. (2000). Context-dependent and invariant associations between APOE genotype and levels of lipoproteins and risk of ischemic heart disease: a review. *Scand J Clin Lab Invest*. 60 (Suppl. 233):3±26.

Gillies, P J. (2003). Nutrigenomics : the Rubicon of molecular nutrition. *J am Diet Ass*. 103 (12 suppl 2):50-55.

Gregori, D. & Foltran, F. & Verduci, E. & Ballali, S. & Franchin, L. & Ghidina, M. &. Halpern, G M. & Giovannini, M. (2011) A Genetic Perspective on Nutritional Profiles: Do We Still Need Them?. *J Nutrigenet Nutrigenomic*. 4 (1):25-35.

Hank Juo, S-H. & Wyszynski, D F. & Beaty, T H. & Huang, H-Y. & Bailey-W, J E. (1999). Mild association between the A/G polymorphism in the promoter of the apolipoprotein A-I gene and apolipoprotein A-I levels: A meta- analysis. *American Journal of Medical Genetics*. 82 (3):235-241.

Heilbronn a, L. K., & Noakes b, M. & Morris a, A. M. & Kind b, K. L. & Clifton, P. M. (2000). 360His polymorphism of the apolipoproteinA-IV gene and plasma lipid response to energy restricted diets in overweight subjects. *Atherosclerosis*. 150: 187–192.

Hernell, O. & West. C. (2008). Do we need personalized recommendations for infants at risk of developing disease? *Nestle Nutr Workshop ser Pediatr Program*. 62:239-49; discussion 249-52.

Hockey, K. J. & Anderson, R. A. & Cook, V. R. & Hantgan, R. R. & Weinberg R. B. (2001)Effect of the apolipoprotein A-IV Q360H polymorphism on postprandial plasma triglyceride clearance. *J. Lipid Res.* . 42: 211–217.

Isasi, CR. & Couch, SC. & Deckelbaum, RJ. et al. (2000). The apolipoprotein e2 allele is associated with an anti- atherogenic lipoprotein profile in children: the Columbia University Biomarkers Study. *Pediatrics*; 106:568±575.

Jarvik, GP., & Goode, EL. & Austin, MA, et al. (1997). Evidence that the apolipoprotein Egenotype effects on lipid levels can change with age in males: a longitudinal analysis. *Am J Hum Genet*; 61:171±181.

Kobayashi, J. & Saito, Y. & Taira, K. & Hikita, M. & , Takahashi, K. & Bujo, H. & Morisaki, N. & Saito, Y. (2001). Effect of apolipoprotein E3:4 phenotype on postprandial triglycerides and retinyl palmitate metabolism in plasma from hyperlipidemic subjects in Japan. *Atherosclerosis*. 154; 539–546.

Kusmann, M. & Fsy, L B. (2008). nutrigenomics and personalized nutrition:science and concept. *Personalized Medicine*. 5 (5):447-455.

Loktionov, A. & Scollen, S. & McKeown, N. & Bingham S. (2000). Gene±nutrient interactions: dietary behavior associated with high coronary heart disease risk particularly affects serum LDL cholesterol in apolipoprotein E (4-carrying free-living individuals. *Br J Nutr*. 84:885±890.

Lopez-Miranda, J. & Ordovas, JM. & Mata, P, et al. (1994). Effect of apolipoprotein E phenotype on diet-induced lowering of plasma low density lipoprotein cholesterol. *J Lipid Res.* 35:1965–75.

Lovegrove, J. A. & Gitau, R. (2008). Personalized nutrition for the prevention of cardiovascular disease: a future perspective. *Journal of Human Nutrition and Dietetics.* 21 (4) : 306–316.

Mahley, RW. & PeÂ, pin J. & Erhan, Paraoglu K, et al. (2000). Low levels of high density lipoproteins in Turks, a population with elevated hepatic lipase: high density lipoprotein characterization and gender-specific effects of apolipoprotein E genotype. *J Lipid Res.* 41:1290±1301.

Masson, L F. & McNeill, G. & Avenell, A. (2003). Genetic variation and the lipid response to dietary intervention: a systematic review· *American Journal of Clinical Nutrition.* 77 (5): 1098-1111.

Masson, L F. & McNeill, G. (2005). The effect of genetic variation on the lipid response to dietary change: recent findings. *Current Opinion in Lipidology.* 16 (1):61-67.

McCluskey, S. & Baker, D. & Perey, D. & Lewis, P. & Middleton, E. (2007). Reduction in cardiovascular risk in association with population screening : a 10- year longitudinal study. *J Public Heaht (oxf).* 29:379-387.

Merkel, M. & Eckel, R H. & Goldberg, I J. (2011). Lipoprotein lipase: genetics, lipid uptake and regulation
URL:www. jlr. org. on July 26.

Miggiano, GA. & De Sanctis, R. (2006). Nutritional genomics: toward a personalized diet. *Clin Ter.* 157 (4):355-61.

Musunuru, K. (2010). Atherogenic Dyslipidemia: Cardiovascular Risk and Dietary Intervention. *Lipids.* 45:907–914.

Mutch, D M. & Wahli, W. & Gary, W. (2005). Nutrigenomics and nutrigenetics: the emerging faces of nutrition. *The FASEB Journal.* 19:1602-1616.

Ordovas, J. M. (2002). Gene-diet interaction and plasma lipid responses to dietary intervention. *Biochemical Society Transactions.* 30: (68–73).

a.Ommen, B V. (2004). Nutrigenomics: Exploiting Systems Biology in the Nutrition and Health Arenas. *Nutrition.* 20:4–8.

b.Ordovas, JM. (2004). The quest for cardiovascular health in the genomic era : nutrigenetics and plasma lipoproteins. *Proc Nutr Soc.* 63 (1):145-152.

Ordovas JM, Corella D. (2004). Nutritional genomics. *Annu Rev Genomics Hum Genet.* 5:71-118.

Ordovas JM, Mooser V. (2004). Nutrigenomics and nutrigenetics. *Curr Opin Lipidol.* 15 (2):101-8.

Ordovas, J. M. (2006). Nutrigenetics, plasma lipids and cardiovascular risk. *Journal Of The American Dietetic Association.* 106 (7):1074-81.

Ordovas. J M. & Kaput, J. & Corella, D. (2007). Nutrition in the genomics era: Cardiovascular disease risk and the Mediterranean diet. *Molecular Nutrition & Food Research.* 51 (10) :1293–1299.

Ordovas, J M. (2009). Genetic influences on blood lipids and cardiovascular disease risk: tools for primary prevention. *American Journal of Clinical Nutrition.* 89 (5):1509S-1507S.

Perez-Martinez, P. & Garcia-Rios, A. & Delgado-Lista, J. & Perez-Jimenez, F. & Lopez-Miranda, J. (2011). Nutrigenetics of the postprandial lipoprotein metabolism: evidences from human intervention studies. *Curr Vasc Pharmacol.* 9 (3):287-91.

Rantala, M. & Rantala, TT. & Savolainen, MJ. & Friedlander, Y. & Kesaniemi, YA. (2000). Apolipoprotein B gene polymorphisms and serum lipids: meta-analysis of the role of genetic variation in responsiveness to diet. *Am J Clin Nutr.* 71:713-24.

Rideout, T C. (2011). Getting personal: considering variable interindividual responsiveness to dietary lipid-lowering therapies. *Current Opinion in Lipidology.* 22 (1): 37–42 .

Rimbach, G. & Minihane, A M. (2009). nutrigenetics and personalized nutrition:how far have we progressed and are we likely to get there? *Proceedings of the Nutrition Society.* 68 (2): 162-172.

Rubin, J. & Berglund, L. (2002). Apolipoprotein E and diets: a case of gene-nutrient interaction? *Current Opinion in Lipidology.* 13:25±32.

Ryan-Harshman, M. & Vogel, E. & Jones-Taggart, H. & Green-Johnson, J. & Castle, D. & Austin, Z. & Anderson, K. (2008). Nutritional genomics and dietetic professional practice. Kristin Anderson Can J Diet Pract Res. 69 (4):177-82.

Shalileh, M. & , Shidfar, F. & Eghtesadi, SH. & Haghani, H. & Heidari, I. (2009). The Effects of Calcium Supplement on Serum Lipoprotein in Obese Adults Receiving Energy Restricted Diet. *Iranian J Publ Health.* 38 (4):10-20.

Shalileh, M. & , Shidfar, F. & Haghani, H. & Eghtesadi, SH. & Heidari, I. (2010). The influence of calcium supplement on body composition, weight loss and insulin resistance in obese adults receiving low calorie diet. JRMS; 15 (4):1-11.

Sheweta, B. & Deepak, M. & BS Khatkar. (2011). Nutrigenomics :The emerging face of nutrition. *International Journal of Current Research and Review.* 3 (6) :108-113.

Subbiah, M T R. (2007). Nutrigenetics and nutraceuticals: the next wave riding on personalized medicine. *Transl res.* 149 (2):55-61.

Sutton, A J. & Duval, S J. & Tweedie, R L. & Abrams, K R. & Jones, D R. *(2000).* Empirical assessment of effect of publication bias on meta-analyse. *BMJ.* 320 : 1574

Svacina, S. (2007)Nutrigenetics and nutrigenomics. *Cas Lek Cesk.* 146 (11):837-9.

Tai, E S. & Corella, D. & Deurenberg-Yap, M. & Cutter, J. & Chew Kai, S. & Tan, C E. & Ordovas, J M. (2003). Dietary Fat Interacts with the -514C>T Polymorphism in the Hepatic Lipase Gene Promoter on Plasma Lipid Profiles in a Multiethnic Asian Population: The 1998 Singapore National Health Survey. *J Nutr.* 133:3399-3408.

Tikkanen, M. & Huttunen, JK. & Pajukanta, PE. & Pietinen, P. (1995). Apolipoprotein E polymorphism and dietary plasma cholesterol response. *Can J Cardiol.* 11:93G-96G.

URL: en. wikipedia. org/wiki/Dyslipidemia.

URL : http://www. who. int/mediacentre/factsheets/fs317/en/index. html

Wallace, A J. & E Humphries, S. & Fisher, R M. & Mann, J I. & Chisholm, A. & Sutherland, W H F. (2000). Genetic factors associated with response of LDL subfractions to change in the nature of dietary fat. *Atherosclerosis.* ; 149 (2) : 387-394.

Weggemans, RM. & Zock, PL. & Ordovas JM, et al. (2001). Apoprotein E genotype and the response of serum cholesterol to dietary fat, cholesterol and cafestol. *Atherosclerosis.* 154:547±555.

Weinberg, R B. & Geissinger, B W. & Kasala, K. & Hockey, K J. & James G, T. & Easter, L. & Crouse, R. (2000). Effect of apolipoprotein A-IV genotype and dietary fat on cholesterol absorption in humans. *J Lipid Res.* 41: 2035-2041.

Weinberg RB. (2002). Apolipoprotein A-IV polymorphisms and diet-gene interactions. *Curr Opin Lipidol*. 13 (2):125-34.

Wood, Philip A. (2008). Potential of nutrigenetics in the treatment of metabolic disorders. Expert Review of Endocrinology and Metabolism. 3 (6): 705-713.

Xacur-García F, Castillo-Quan JI, Hernández-Escalante VM, Laviada-Molina H. (2008). Nutritional genomics: an approach to the genome-environment interaction. *Rev Med Chil*. Nov. 136 (11):1460-7.

Xu, CF. & Boerwinkle, E. & Tikkanen, MJ. & Huttunen, JK. & Humphries, SE. & Talmud, PJ. (1990). Genetic variation at the apolipoprotein gene loci contribute to response of plasma lipids to dietary change. *Genet Epidemiol*; 7:261–75.

Zak, A. & Slaby, A. (2007). Gene – diet interactions in atherogenic dyslipidemias (part1). *Cas Lek Cesk*. 146 (12):896-901.

Zhang, C. & Lopez-Ridaura, R. & Rimm, E B. & Rifai, Nr. & Hunter, D J. & Hu, F B. (2005). Interactions between the –514C→T polymorphism of the hepatic lipase gene and lifestyle factors in relation to HDL concentrations among US diabetic men. *American Journal of Clinical Nutrition*. 81 (6):1429-1435.

Ethnic Difference in Lipid Profiles

Lei Zhang[1,2,3,4], Qing Qiao[1,4] and Yanhu Dong[2,3]
[1]*Hjelt Institute, University of Helsinki, Helsinki,*
[2]*Qingdao Endocrine & Diabetes Hospital, Qingdao,*
[3]*Weifang Medical University, Weifang,*
[4]*National Institute for Health and Welfare, Helsinki,*
[1,4]*Finland*
[2,3]*China*

1. Introduction

Dyslipidaemia is a major cardiovascular disease (CVD) risk factor that plays an important role in the progress of atherosclerosis, the underlying pathology of CVD. To keep lipids and lipoproteins levels within ideal range has been recommended by different national, regional, or global (2001; Graham et al. 2007; World Health Organization 2007) guidelines on the prevention and management of CVD. The prevalence and pattern of lipid disorder, however, differ between ethnicities and populations.

As a component of the metabolic syndrome, dyslipidaemia often coexists with diabetes, the coronary heart disease (CHD) risk equivalent. An atherogenic lipid profiles consists of high triglycerides (TG) and small dense low-density lipoprotein cholesterol (LDL-C) and low high-density lipoprotein cholesterol (HDL-C). The importance of dyslipidaemia on risk of CVD in patients with diabetes has been extensively studied in numerous studies. Reduced HDL-C is well documented as an independent predictor of CVD events (Wilson et al. 1988; Cooney et al. 2009). In contrast, the role of TG as an independent risk factor for CVD is more controversial (Patel et al. 2004; Psaty et al. 2004; Barzi et al. 2005; Sarwar et al. 2007; Wang et al. 2007). Recently, the interest to use novel parameters such as total cholesterol (TC) to HDL ratio (TC/HDL-C), non-HDL-cholesterol (non-HDL-C), apolipoprotein B (apoB) and apolipoprotein A (apoA) to assess CVD risk has increased (Barzi et al. 2005; Pischon et al. 2005; Charlton-Menys et al. 2009). As a CVD risk predictor, the non-HDL-C has been considered to be superior to LDL-C (Cui et al. 2001; Schulze et al. 2004; Liu et al. 2005; Ridker et al. 2005). However, there are racial and geographic disparities in lipid profiles not only in general populations but also in individuals with different glucose categories. The Third Report of the National Cholesterol Education Program Expert Panel on Detection, Evaluation, and Treatment of High Blood Cholesterol in Adults (NCEP-ATP III) has recommended that certain factors be recognized when clinicians evaluate the lipid profile of different population groups (Adult Treatment Panel III 2002). Although management of lipids using NCEP-ATP III guidelines is applicable to all populations, unique aspects of risk factor profile call for special attention to certain features in different racial/ethnic groups.

2. Ethnic differences in lipid profiles in general populations

The prevalence of dyslipidaemia varies depending on the population studied, geographic location, socioeconomic development and the definition used (Wood et al. 1972; Mann et al. 1988; Onat et al. 1992; Berrios et al. 1997; Ezenwaka et al. 2000; Foucan et al. 2000; Hanh et al. 2001; Zaman et al. 2001; Azizi et al. 2003; Florez et al. 2005; Li et al. 2005; Hertz et al. 2006; Pang et al. 2006; Pongchaiyakul et al. 2006; Tekes-Manova et al. 2006; Zhao et al. 2007; Erem et al. 2008; Steinhagen-Thiessen et al. 2008). Caucasians generally have higher mean TC concentrations than do populations of Asian or African origin (Fuentes et al. 2003; Tolonen et al. 2005). In general populations, the highest prevalence of hypercholesterolaemia (TC ≥ 6.5mmol/l) has been seen in Malta (up to 50% in women) and the lowest in China (2.7% in men) in the World Health Orgnization (WHO) Inter-Health Programme (Berrios et al. 1997). However, inhabitants of the developing world now have had access to more fats in their diets and more sedentary lives; therefore the disease is becoming an increasing problem there.

Ethnic differences in the risk of CVD and type 2 diabetes have consistently been identified, with the most studies comparing the risk between African-Americans and Whites. African-Americans usually display a more favorable lipid profile compared with Whites, despite having the highest overall mortality rates from CVD. In general, African-American men have similar or lower LDL-C and TG but higher HDL-C levels compared with White men. There is evidence that the difference in HDL-C between African-American and White men may be due to a relatively lower hepatic lipase activity in African-Americans (Vega GL 1998). The difference in TG may be related to increased activity of lipoprotein lipase in African-Americans (Sumner AE 2005). However, compared with Whites, Hispanics and Asians, African-Americans have less favorable levels of lipoprotein(a) (Lp[a]), which is structurally similar to LDL-C, with an additional disulfide linked glycoprotein termed ApoA. A number of studies have suggested that Lp(a) may be an important risk factor for CVD (Danesh J 2000; The Emerging Risk Factors C 2009).

Compared to non-Hispanic Whites, Hispanics, specifically Mexican-Americans, have demonstrated lower HDL-C and higher TG levels (Sundquist J 1999). Data from the Dallas Heart Study and a smaller cross-sectional analysis of healthy individuals confirm that levels of Lp(a) are likely similar or even lower in Hispanics compared with Whites (Tsimikas S 2009). Although Lp(a) levels have been associated with endothelial dysfunction in Hispanics, the relationship with coronary artery disease in this population is less clear.

Asian Indians exhibit a higher prevalence of diabetes mellitus than Chinese and Malays (Tan et al. 1999). They also have higher serum TG concentrations and lower HDL-C concentrations than Chinese (Gupta M 2006). In the HeartSCORE and IndiaSCORE studies (Mulukutla et al. 2008) where lipids were measured with the same assay procedures for Asian Indians as for Whites and Blacks, Asian Indians had lowest TC and HDL-C and highest TG among all the ethnic groups studied. In another multi-ethnic study of the 1992 Singapore National Health Survey (Tan et al. 1999), Asian Indians appeared to have lower HDL-C but higher TG levels compared with the Chinese group. Data in other racial/ethnic groups are somewhat limited. Mean total cholesterol and LDL-C levels are lower in American Indians compared with the US average, and levels of Lp(a) are reported to be lower than in Whites (Wang W 2002). East Asians tend to have lower LDL-C, HDL-C and TG as compared with non-Asians (Karthikeyan et al. 2009). East Asians have been reported to have low Lp(a) levels, whereas south Asians have higher mean Lp(a) levels (Geethanjali FS 2003; Berglund L 2004).

Globalization of the western lifestyle contribute to worldwide increases of adiposity and type 2 diabetes not only in adults but also in children and adolescents (Kelishadi et al. 2006; Schwandt et al. 2010). In the BIG Study comparing the prevalence of the metabolic syndrome components in children and adolescents of European, Asian and South-American ethnicities, Iranian and Brazilian youths had considerably higher prevalence of dyslipidaemia than German youths. The most remarkable ethnic difference detected in this study is the high prevalence of low HDL-C levels in Iranian children and adolescents (38%) compared with German youths (7%) (Schwandt et al. 2010). Future longitudinal studies should seek the clinical importance of these ethnic differences.

3. Ethnic differences in lipid profiles in the state of hyperglycaemia

3.1 Lipid disorder and CVD risk in individuals with hyperglycaemia

Lipids and lipoproteins abnormalities are major metabolic disorders, commonly including elevated levels of TC, LDL-C, Lp(a) and TG and reduced levels of HDL-C. In patients with type 2 diabetes, a CHD equivalent (Juutilainen et al. 2005), it is most commonly characterized by elevated TG and reduced HDL-C (Goldberg, I. J. 2001; Krauss 2004; Kendall 2005). There is increasing evidence that the diabetic dyslipidaemia pattern is common not only in patients with overt diabetes (Barrett-Connor et al. 1982) but also in individuals with different glucose categories, i.e., impaired glucose tolerance (IGT) or impaired fasting glucose (IFG) (Meigs et al. 2002; Novoa et al. 2005; Chen et al. 2006; Pankow et al. 2007). These abnormalities can be present alone or in combination with other metabolic disorders. It is well known that the risk of morbidity and mortality from CVD is increased by two- to four-fold in diabetic patients compared with the general population (Kannel 1985; Morrish et al. 1991; Almdal et al. 2004). A number of studies have determined the association of dyslipidaemia with cardiovascular risk in people with hyperglycaemia, and most of them were conducted in patients with diabetes. There is a large body of evidence linking dyslipidaemia and cardiovascular risk in patients with diabetes against quite few negative reports (Vlajinac et al. 1992; Roselli della Rovere et al. 2003) on this issue. Cross-sectional studies have found positive associations of atherosclerotic vascular disease with TC (Ronnemaa et al. 1989; Jurado et al. 2009), LDL-C (Reckless et al. 1978; Agarwal et al. 2009; Jurado et al. 2009), non-HDL-C (Jurado et al. 2009), TG (Santen et al. 1972; Ronnemaa et al. 1989; Gomes et al. 2009), apoB (Ronnemaa et al. 1989) and Lp(a) (Mohan et al. 1998; Murakami et al. 1998; Smaoui et al. 2004), but inverse associations with HDL-C (Reckless et al. 1978; Ronnemaa et al. 1989; Smaoui et al. 2004; Grant and Meigs 2007; Gomes et al. 2009; Jurado et al. 2009) and apoA-I (Seviour et al. 1988; Ronnemaa et al. 1989).

Prospective data have provided with further evidence. The UKPDS study (Turner et al. 1998) has demonstrated that high LDL-C and low HDL-C are potentially modifiable risk factors for coronary artery disease (CAD) in patients with type 2 diabetes. TG, however, was not independently associated with CAD risk in this study, possibly because of its close inverse relationship with HDL-C. Results from the MRFIT (Stamler et al. 1993), in which 356,499 nondiabetic and 5163 diabetic men without CHD at baseline were followed for 12 years, indicated that serum cholesterol is an independent predictor of CHD mortality in men with diabetes. Rosengren et al. (Rosengren et al. 1989) showed similar results in a prospective study of 6897 middle aged diabetic men. Patients with TC > 7.3 mmol/l had a significantly higher incidence of CHD during the 7-year follow up than those with TC ≤ 5.5 mmol/l (28.3% vs. 5.4%, p<0.05). Long term follow-up of the London cohort of the WHO

Multinational Study of Vascular Disease in Diabetics, consisting of 254 type 2 diabetic patients, has showed that TC was associated with incidence of MI (Morrish et al. 1991) and overall cardiovascular mortality (Morrish et al. 1990). The role of TC in predicting CHD was also confirmed in women patients with diabetes (Schulze et al. 2004).

3.2 Ethnic difference in lipid profiles across glucose categories

Although the ethnic variation in lipid patterns has been wided studied in general populations, the ethnic differences in lipid profiles given the same glucose levels have not been well investigated. This issue has been recently studied in the DECODE (Diabetes Epidemiology: Collaborative analysis Of Diagnostic criteria in Europe) and DECODA (Diabetes Epidemiology: Collaborative analysis Of Diagnostic criteria in Asia) study, which consisted of 64 cohorts of mainly population-based from 24 countries and regions around the world, with about 84 000 Europeans and 84 207 Asians of Chinese, Japanese, Indians, Mongolians and Filipinos.

In the collaborative analysis of seven ethnic groups of European and Asian populations (studies included see Appendix 1), considerable ethnic differences in lipid profiles were observed within each glucose category. Asian Indians exhibited an adverse lipid pattern consisting of low HDL-C and high TG across all glucose categories as compared with other ethnic groups. Reduced HDL-C is prevalent even in Asian Indians with desirable LDL-C levels regardless of the diabetic status. In addition, in most of the ethnic groups, individuals detected with undiagnosed diabetes had a worse lipid profile than did diagnosed cases. Age-, cohort- and BMI adjusted mean TC, LDL-C and TG increased while the mean HDL-C decreased with more pronounced glucose intolerance in most of the ethnic groups in individuals without a prior history of diabetes (Fig. 1 a-h). Subjects with undiagnosed diabetes, however, had a worse lipid profile than those with known disease. Within individuals with normoglycaemia, mean lipid and lipoprotein concentrations differed among the ethnic groups. The Europeans had highest TC (Fig. 1 a-b) and LDL-C (Fig. 1 c-d), while Qingdao Chinese had highest HDL-C levels among all ethnic groups (Fig. 1 e-f). In contrast, Asian Indians had the lowest TC (Fig. 1 a-b), LDL-C (Fig. 1 c-d) and HDL-C (Fig. 1 e-f) but the highest TG (Fig. 1 g-h) among the ethnic groups ($p < 0.05$ for all comparisons). These ethnic differences were consistently found in all glucose categories.

The multivariate-adjusted odds ratio (95% CI) of having low HDL-C was significantly higher for Asian Indians, Mauritian Indians, Hong Kong Chinese and Southern Europeans but lower for Qingdao Chinese compared with Central & North (C&N) Europeans, across all glucose categories from normal to diabetes (Table 1). Asian Indians and Mauritian Indians tended to have higher but Southern Europeans lower odds ratios for having high-TG compared with the reference group. Unlike that for HDL-C or TG, the odds ratio for having high LDL-C was consistently lower in all Asian ethnic groups compared with the reference, across most of the glucose categories.

In the HeartSCORE and IndiaSCORE studies (Mulukutla et al. 2008) where lipids were measured with the same assay procedures for Asian Indians as for whites and blacks, Asian Indians had lowest TC and HDL-C and highest TG among all the ethnic groups studied. In another multi-ethnic study of the 1992 Singapore National Health Survey (Tan et al. 1999), Asian Indians appeared to have lower HDL-C but higher TG levels compared with Chinese. The findings of these previous studies are consistent with ours although glucose status was not controlled in the previous studies.

Similar to others (Harris and Eastman 2000; Hadaegh et al. 2008), we observed a worse lipid profile in individuals with undiagnosed diabetes than that of previously diagnosed patients in most of the ethnic groups, indicating individuals with undiagnosed diabetes are at increased CVD risk and need to be identified and treated early. On the other hand, glycaemic control is shown to be an important determinant of diabetic dyslipidaemia (Ismail et al. 2001). The better lipid profile in diagnosed diabetes as compared with undiagnosed diabetes might imply a benefit of lifestyle intervention or drug treatment targeting favorable metabolic profiles and hemoglobin A1c (HbA1c), a surrogate measure for average blood glucose. However, to what extent the levels of HbA1c have contributed to the differences is unknown due to the lack of information in the current study. In addition, the data on lipid-lowering treatment is not available for most of the earlier studies conducted in the 1990s because the statins were not widely prescribed at that time. These deserve further investigation in future studies.

In contrast to the lower HDL-C and higher TG profiles, Asian Indians had considerably lower TC and LDL-C concentrations than others. As shown in Table 2, 71% non-diabetic and 57.6% diabetic Asian Indians had low LDL-C (< 3.0 mmol/l), while the corresponding figures were 19.2% and 24.6% (p < 0.01) for C&N Europeans and 46.6% and 38.8% (p < 0.01) for Qingdao Chinese. However, even within the low LDL-C category, there was still a higher proportion of Asian Indians having low HDL-C compared with others (Table 2). The results were confirmed in the same analysis conducted separately for men and women.

There is a large body of evidence showing that diabetes is associated with a high prevalence of dyslipidaemia (Kannel 1985; Cowie et al. 1994; 1997; Jacobs et al. 2005; Bruckert et al. 2007; Abdel-Aal et al. 2008; Ahmed et al. 2008; Okafor et al. 2008; Surana et al. 2008; Agarwal et al. 2009; Jurado et al. 2009; Papazafiropoulou et al. 2009; Roberto Robles et al. 2009; Temelkova-Kurktschiev et al. 2009; Zhang et al. 2009; Seyum et al. 2010). In the Framingham Heart Study (Kannel 1985), the prevalence of low HDL-C (21% vs. 12% in men and 25% vs. 10% in women, respectively) and high TG levels (19% vs. 9% in men and 17% vs. 8% in women, respectively) in people with diabetes was almost twice as high as the prevalence in non-diabetic individuals. By contrast, TC and LDL-C levels did not differ from those of non-diabetic counterparts. A similar pattern of lipid profiles was observed in the UK Prospective Diabetes Study (UKPDS) (1997). In this study, the plasma TG levels were substantially increased whereas HDL-C levels were markedly reduced in both men and women with diabetes compared with the non-diabetic controls. Higher prevalence has been reported in other studies. Data from a primary care-based 7692 patients with type 2 diabetes in the United States showed nearly half of the patients had low HDL-C (Grant and Meigs 2007). The figure was even worse in an urban Indian cohort of 5088 type 2 diabetes patients, with more than half having low HDL-C (52.3%) or high TG (57.9%) (Surana et al. 2008). In addition to the traditional lipid measurement, increased levels of apoB were also seen in patients with diabetes compared with non-diabetic individuals (Bangou-Bredent et al. 1999). It has been shown that the prevalence of lipid and/or glucose abnormality differs between ethnic groups. It is clear that certain ethnic groups have differences in lipid profiles in general. Elevated TG and reduced HDL-C, as the components of the metabolic syndrome and atherogenic dyslipidaemia, was seen more common in Asian Indians than in the Whites (Anand et al. 2000; Razak et al. 2005; Chandalia et al. 2008; Mulukutla et al. 2008), Chinese (Tan et al. 1999; Anand et al. 2000; Razak et al. 2005; The DECODA Study Group 2007; Karthikeyan et al. 2009), Japanese (The DECODA Study Group 2007; Karthikeyan et al. 2009) or Africans (Mulukutla et al. 2008). In a nationally representative sample of seven ethnic groups in the UK (Zaninotto et al. 2007), the prevalence of low HDL-C was highest in south Asian groups such as Bangladeshi, Indian and Pakistani, followed by Chinese, Irish and those from the general population living in private households; In contrast, the lowest prevalence was seen in Black Caribbean. Similar finding was reported in another study where the comparison was made between non-South-Asians and South Asians (France et al. 2003). In addition, African Americans have been reported to have less adverse lipid profiles than Whites or Hispanics despite the presence of diabetes (Werk et al. 1993; Cowie et al. 1994; Sharma and Pavlik 2001). The causes of ethnic difference in levels of CVD risk factor are complex and may include genetic, environmental and cultural factors (Zaninotto et al. 2007). However, little is known about such ethnic differences in lipid profiles at comparable glucose tolerance status.

4. Causes of ethnic differences

There are several factors that contribute to the development of dyslipidaemia (2001), including genetic factors (Cohen et al. 1994) and acquired factors (Chait and Brunzell 1990; Devroey et al. 2004; Ruixing et al. 2008) such as overweight and obesity (Denke et al. 1993; Denke et al. 1994; Brown et al. 2000), physical inactivity (Berg et al. 1997; Hardman 1999), cigarette smoking (Criqui et al. 1980; Cade and Margetts 1989; Umeda et al. 1998; Fisher et al. 2000; Wu et al. 2001; Maeda et al. 2003; Mammas et al. 2003; Venkatesan et al. 2006; Grant and Meigs 2007; Arslan et al. 2008; Batic-Mujanovic et al. 2008), high fat intake (Hennig et al. 2001; Millen et al. 2002; Tanasescu et al. 2004), very high carbohydrate diets (> 60 percent of total energy) (McNamara and Howell 1992) and certain drugs (Lehtonen 1985; Fogari et al. 1988; Roberts 1989; Middeke et al. 1990; Stone 1994) (such as beta-blockers, anabolic steroids, progestational agents, et al.). Excess alcohol intake is also documented as a risk factor (Umeda et al. 1998; Wu et al. 2001; Mammas et al. 2003) despite that moderate alcohol consumption may have a beneficial effect on improving HDL-C concentrations (De Oliveira et al. 2000; Shai et al. 2004). In addition, glycaemic control is an important determinant of dyslipidaemia in patients with diabetes (Ismail et al. 2001; Grant and Meigs 2007; Ahmed et al. 2008; Gatti et al. 2009). Among these acquired factors, overweight, obesity and physical inactivity appear to be most important (Denke et al. 1993; Denke et al. 1994; Berg et al. 1997; Hardman 1999; Brown et al. 2000). They are also the most important lifestyle variables that decrease insulin action and increase the risk of diabetes.

The causes of ethnic difference in cardiovascular risk profile are complex. Possible contributors include genetic, environmental, psychosocial, cultural and unmeasured factors and many are not well clarified (Zaninotto et al. 2007). It is clear that the observed ethnic differences in lipid profiles cannot be explained by genetics alone and may be more indicative of lifestyle-related factors such as dietary pattern and physical activity (Ruixing et al. 2008; McNaughton et al. 2009; Sisson et al. 2009). To what extent is ethnic-specific lifestyle pattern associated with different lipid profiles deserves further investigation.

4.1 Genetic factors

An adverse lipid profile in Asian Indians has been reported to be associated with the greater susceptibility to insulin resistance (Tan et al. 1999; Anand et al. 2000; Bhalodkar et al. 2005; Palaniappan et al. 2007), and a higher percentage of body fat for the same BMI as compared with Whites (McKeigue et al. 1991), which may contribute to the high prevalence of CVD

(Kuller 2004) and diabetes (Ramachandran et al. 2008; Snehalatha and Ramachandran 2009) in this ethnic group. In addition, it may also reflect the genetic variation, for example, at the apoE locus (Tan et al. 2003) and an excess of other risk factors such as homocysteine, Lp(a) or dietary fat (France et al. 2003).

4.2 Environmental factors

As suggested by previous research, dietary factors may play a role in both lipid and insulin profiles, although these patterns may be mediated by body fat content (Ku CY 1998). Total fat (and saturated fat) intake has been shown to adversely affect total cholesterol concentrations in children, adolescents, and young adults (Post GB 1997). The difference in HDL-C concentrations between Qingdao and Hong Kong Chinese subgroups observed in the DECODA study cannot be simply explained by the difference in assay methods. It may largely attribute to the differences in dietary structure and preference, geographic and environmental factors. Shellfish and beer, for example, are commonly consumed all the year round in Qingdao. Nevertheless, whether other factors exist and contribute to the high HDL-C in Qingdao needs to be further investigated.

Mexican Americans have been previously reported to have greater adiposity, higher TG levels and lower HDL-C levels than Anglos. The relationship between behavioral variables (caloric balance, cigarette and alcohol consumption, exercise, post-menopausal estrogen or oral contraceptive use) and lipid pattern has been investigated in the San Antonio Heart Study (1979–1982) (n=2,102) to explain the ethnic difference in lipids and lipoproteins. Adjustment for caloric balance (as reflected by body mass index) narrowed the ethnic difference in TG and HDL-C levels for both sexes, while adjustment for smoking widened the ethnic difference. For females, the ethnic difference was also decreased by adjustment for alcohol and estrogen use. However, adjustment for these behavioral variables did not completely eliminate the ethnic difference in lipids and lipoproteins in either sex. Increased central adiposity, more characteristic of Mexican Americans than Anglos, was positively associated with triglycerides and negatively associated with HDL-C levels, especially in females. Fat patterning made a more important contribution to the prediction of TG and HDL-C levels than did the other behavioral variables (except for caloric balance) and, in general, eliminated ethnic differences in lipids and lipoproteins (Steven H 1986). Epidemiologists should consider the use of a centrality index to distinguish different types of adiposity since it is easy and inexpensive to measure.

5. Implications for management and prevention of dyslipidaemia

Epidemiological investigations of human populations have revealed a robust relationship between lipids and CVD risk. Furthermore, the benefit of lipid-modifying strategy on cardiovascular events has been demonstrated from a large number of randomized clinical trials (Thavendiranathan et al. 2006; Mills et al. 2008), especially from those using 3-hydroxy-3-methyl-glutaryl-CoA (HMG-CoA) reductase inhibitors (i.e., statins) (Goldberg, R. B. et al. 1998; Collins et al. 2003; Colhoun et al. 2004; Pyorala et al. 2004; Sever et al. 2005; Knopp et al. 2006; Shepherd et al. 2006). Intensive control of dyslipidaemia has been greatly emphasized in the prevention and management of CVD. Current guidelines from the National Cholesterol Education Program Adult Treatment Panel III (ATP III) (Adult Treatment Panel III 2002), the European Society of Cardiology (Graham et al. 2007) and the American Diabetes Association (American Diabetes Association 2009) consistently

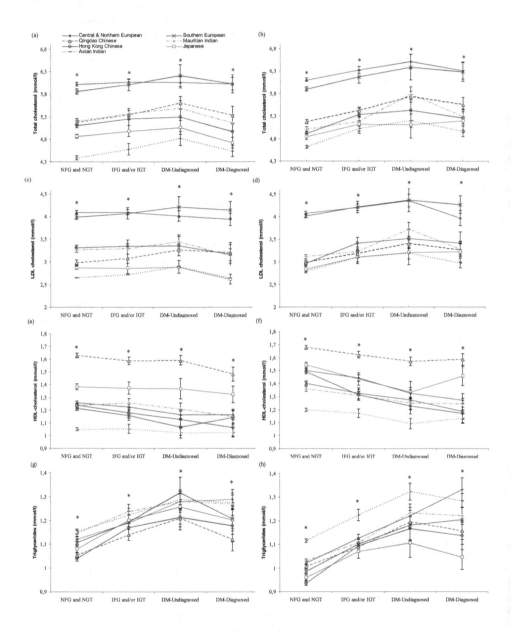

Fig. 1. Age-, study cohort- and body mass index-adjusted mean lipid (geometric means for triglycerides) and lipoprotein concentrations and 95% CIs (vertical bars) in men (figure 1-a, c, e and g) and women (figure 1-b, d, f and h) by ethnicities and glucose categories.* p for trend < 0.05 within each glucose category.

	HDL-C < 1.03 in men and < 1.29 in women (mmol/l)				TG ≥ 1.7 mmol/l				LDL-C ≥ 3 mmol/l			
	NFG and NGT	IFG and/or IGT	Undiagnosed diabetes	Diagnosed diabetes	NFG and NGT	IFG and/or IGT	Undiagnosed diabetes	Diagnosed Diabetes	NFG and NGT	IFG and/or IGT	Undiagnosed diabetes	Diagnosed diabetes
Men												
Central & Northern European [a]	1	1	1	1	1	1	1	1	1	1	1	1
Hong Kong Chinese	1.63 (1.41-1.87)	2.75 (2.09-3.62)	1.82 (1.20-2.76)	2.57 (1.48-4.46)	0.75 (0.64-0.87)	1.16 (0.88-1.53)	1.05 (0.70-1.58)	0.63 (0.36-1.12)	0.51 (0.44-0.58)	0.61 (0.46-0.82)	0.51 (0.33-0.78)	0.86 (0.49-1.52)
Qingdao Chinese	0.12 (0.09-0.16)	0.07 (0.04-0.13)	0.11 (0.07-0.20)	0.16 (0.08-0.32)	0.68 (0.58-0.79)	0.81 (0.66-1.00)	0.81 (0.61-1.09)	0.40 (0.26-0.63)	0.23 (0.20-0.26)	0.30 (0.24-0.37)	0.44 (0.32-0.60)	0.57 (0.37-0.86)
Asian Indian	4.74 (4.19-5.37)	5.05 (3.88-6.56)	3.07 (2.15-4.40)	2.37 (1.67-3.35)	1.40 (1.23-1.58)	1.53 (1.19-1.97)	1.24 (0.88-1.75)	1.42 (1.01-2.00)	0.12 (0.10-0.13)	0.17 (0.13-0.22)	0.23 (0.16-0.33)	0.29 (0.20-0.41)
Mauritian Indian	1.82 (1.58-2.09)	2.04 (1.58-2.63)	1.27 (0.89-1.81)	1.16 (0.78-1.74)	1.47 (1.28-1.69)	1.55 (1.23-1.98)	1.18 (0.85-1.65)	1.06 (0.72-1.57)	0.39 (0.34-0.45)	0.38 (0.30-0.49)	0.49 (0.34-0.70)	0.75 (0.50-1.12)
Japanese	0.87 (0.73-1.03)	1.29 (0.98-1.70)	0.73 (0.44-1.20)	0.57 (0.36-0.90)	0.99 (0.84-1.15)	1.31 (1.02-1.68)	1.36 (0.88-2.09)	1.02 (0.68-1.53)	0.26 (0.23-0.30)	0.35 (0.27-0.44)	0.36 (0.23-0.57)	0.77 (0.51-1.16)
Southern European	1.21 (1.06-1.37)	1.49 (1.15-1.93)	1.79 (1.19-2.70)	1.13 (0.78-1.63)	0.78 (0.69-0.88)	0.83 (0.65-1.07)	1.16 (0.77-1.75)	0.58 (0.40-0.84)	0.87 (0.75-1.00)	0.99 (0.73-1.36)	1.80 (1.01-3.23)	1.52 (0.99-2.31)
Women												
Central & Northern European [a]	1	1	1	1	1	1	1	1	1	1	1	1
Hong Kong Chinese	2.23 (1.93-2.57)	3.79 (2.88-4.98)	3.02 (1.88-4.85)	3.03 (1.68-5.48)	0.86 (0.69-1.08)	1.16 (0.85-1.58)	0.98 (0.61-1.57)	0.69 (0.39-1.21)	0.41 (0.35-0.47)	0.64 (0.48-0.86)	0.61 (0.36-1.04)	1.21 (0.66-2.22)
Qingdao Chinese	0.66 (0.57-0.76)	0.52 (0.41-0.65)	0.27 (0.19-0.38)	0.20 (0.13-0.31)	1.29 (1.11-1.50)	1.06 (0.87-1.30)	0.99 (0.73-1.36)	0.57 (0.39-0.84)	0.40 (0.36-0.45)	0.45 (0.37-0.55)	0.48 (0.33-0.69)	0.67 (0.45-0.99)
Asian Indian	10.91 (9.68-12.30)	7.80 (5.99-9.94)	8.64 (5.62-13.29)	4.34 (2.93-6.44)	2.76 (2.39-3.18)	2.21 (1.71-2.87)	3.13 (2.15-4.55)	1.29 (0.90-1.85)	0.22 (0.20-0.25)	0.36 (0.28-0.47)	0.36 (0.24-0.54)	0.41 (0.28-0.60)
Mauritian Indian	4.41 (3.88-5.02)	3.80 (3.05-4.74)	2.65 (1.82-3.88)	2.26 (1.53-3.35)	1.38 (1.16-1.65)	1.15 (0.91-1.47)	1.54 (1.07-2.23)	0.81 (0.56-1.19)	0.48 (0.42-0.55)	0.50 (0.40-0.63)	0.78 (0.51-1.21)	0.85 (0.57-1.27)
Japanese	2.40 (2.12-2.73)	3.07 (2.44-3.87)	2.65 (1.62-4.34)	1.07 (0.67-1.72)	0.92 (0.77-1.09)	1.19 (0.93-1.53)	0.72 (0.43-1.21)	0.41 (0.25-0.68)	0.58 (0.51-0.66)	0.67 (0.52-0.87)	0.56 (0.31-0.99)	2.24 (1.27-3.93)
Southern European	1.50 (1.34-1.68)	1.62 (1.26-2.08)	0.93 (0.56-1.52)	1.70 (1.13-2.56)	0.70 (0.60-0.81)	0.80 (0.61-1.05)	0.60 (0.36-1.01)	0.53 (0.35-0.79)	0.98 (0.87-1.11)	1.39 (1.01-1.93)	1.38 (0.70-2.72)	2.67 (1.62-4.42)

Model adjusted for age, study cohort, body mass index, systolic blood pressure and smoking status. NFG, normal fasting glucose; NGT, normal glucose tolerance. [a] Reference group

Table 1. Odds ratio (95% confidence interval) of having dyslipidaemia in relation to ethnicity by glucose categories.

	LDL-C < 3 mmol/l				LDL-C ≥ 3 mmol/l			
	Normal HDL-C and normal TG, %	Low HDL-C [a] alone, %	High TG [b] alone, %	both, %	Normal HDL-C and normal TG, %	Low HDL-C [a] alone, %	High TG [b] alone, %	both, %
Non-diabetic population								
Hong Kong Chinese	29.3	9.9	1.6	4.2	32.1	12.9	3.7	6.2
Qingdao Chinese	31.0	5.4	8.3	1.9	40.5	2.4	9.8	0.7
Asian Indian	23.2	33.6	3.2	11.0	9.2	10.7	2.8	6.4
Mauritian Indian	23.9	15.8	5.0	4.7	23.2	14.7	5.7	7.0
Japanese	25.2	6.4	3.4	3.5	38.2	13.0	5.0	5.3
Central & Northern European	13.3	2.3	2.0	1.6	48.6	9.7	12.6	10.0
Southern European	14.2	4.3	1.1	2.1	45.5	15.1	7.8	10.0
Diabetic population								
Hong Kong Chinese	12.4	9.6	1.4	11.0	22.6	18.1	7.6	17.2
Qingdao Chinese	21.1	3.5	11.1	3.1	37.9	2.7	19.1	1.5
Asian Indian	12.8	17.4	6.0	21.4	8.1	12.4	7.2	14.7
Mauritian Indian	12.4	8.6	6.4	10.2	21.2	15.5	10.2	15.5
Japanese	14.3	6.0	7.1	5.1	34.3	11.6	12.2	9.4
Central & Northern European	10.5	2.8	4.9	6.4	30.4	9.3	16.4	19.4
Southern European	7.5	3.3	6.0	10.2	24.4	11.2	12.8	14.8

a < 1.03 mmol/l in men and < 1.29 mmol/l in women
b ≥ 1.70 mmol/l

Table 2. Proportions (%) of individuals according to lipid levels stratified by diabetic status in each ethnic group.

recommend that LDL-C should be the primary target of therapy not only in patients with CHD or diabetes but also in individuals with increased cardiovascular risk. In addition, non-HDL-C is set by ATP III as a secondary target of therapy and HDL-C and TG as potential target. The Current guideline, mainly based on the data of Whites, consistently recommend that LDL-C < 2.6 mmol/l should be the primary target of therapy in patients with diabetes. As shown in our study and others' (Mulukutla et al. 2008; Karthikeyan et al. 2009), the Asian Indian population had significantly lower TC and LDL-C than did Whites. The threshold of LDL-C for treatment target for Whites may be too high for Asian Indians. Further studies are warranted to verify this hypothesis and determine the threshold applicable to this ethnic group.

In contrast to LDL-C, HDL-C has been either dropped from (Graham et al. 2007) or set as a secondary (American Diabetes Association 2010) or tertiary (Expert Panel on Detection 2001) target in the major guidelines despite the strong evidence of reduced HDL-C as an independent risk factor for CVD (Boden 2000). This may change if more therapy choices developed to increase HDL-C levels and improve HDL function are shown to prevent CVD (Singh et al. 2007; Duffy and Rader 2009; Sorrentino et al. 2010) or reduce the residual cardiovascular risk (Fruchart J 2008). Most recently, the ARBITER 6-HALTS (Arterial Biology for the Investigation of the Treatment Effects of Reducing Cholesterol 6-HDL and LDL Treatment Strategies in Atherosclerosis) trial has shown a significant improvement in serum HDL-C levels and regression of carotid intima-media thickness when ERN was conbined with statin therapy in patients with CHD or CHD equivalent (Taylor et al. 2009; Villines et al. 2010). Considering the high proportion of Asian Indians with adverse HDL-C levels, appropriate approaches to increasing HDL-C and/or improving HDL function may become an important treatment target in Asian Indians in order to reduce their excess CVD risks.

6. Appendix 1

Countries and studies	Blood sample	Total cholesterol	High-density lipoprotein cholesterol	Triglycerides
China				
Hong Kong Cardiovascular DiseaseRisk Factor Prevalence Study	Plasma	Cholesterol oxidase (CHOD) method; Hitachi 717 analyser (Hitachi Instruments, California, USA).	Measured after precipitation of very-low density lipoprotein (VLDL) and low-density lipoprotein (LDL) by polyethylene glycol PEG 6000.	Lipase/glycerol kinase method;
Hong Kong Workforce Survey on CVD Risk Factors	Venous Plasma	Enzymatic method, with reagents (Baker Instruments Corporation, Allentown, PA 18103, USA) with Cobas Mira analyzer (Hoffman-La Roche and Co., Basle Switzerland).	Enzymatic method after precipitation with dextran sulphate-MgCl$_2$ on Cobas Mira analyzer (Hoffman-La Roche and Co., Basle Switzerland)	Enzymatic method, with reagents (Baker Instruments Corporation, Allentown, PA 18103, USA) with Cobas Mira analyzer (Hoffman-La Roche and Co., Basle Switzerland)
Qingdao Diabetes Survey 2002	Venous Plasma	Enzymatic method (AMS Analyzer Medical System, SABA-18, Rome, Italy)	Enzymatic method after precipitation (AMS Analyzer Medical System, SABA-18, Rome, Italy)	Enzymatic method (AMS Analyzer Medical System, SABA-18, Rome, Italy)
Qingdao Diabetes Study 2006	Serum	Enzymatic method (Olympus reagent) With OLYMPUS-AU640 Automatic Analyzers (Olympus Optical. Tokyo, Japan)	Direct method (Olympus reagent) with OLYMPUS-AU640 Automatic Analyzers (Olympus Optical. Tokyo, Japan)	Enzymatic method (Olympus reagent) with OLYMPUS-AU640 Automatic Analyzers (Olympus Optical. Tokyo, Japan)

Finland

East-West men	Serum	Enzymatic techniques (Monotest, Boehringer Mannheim GmbH, FRG) Olli C3000 photometer (Kone Oy, Finland)	Enzymetic method after precipitation of VLDL and LDL by means of dextran-magnesium-chloride, with Olli C3000 photometer (Kone Oy, Finland)	Enzymatic techniques (Monotest, Boehringer Mannheim GmbH, FRG) Olli C3000 photometer (Kone Oy, Finland)
National FINRISK Study 87, 92	Serum	Enzymatic techniques (Cholesterol oxidase-peroxidase-amidopyrine, CHOD-PAP, Boehringer-Mannheim, Mannheim, Germany)	Enzymatic method after dextran sulfate magnesium chloride precipitation of apolipoprotein B (apoB)-containing lipoproteins	Enzymatic techniques (CHOD-PAP, Boehringer-Mannheim, Mannheim, Germany)
National FINRISK Study 2002	Serum	Enzymatic method (CHOD-PAP; Thermo Elektron Oy, Finland);	Enzymatic method (CHOD-PAP; Thermo Elektron Oy, Finland) after precipitation by the PTA-precipitation method	Enzymatic techniques (Glycerol phosphate oxidase-peroxidase-amidopyrine, GPO-PAP; Thermo Elektron Oy)
Oulu Study	Serum	Enzymatic method (CHOD-PAP, Boehringer Mannheim, Mannheim, Germany).	Enzymatic CHOD-PAP method after precipitation of LDL and VLDL with a reagent containing phosphotungstic acid and $MgCl_2$ (Boehringer Mannheim)	Enzymatic method (CHOD-PAP, Boehringer Mannheim, Mannheim, Germany)
Savitaipale Study	Plasma	Enzymatic colorimetric method (CHOD-PAP) Cobas Integra 400/700 analyzer	Enzymatic colorimetric method (CHOD-PAP) Cobas Integra 400/700 analyzer	Enzymatic colorimetric method (CHOD-PAP) Cobas Integra 400/700 analyzer
Vantaa Study	Serum	Enzymatic techniques (Boehringer-Mannheim)	Enzymatic method after precipitation with polyethylenglycol	Enzymatic techniques (Boehringer-Mannheim)

India

Chennai 94	Serum	Enzymatic method; Hitachi 704 autoanalyser, using Boehringer Mannheim (Mannheim, Germany) reagents	Phosphotungstate-magnesium precipitation method. Hitachi 704 autoanalyser, using Boehringer Mannheim (Mannheim, Germany) reagents	Enzymatic method. Hitachi 704 autoanalyser, using Boehringer Mannheim (Mannheim, Germany) reagents

Chennai 97	Venous Plasma	CHOD-PAP method (Boehringer Mannheim, Germany); Corning Express Plus Auto Analyser (Corning, medfied, MA, USA)	Phosphotungstic acid method after precipitation of LDL and chylomicrons (Boehringer Mannheim, Germany); Corning Express Plus Auto Analyser (Corning, medfied, MA, USA)	GPO-PAP method (Boehringer Mannheim, Germany); Corning Express Plus Auto Analyser (Corning, medfied, MA, USA)
CURES	Serum	CHOD-PAP method with Hitachi-912 Autoanalyser (Hitachi, Mannheim, Germany) using kits supplied by Roche Diagnostics (Mannheim, Germany).	Direct method (polyethylene glycol–pretreated enzymes) with Hitachi-912 Autoanalyser (Hitachi, Mannheim, Germany) using kits supplied by Roche Diagnostics (Mannheim, Germany).	GPO-PAP method; Hitachi-912 Autoanalyser (Hitachi, Mannheim, Germany) using kits supplied by Roche Diagnostics (Mannheim, Germany).
Chennai 2006	Serum	Standard enzymatic procedures (Roche Diagnostics, Mannheim, Germany)	Direct assay method (Roche Diagnostics, Mannheim, Germany)	Standard enzymatic procedures (Roche Diagnostics, Mannheim, Germany)
Italy				
Cremona Study	Plasma	Enzymatic techniques (Boehringer-Mannheim, Mannheim, Germany) with CIBA Corning 550 Express Auto-analyser	Precipitation with PEG using a Colortest kit (Roche, Basel, Switzerland).	Enzymatic techniques (Boehringer-Mannheim, Mannheim, Germany) with CIBA Corning 550 Express Auto-analyser
Japan				
Funagata Study	Plasma	Cholesterol oxidase method (L-type Wako CHO-H [Wako Pure Chemical Industries, Osaka, Japan]) with TBA 80FR (Toshiba medical system corporation, Tokyo)	Direct method (Cholesterol N HDL [Daiichi Pure Chemicals, Tokyo, Japan]) with TBA 80FR (Toshiba medical system corporation, Tokyo)	GPO HDAOS method (Pureauto S TG-N [Daiichi Pure Chemicals, Tokyo, Japan]) with TBA 80FR (Toshiba medical system corporation, Tokyo)
Hisayama Study	Serum	Enzymatic techniques (TBA-80S; Toshiba Inc., Tokyo, Japan)	Enzymatic method after precipitation of of VLDL and LDL with dextran sulfate and magnesium (TBA-80S; Toshiba Inc., Tokyo, Japan)	Enzymatic techniques (TBA-80S; Toshiba Inc., Tokyo, Japan)
Mauritius				

Mauritius 1987	Venous plasma	Manual enzymatic colorimetric method (Coulter Minikem Spectrophotometer), (Boeringer Cat no 701912)	Manual enzymatic colorimetric method (Coulter Minikem Spectrophotometer), (Boeringer Cat no 701912) Precipitation method (Biomerieux)	Manual enzymatic colorimetric method(Coulter Minikem Spectrophotometer) (Boeringer Cat nr 400971)
Mauritius 1992	Venous plasma	Automated enzymatic method with Chemistry Profile Analyser Model LS (Coulter- France)	Automated enzymatic method, Chemistry Profile Analyser Model LS (Coulter- France) Precipitation method (Biomerieux)	Automated enzymatic method with Chemistry Profile Analyser Model LS (Coulter- France)
Mauritius 1998	Venous plasma	Automated enzymatic methods; Cobas Mira analyzer (Roche Diagnostics, France)	Automated enzymatic methods; Cobas Mira analyzer (Roche Diagnostics, France) Direct method (Biomerieux)	Automated enzymatic methods; Cobas Mira analyzer (Roche Diagnostics, France)
Poland				
POLMONICA	Serum	Direct Liebermann- Burchard method (Boehringer- Mannheim)	Determined in the supernatant after precipitation with heparin manganese (Boehringer- Mannheim)	Enzymatic method (Boehringer- Mannheim)
Republic of Cyprus				
Nicosia Diabetes Study	Whole Blood	Cobas Micra Plus Roche	Cobas Micra Plus Roche	Cobas Micra Plus Roche
Spain				
The Guía Study	Plasma	Standard enzymatic methods (Boehringer- Mannheim Hitachi 717 autoanalyser, Tokyo, Japan)	Phosphotungstate precipitation (Boehringer- Mannheim Hitachi 717 autoanalyser, Tokyo, Japan)	Standard enzymatic methods (Boehringer- Mannheim Hitachi 717 autoanalyser, Tokyo, Japan)
The Viva Study	Plasma	Enzymatic techniques (Boehringer- Mannheim)	Enzymatic techniques (Boehringer-Mannheim)	Enzymatic techniques (Boehringer- Mannheim)
Sweden				
MONICA	Serum	Enzymatic techniques (Boehringer- Mannheim GmbH, Germany)	Phosphotungstate-Mg^{2+} precipitation method	Enzymatic method (CHOD-PAP, Boehringer- Mannheim GmbH, Germany)
The Uppsala Longitudinal Study of Adult	Serum	Enzymatic techniques using IL Test Cholesterol Trinders's	Separated by precipitation with magnesium chloride/	Enzymatic techniques using IL Test Cholesterol

Men (ULSAM)		Method and IL Test Enzymatic-colorimetric Method for use in a Monarch apparatus (Instrumentation Laboratories, Lexington, USA). (http://www.pubcare.uu.se/ULSAM/invest/70yrs/meth70.htm#09)	phosphotumgstate.	Trinders's Method and IL Test Enzymatic-colorimetric Method for use in a Monarch apparatus (Instrumentation Laboratories, Lexington, USA).
The Netherlands				
The Hoorn Study	Serum	Enzymatic techniques (Boehringer-Mannheim, Mannheim, Germany);	Enzymatic techniques after precipitation of the low and very low-density lipoproteins (Boehringer-Mannheim, Mannheim, Germany)	Enzymatic techniques (Boehringer-Mannheim, Mannheim, Germany);
Zutphen	Serum	Enzymatic techniques (CHOD-PAP mono-test kit,Boehringer-Mannheim)	Enzymatic method after precipitation of apoB-containing particles by means of dextran magnesium sulphate.	Enzymatic techniques (CHOD-PAP mono-test kit,Boehringer-Mannheim)
U.K.				
Isle of ELY Diabetes Project	Plasma	Enzymatic techniques, RA 1000 (Bayer Diagnostics, Basingstoke, Hants, UK)	Enzymatic methods	Standard automated enzymatic method with the RA1000 (Bayer Diagnostics, Suffolk, U.K.),
Newcastle Heart Project	Plasma	Cholesterol oxidase/peroxidase method with Cobas Bio centrifugal analyzer (Roche Products Ltd, Welwyn Garden City, UK)	Measuring the supernatant cholesterol concentration after precipitation of apoB-containing lipoproteins with heparin and manganese. Cobas Bio centrifugal analyzer (Roche Products Ltd, Welwyn Garden City, UK)	Lipase/glycerol kinase method. Cobas Bio centrifugal analyzer (Roche Products Ltd, Welwyn Garden City, UK)
The Goodinge Study	Plasma	Cholesterol esterase method (Boehringer Mannheim, Lewes, Sussex, U.K.)	Enzymatic spectrophotometric method (Roche Diagnostics, Hatfield, Herts, U.K.) after precipitation of LDL by the addition of phosphotungstic acid in the presence of magnesium ions.	Enzymatic spectrophotometric method (Roche Diagnostics, Hatfield, Herts, U.K.).

Measures of lipid components in each study.

7. References

Abdel-Aal, N. M., A. T. Ahmad, E. S. Froelicher, A. M. Batieha, M. M. Hamza, et al. (2008). "Prevalence of dyslipidemia in patients with type 2 diabetes in Jordan." Saudi Med J 29(10): 1423-1428.

Adult Treatment panel III (2002). "Third Report of the National Cholesterol Education Program (NCEP) Expert Panel on Detection, Evaluation, and Treatment of High Blood Cholesterol in Adults (Adult Treatment Panel III) final report." Circulation 106(25): 3143-3421.

Agarwal, A. K., S. Singla, R. Singla, A. Lal, H. Wardhan, et al. (2009). "Prevalence of coronary risk factors in type 2 diabetics without manifestations of overt coronary heart disease." J Assoc Physicians India 57: 135-142.

Ahmed, N., J. Khan and T. S. Siddiqui (2008). "Frequency of dyslipidaemia in type 2 diabetes mellitus in patients of Hazara division." J Ayub Med Coll Abbottabad 20(2): 51-54.

Almdal, T., H. Scharling, J. S. Jensen and H. Vestergaard (2004). "The independent effect of type 2 diabetes mellitus on ischemic heart disease, stroke, and death: a population-based study of 13,000 men and women with 20 years of follow-up." Arch Intern Med 164(13): 1422-1426.

American Diabetes Association (2009). "Standards of medical care in diabetes--2009." Diabetes Care 32 Suppl 1: S13-61.

American Diabetes Association (2010). "Standards of medical care in diabetes--2010." Diabetes Care 33 Suppl 1: S11-61.

Anand, S. S., S. Yusuf, V. Vuksan, S. Devanesen, K. K. Teo, et al. (2000). "Differences in risk factors, atherosclerosis, and cardiovascular disease between ethnic groups in Canada: the Study of Health Assessment and Risk in Ethnic groups (SHARE)." Lancet 356(9226): 279-284.

Arslan, E., T. Yakar and I. Yavasoglu (2008). "The effect of smoking on mean platelet volume and lipid profile in young male subjects." Anadolu Kardiyol Derg 8(6): 422-425.

Azizi, F., M. Rahmani, A. Ghanbarian, H. Emami, P. Salehi, et al. (2003). "Serum lipid levels in an Iranian adults population: Tehran Lipid and Glucose Study." Eur J Epidemiol 18(4): 311-319.

Bangou-Bredent, J., V. Szmidt-Adjide, P. Kangambega-Nouvier, L. Foucan, A. Campier, et al. (1999). "Cardiovascular risk factors associated with diabetes in an Indian community of Guadeloupe. A case control study." Diabetes Metab 25(5): 393-398.

Barrett-Connor, E., S. M. Grundy and M. J. Holdbrook (1982). "Plasma lipids and diabetes mellitus in an adult community." Am J Epidemiol 115(5): 657-663.

Barzi, F., A. Patel, M. Woodward, C. M. Lawes, T. Ohkubo, et al. (2005). "A comparison of lipid variables as predictors of cardiovascular disease in the Asia Pacific region." Ann Epidemiol 15(5): 405-413.

Batic-Mujanovic, O., A. Beganlic, N. Salihefendic, N. Pranjic and Z. Kusljugic (2008). "Influence of smoking on serum lipid and lipoprotein levels among family medicine patients." Med Arh 62(5-6): 264-267.

Berg, A., M. Halle, I. Franz and J. Keul (1997). "Physical activity and lipoprotein metabolism: epidemiological evidence and clinical trials." Eur J Med Res 2(6): 259-264.

Berglund L, R. R. (2004). "Lipoprotein(a): an elusive cardiovascular risk factor." Arterioscler. Thromb. Vasc. Biol 24(12): 2219-2226.

Berrios, X., T. Koponen, T. Huiguang, N. Khaltaev, P. Puska, et al. (1997). "Distribution and prevalence of major risk factors of noncommunicable diseases in selected countries: the WHO Inter-Health Programme." Bull World Health Organ 75(2): 99-108.

Bhalodkar, N. C., S. Blum, T. Rana, R. Kitchappa, A. N. Bhalodkar, et al. (2005). "Comparison of high-density and low-density lipoprotein cholesterol subclasses and sizes in Asian Indian women with Caucasian women from the Framingham Offspring Study." Clin Cardiol 28(5): 247-251.

Boden, W. E. (2000). "High-density lipoprotein cholesterol as an independent risk factor in cardiovascular disease: assessing the data from Framingham to the Veterans Affairs High--Density Lipoprotein Intervention Trial." Am J Cardiol 86(12A): 19L-22L.

Brown, C. D., M. Higgins, K. A. Donato, F. C. Rohde, R. Garrison, et al. (2000). "Body mass index and the prevalence of hypertension and dyslipidemia." Obes Res 8(9): 605-619.

Bruckert, E., M. Baccara-Dinet and E. Eschwege (2007). "Low HDL-cholesterol is common in European Type 2 diabetic patients receiving treatment for dyslipidaemia: data from a pan-European survey." Diabet Med 24(4): 388-391.

Cade, J. and B. Margetts (1989). "Cigarette smoking and serum lipid and lipoprotein concentrations." Bmj 298(6683): 1312.

Chait, A. and J. D. Brunzell (1990). "Acquired hyperlipidemia (secondary dyslipoproteinemias)." Endocrinol Metab Clin North Am 19(2): 259-278.

Chandalia, M., V. Mohan, B. Adams-Huet, R. Deepa and N. Abate (2008). "Ethnic difference in sex gap in high-density lipoprotein cholesterol between Asian Indians and Whites." J Investig Med 56(3): 574-580.

Charlton-Menys, V., D. J. Betteridge, H. Colhoun, J. Fuller, M. France, et al. (2009). "Apolipoproteins, cardiovascular risk and statin response in type 2 diabetes: the Collaborative Atorvastatin Diabetes Study (CARDS)." Diabetologia 52(2): 218-225.

Chen, L. K., M. H. Lin, Z. J. Chen, S. J. Hwang, S. T. Tsai, et al. (2006). "Metabolic characteristics and insulin resistance of impaired fasting glucose among the middle-aged and elderly Taiwanese." Diabetes Res Clin Pract 71(2): 170-176.

Cohen, J. C., Z. Wang, S. M. Grundy, M. R. Stoesz and R. Guerra (1994). "Variation at the hepatic lipase and apolipoprotein AI/CIII/AIV loci is a major cause of genetically determined variation in plasma HDL cholesterol levels." J Clin Invest 94(6): 2377-2384.

Colhoun, H. M., D. J. Betteridge, P. N. Durrington, G. A. Hitman, H. A. Neil, et al. (2004). "Primary prevention of cardiovascular disease with atorvastatin in type 2 diabetes in the Collaborative Atorvastatin Diabetes Study (CARDS): multicentre randomised placebo-controlled trial." Lancet 364(9435): 685-696.

Collins, R., J. Armitage, S. Parish, P. Sleigh and R. Peto (2003). "MRC/BHF Heart Protection Study of cholesterol-lowering with simvastatin in 5963 people with diabetes: a randomised placebo-controlled trial." Lancet 361(9374): 2005-2016.

Cooney, M. T., A. Dudina, D. De Bacquer, L. Wilhelmsen, S. Sans, et al. (2009). "HDL cholesterol protects against cardiovascular disease in both genders, at all ages and at all levels of risk." Atherosclerosis 206(2): 611-616.

Cowie, C. C., B. V. Howard and M. I. Harris (1994). "Serum lipoproteins in African Americans and whites with non-insulin-dependent diabetes in the US population." Circulation 90(3): 1185-1193.

Criqui, M. H., R. B. Wallace, G. Heiss, M. Mishkel, G. Schonfeld, et al. (1980). "Cigarette smoking and plasma high-density lipoprotein cholesterol. The Lipid Research Clinics Program Prevalence Study." Circulation 62(4 Pt 2): IV70-76.

Cui, Y., R. S. Blumenthal, J. A. Flaws, M. K. Whiteman, P. Langenberg, et al. (2001). "Non-high-density lipoprotein cholesterol level as a predictor of cardiovascular disease mortality." Arch Intern Med 161(11): 1413-1419.

Danesh J, C. R., Peto R. (2000). "Lipoprotein(a) and coronary heart disease: meta-analysis of prospective studies." Circulation 102(10): 1082-1085.

De Oliveira, E. S. E. R., D. Foster, M. McGee Harper, C. E. Seidman, J. D. Smith, et al. (2000). "Alcohol consumption raises HDL cholesterol levels by increasing the transport rate of apolipoproteins A-I and A-II." Circulation 102(19): 2347-2352.

Denke, M. A., C. T. Sempos and S. M. Grundy (1993). "Excess body weight. An underrecognized contributor to high blood cholesterol levels in white American men." Arch Intern Med 153(9): 1093-1103.

Denke, M. A., C. T. Sempos and S. M. Grundy (1994). "Excess body weight. An under-recognized contributor to dyslipidemia in white American women." Arch Intern Med 154(4): 401-410.

Devroey, D., N. De Swaef, P. Coigniez, J. Vandevoorde, J. Kartounian, et al. (2004). "Correlations between lipid levels and age, gender, glycemia, obesity, diabetes, and smoking." Endocr Res 30(1): 83-93.

Duffy, D. and D. J. Rader (2009). "Update on strategies to increase HDL quantity and function." Nat Rev Cardiol 6(7): 455-463.

Erem, C., A. Hacihasanoglu, O. Deger, M. Kocak and M. Topbas (2008). "Prevalence of dyslipidemia and associated risk factors among Turkish adults: Trabzon lipid study." Endocrine 34(1-3): 36-51.

Expert Panel on Detection, E., and Treatment of High Blood Cholesterol in Adults (2001). "Executive Summary of The Third Report of The National Cholesterol Education Program (NCEP) Expert Panel on Detection, Evaluation, And Treatment of High Blood Cholesterol In Adults (Adult Treatment Panel III)." Jama 285(19): 2486-2497.

Ezenwaka, C. E., N. Premanand and F. A. Orrett (2000). "Studies on plasma lipids in industrial workers in central Trinidad and Tobago." J Natl Med Assoc 92(8): 375-381.

Fisher, S. D., W. Zareba, A. J. Moss, V. J. Marder, C. E. Sparks, et al. (2000). "Effect of smoking on lipid and thrombogenic factors two months after acute myocardial infarction." Am J Cardiol 86(8): 813-818.

Florez, H., E. Silva, V. Fernandez, E. Ryder, T. Sulbaran, et al. (2005). "Prevalence and risk factors associated with the metabolic syndrome and dyslipidemia in White, Black, Amerindian and Mixed Hispanics in Zulia State, Venezuela." Diabetes Res Clin Pract 69(1): 63-77.

Fogari, R., A. Zoppi, C. Pasotti, L. Poletti, F. Tettamanti, et al. (1988). "Effects of different beta-blockers on lipid metabolism in chronic therapy of hypertension." Int J Clin Pharmacol Ther Toxicol 26(12): 597-604.

Foucan, L., P. Kangambega, D. Koumavi Ekouevi, J. Rozet and J. Bangou-Bredent (2000). "Lipid profile in an adult population in Guadeloupe." Diabetes Metab 26(6): 473-480.

France, M. W., S. Kwok, P. McElduff and C. J. Seneviratne (2003). "Ethnic trends in lipid tests in general practice." QJM 96(12): 919-923.

Fruchart J, S. F., Hermans M, Assmann, G, Brown W, Ceska R, Chapman M, Dodson P, Fioretto P, Ginsberg H (2008). "The residual risk reduction initiative: a call to action to reduce residual vascular risk in dyslipidaemic patients." Diabetes&Vascular Disease Research 5(4): 319-335.

Fuentes, R., T. Uusitalo, P. Puska, J. Tuomilehto and A. Nissinen (2003). "Blood cholesterol level and prevalence of hypercholesterolaemia in developing countries: a review of population-based studies carried out from 1979 to 2002." Eur J Cardiovasc Prev Rehabil 10(6): 411-419.

Gatti, A., M. Maranghi, S. Bacci, C. Carallo, A. Gnasso, et al. (2009). "Poor glycemic control is an independent risk factor for low HDL cholesterol in patients with type 2 diabetes." Diabetes Care 32(8): 1550-1552.

Geethanjali FS, L. K., Lingenhel A. (2003). "Analysis of the apo(a) size polymorphism in Asian Indian populations: association with Lp(a) concentration and coronary heart disease." Atherosclerosis 169(1): 121-130.

Goldberg, I. J. (2001). "Clinical review 124: Diabetic dyslipidemia: causes and consequences." J Clin Endocrinol Metab 86(3): 965-971.

Goldberg, R. B., M. J. Mellies, F. M. Sacks, L. A. Moye, B. V. Howard, et al. (1998). "Cardiovascular events and their reduction with pravastatin in diabetic and glucose-intolerant myocardial infarction survivors with average cholesterol levels: subgroup analyses in the cholesterol and recurrent events (CARE) trial. The Care Investigators." Circulation 98(23): 2513-2519.

Gomes, M. B., D. Giannella-Neto, M. Faria, M. Tambascia, R. M. Fonseca, et al. (2009). "Estimating cardiovascular risk in patients with type 2 diabetes: a national multicenter study in Brazil." Diabetol Metab Syndr 1(1): 22.

Graham, I., D. Atar, K. Borch-Johnsen, G. Boysen, G. Burell, et al. (2007). "European guidelines on cardiovascular disease prevention in clinical practice: executive summary. Fourth Joint Task Force of the European Society of Cardiology and other societies on cardiovascular disease prevention in clinical practice (constituted by representatives of nine societies and by invited experts)." Eur J Cardiovasc Prev Rehabil 14 Suppl 2: E1-40.

Grant, R. W. and J. B. Meigs (2007). "Prevalence and treatment of low HDL cholesterol among primary care patients with type 2 diabetes: an unmet challenge for cardiovascular risk reduction." Diabetes Care 30(3): 479-484.

Gupta M, S. N., Verma S. (2006). "South Asians and cardiovascular risk: what clinicians should know." Circulation 113(25): E924-E929.

Hadaegh, F., M. R. Bozorgmanesh, A. Ghasemi, H. Harati, N. Saadat, et al. (2008). "High prevalence of undiagnosed diabetes and abnormal glucose tolerance in the Iranian urban population: Tehran Lipid and Glucose Study." BMC Public Health 8: 176.

Hanh, T. T. M., T. Komatsu, N. T. Hung, V. N. Chuyen, Y. Yoshimura, et al. (2001). "Nutritional status of middle-aged Vietnamese in Ho Chi Minh City." J Am Coll Nutr 20(6): 616-622.

Hardman, A. E. (1999). "Physical activity, obesity and blood lipids." Int J Obes Relat Metab Disord 23 Suppl 3: S64-71.

Harris, M. I. and R. C. Eastman (2000). "Early detection of undiagnosed diabetes mellitus: a US perspective." Diabetes Metab Res Rev 16(4): 230-236.

Hennig, B., M. Toborek and C. J. McClain (2001). "High-energy diets, fatty acids and endothelial cell function: implications for atherosclerosis." J Am Coll Nutr 20(2 Suppl): 97-105.

Hertz, R. P., A. N. Unger and C. M. Ferrario (2006). "Diabetes, hypertension, and dyslipidemia in Mexican Americans and non-Hispanic whites." Am J Prev Med 30(2): 103-110.

Ismail, I. S., W. Nazaimoon, W. Mohamad, R. Letchuman, M. Singaraveloo, et al. (2001). "Ethnicity and glycaemic control are major determinants of diabetic dyslipidaemia in Malaysia." Diabet Med 18(6): 501-508.

Jacobs, M. J., T. Kleisli, J. R. Pio, S. Malik, G. J. L'Italien, et al. (2005). "Prevalence and control of dyslipidemia among persons with diabetes in the United States." Diabetes Res Clin Pract 70(3): 263-269.

Jurado, J., J. Ybarra, P. Solanas, J. Caula, I. Gich, et al. (2009). "Prevalence of cardiovascular disease and risk factors in a type 2 diabetic population of the North Catalonia diabetes study." J Am Acad Nurse Pract 21(3): 140-148.

Juutilainen, A., S. Lehto, T. Ronnemaa, K. Pyorala and M. Laakso (2005). "Type 2 diabetes as a "coronary heart disease equivalent": an 18-year prospective population-based study in Finnish subjects." Diabetes Care 28(12): 2901-2907.

Kannel, W. B. (1985). "Lipids, diabetes, and coronary heart disease: insights from the Framingham Study." Am Heart J 110(5): 1100-1107.

Karthikeyan, G., K. K. Teo, S. Islam, M. J. McQueen, P. Pais, et al. (2009). "Lipid profile, plasma apolipoproteins, and risk of a first myocardial infarction among Asians: an analysis from the INTERHEART Study." J Am Coll Cardiol 53(3): 244-253.

Kelishadi, R., G. Ardalan, R. Gheiratmand and A. Ramezani (2006). "Is family history of premature cardiovascular diseases appropriate for detection of dyslipidemic children in population-based preventive medicine programs? CASPIAN study." Pediatr Cardiol 27(6): 729-736.

Kendall, D. M. (2005). "The dyslipidemia of diabetes mellitus: giving triglycerides and high-density lipoprotein cholesterol a higher priority?" Endocrinol Metab Clin North Am 34(1): 27-48.

Knopp, R. H., M. d'Emden, J. G. Smilde and S. J. Pocock (2006). "Efficacy and safety of atorvastatin in the prevention of cardiovascular end points in subjects with type 2 diabetes: the Atorvastatin Study for Prevention of Coronary Heart Disease Endpoints in non-insulin-dependent diabetes mellitus (ASPEN)." Diabetes Care 29(7): 1478-1485.

Krauss, R. M. (2004). "Lipids and lipoproteins in patients with type 2 diabetes." Diabetes Care 27(6): 1496-1504.

Ku CY, G. B., Nagy TR, Goran MI. (1998). "Relationships between dietary fat, body fat, and serum lipid profile in prepubertal children." Obes Res(6): 400-407.

Kuller, L. H. (2004). "Ethnic differences in atherosclerosis, cardiovascular disease and lipid metabolism." Curr Opin Lipidol 15(2): 109-113.

Lehtonen, A. (1985). "Effect of beta blockers on blood lipid profile." Am Heart J 109(5 Pt 2): 1192-1196.

Li, Z., R. Yang, G. Xu and T. Xia (2005). "Serum lipid concentrations and prevalence of dyslipidemia in a large professional population in Beijing." Clin Chem 51(1): 144-150.

Liu, J., C. Sempos, R. P. Donahue, J. Dorn, M. Trevisan, et al. (2005). "Joint distribution of non-HDL and LDL cholesterol and coronary heart disease risk prediction among individuals with and without diabetes." Diabetes Care 28(8): 1916-1921.

Maeda, K., Y. Noguchi and T. Fukui (2003). "The effects of cessation from cigarette smoking on the lipid and lipoprotein profiles: a meta-analysis." Prev Med 37(4): 283-290.

Mammas, I. N., G. K. Bertsias, M. Linardakis, N. E. Tzanakis, D. N. Labadarios, et al. (2003). "Cigarette smoking, alcohol consumption, and serum lipid profile among medical students in Greece." Eur J Public Health 13(3): 278-282.

Mann, J. I., B. Lewis, J. Shepherd, A. F. Winder, S. Fenster, et al. (1988). "Blood lipid concentrations and other cardiovascular risk factors: distribution, prevalence, and detection in Britain." Br Med J (Clin Res Ed) 296(6638): 1702-1706.

McKeigue, P. M., B. Shah and M. G. Marmot (1991). "Relation of central obesity and insulin resistance with high diabetes prevalence and cardiovascular risk in South Asians." Lancet 337(8738): 382-386.

McNamara, D. J. and W. H. Howell (1992). "Epidemiologic data linking diet to hyperlipidemia and arteriosclerosis." Semin Liver Dis 12(4): 347-355.

McNaughton, S. A., G. D. Mishra and E. J. Brunner (2009). "Food patterns associated with blood lipids are predictive of coronary heart disease: the Whitehall II study." Br J Nutr 102(4): 619-624.

Meigs, J. B., D. M. Nathan, R. B. D'Agostino, Sr. and P. W. Wilson (2002). "Fasting and postchallenge glycemia and cardiovascular disease risk: the Framingham Offspring Study." Diabetes Care 25(10): 1845-1850.

Middeke, M., W. O. Richter, P. Schwandt, B. Beck and H. Holzgreve (1990). "Normalization of lipid metabolism after withdrawal from antihypertensive long-term therapy with beta blockers and diuretics." Arteriosclerosis 10(1): 145-147.

Millen, B. E., P. A. Quatromoni, B. H. Nam, C. E. O'Horo, J. F. Polak, et al. (2002). "Dietary patterns and the odds of carotid atherosclerosis in women: the Framingham Nutrition Studies." Prev Med 35(6): 540-547.

Mills, E. J., B. Rachlis, P. Wu, P. J. Devereaux, P. Arora, et al. (2008). "Primary prevention of cardiovascular mortality and events with statin treatments: a network meta-analysis involving more than 65,000 patients." J Am Coll Cardiol 52(22): 1769-1781.

Mohan, V., R. Deepa, S. P. Haranath, G. Premalatha, M. Rema, et al. (1998). "Lipoprotein(a) is an independent risk factor for coronary artery disease in NIDDM patients in South India." Diabetes Care 21(11): 1819-1823.

Morrish, N. J., L. K. Stevens, J. H. Fuller, R. J. Jarrett and H. Keen (1991). "Risk factors for macrovascular disease in diabetes mellitus: the London follow-up to the WHO Multinational Study of Vascular Disease in Diabetics." Diabetologia 34(8): 590-594.

Morrish, N. J., L. K. Stevens, J. H. Fuller, H. Keen and R. J. Jarrett (1991). "Incidence of macrovascular disease in diabetes mellitus: the London cohort of the WHO Multinational Study of Vascular Disease in Diabetics." Diabetologia 34(8): 584-589.

Morrish, N. J., L. K. Stevens, J. Head, J. H. Fuller, R. J. Jarrett, et al. (1990). "A prospective study of mortality among middle-aged diabetic patients (the London Cohort of the WHO Multinational Study of Vascular Disease in Diabetics) II: Associated risk factors." Diabetologia 33(9): 542-548.

Mulukutla, S. R., L. Venkitachalam, O. C. Marroquin, K. C. Kip, A. Aiyer, et al. (2008). "Population variation in atherogenic dyslipidemia: A report from the HeartSCORE and IndiaSCORE Studies." Journal of Clinical Lipidology 2(6): 410-417.

Murakami, K., S. Ishibashi, Y. Yoshida, N. Yamada and Y. Akanuma (1998). "Lipoprotein(a) as a coronary risk factor in Japanese patients with Type II (non-insulin-dependent) diabetes mellitus. Relation with apolipoprotein(a) phenotypes." Diabetologia 41(11): 1397-1398.

Novoa, F. J., M. Boronat, P. Saavedra, J. M. Diaz-Cremades, V. F. Varillas, et al. (2005). "Differences in cardiovascular risk factors, insulin resistance, and insulin secretion in individuals with normal glucose tolerance and in subjects with impaired glucose regulation: the Telde Study." Diabetes Care 28(10): 2388-2393.

Okafor, C. I., O. A. Fasanmade and D. A. Oke (2008). "Pattern of dyslipidaemia among Nigerians with type 2 diabetes mellitus." Niger J Clin Pract 11(1): 25-31.

Onat, A., G. Surdum-Avci, M. Senocak, E. Ornek and Y. Gozukara (1992). "Plasma lipids and their interrelationship in Turkish adults." J Epidemiol Community Health 46(5): 470-476.

Palaniappan, L. P., A. C. Kwan, F. Abbasi, C. Lamendola, T. L. McLaughlin, et al. (2007). "Lipoprotein abnormalities are associated with insulin resistance in South Asian Indian women." Metabolism 56(7): 899-904.

Pang, R. W., S. Tam, E. D. Janus, S. T. Siu, O. C. Ma, et al. (2006). "Plasma lipid, lipoprotein and apolipoprotein levels in a random population sample of 2875 Hong Kong Chinese adults and their implications (NCEP ATP-III, 2001 guidelines) on cardiovascular risk assessment." Atherosclerosis 184(2): 438-445.

Pankow, J. S., D. K. Kwan, B. B. Duncan, M. I. Schmidt, D. J. Couper, et al. (2007). "Cardiometabolic risk in impaired fasting glucose and impaired glucose tolerance: the Atherosclerosis Risk in Communities Study." Diabetes Care 30(2): 325-331.

Papazafiropoulou, A., A. Sotiropoulos, E. Skliros, M. Kardara, A. Kokolaki, et al. (2009). "Familial history of diabetes and clinical characteristics in Greek subjects with type 2 diabetes." BMC Endocr Disord 9: 12.

Patel, A., F. Barzi, K. Jamrozik, T. H. Lam, H. Ueshima, et al. (2004). "Serum triglycerides as a risk factor for cardiovascular diseases in the Asia-Pacific region." Circulation 110(17): 2678-2686.

Pischon, T., C. J. Girman, F. M. Sacks, N. Rifai, M. J. Stampfer, et al. (2005). "Non-high-density lipoprotein cholesterol and apolipoprotein B in the prediction of coronary heart disease in men." Circulation 112(22): 3375-3383.

Pongchaiyakul, C., P. Hongsprabhas and V. Pisprasert (2006). "Rural-urban difference in lipid levels and prevalence of dyslipidemia: a population-based study in Khon Kaen province, Thailand." J Med Assoc Thai 89(11): 1835-1844.

Post GB, K. H., Twisk J, van Mechelen W. (1997). "The association between dietary patterns and cardiovascular disease risk indicators in healthy youngsters: results covering fifteen years of longitudinal development." Eur J Clin Nutr 51: 387-393.

Psaty, B. M., M. Anderson, R. A. Kronmal, R. P. Tracy, T. Orchard, et al. (2004). "The association between lipid levels and the risks of incident myocardial infarction, stroke, and total mortality: The Cardiovascular Health Study." J Am Geriatr Soc 52(10): 1639-1647.

Pyorala, K., C. M. Ballantyne, B. Gumbiner, M. W. Lee, A. Shah, et al. (2004). "Reduction of cardiovascular events by simvastatin in nondiabetic coronary heart disease patients with and without the metabolic syndrome: subgroup analyses of the Scandinavian Simvastatin Survival Study (4S)." Diabetes Care 27(7): 1735-1740.

Ramachandran, A., S. Mary, A. Yamuna, N. Murugesan and C. Snehalatha (2008). "High prevalence of diabetes and cardiovascular risk factors associated with urbanization in India." Diabetes Care 31(5): 893-898.

Razak, F., S. Anand, V. Vuksan, B. Davis, R. Jacobs, et al. (2005). "Ethnic differences in the relationships between obesity and glucose-metabolic abnormalities: a cross-sectional population-based study." Int J Obes (Lond) 29(6): 656-667.

Reckless, J. P., D. J. Betteridge, P. Wu, B. Payne and D. J. Galton (1978). "High-density and low-density lipoproteins and prevalence of vascular disease in diabetes mellitus." Br Med J 1(6117): 883-886.

Ridker, P. M., N. Rifai, N. R. Cook, G. Bradwin and J. E. Buring (2005). "Non-HDL cholesterol, apolipoproteins A-I and B100, standard lipid measures, lipid ratios, and CRP as risk factors for cardiovascular disease in women." Jama 294(3): 326-333.

Roberto Robles, N., S. Barroso, G. Marcos and J. F. Sanchez Munoz-Torrero (2009). "[Lipid control in diabetic patients in Extremadura (Spain)]." Endocrinol Nutr 56(3): 112-117.

Roberts, W. C. (1989). "Recent studies on the effects of beta blockers on blood lipid levels." Am Heart J 117(3): 709-714.

Ronnemaa, T., M. Laakso, V. Kallio, K. Pyorala, J. Marniemi, et al. (1989). "Serum lipids, lipoproteins, and apolipoproteins and the excessive occurrence of coronary heart disease in non-insulin-dependent diabetic patients." Am J Epidemiol 130(4): 632-645.

Roselli della Rovere, G., A. Lapolla, G. Sartore, C. Rossetti, S. Zambon, et al. (2003). "Plasma lipoproteins, apoproteins and cardiovascular disease in type 2 diabetic patients. A nine-year follow-up study." Nutr Metab Cardiovasc Dis 13(1): 46-51.

Rosengren, A., L. Welin, A. Tsipogianni and L. Wilhelmsen (1989). "Impact of cardiovascular risk factors on coronary heart disease and mortality among middle aged diabetic men: a general population study." Bmj 299(6708): 1127-1131.

Ruixing, Y., W. Jinzhen, H. Yaoheng, T. Jing, W. Hai, et al. (2008). "Associations of diet and lifestyle with hyperlipidemia for middle-aged and elderly persons among the Guangxi Bai Ku Yao and Han populations." J Am Diet Assoc 108(6): 970-976.

Santen, R. J., P. W. Willis, 3rd and S. S. Fajans (1972). "Atherosclerosis in diabetes mellitus. Correlations with serum lipid levels, adiposity, and serum insulin level." Arch Intern Med 130(6): 833-843.

Sarwar, N., J. Danesh, G. Eiriksdottir, G. Sigurdsson, N. Wareham, et al. (2007). "Triglycerides and the risk of coronary heart disease: 10,158 incident cases among 262,525 participants in 29 Western prospective studies." Circulation 115(4): 450-458.

Schulze, M. B., I. Shai, J. E. Manson, T. Li, N. Rifai, et al. (2004). "Joint role of non-HDL cholesterol and glycated haemoglobin in predicting future coronary heart disease events among women with type 2 diabetes." Diabetologia 47(12): 2129-2136.

Schwandt, P., R. Kelishadi and G. M. Haas (2010). "Ethnic disparities of the metabolic syndrome in population-based samples of german and Iranian adolescents." Metab Syndr Relat Disord 8(2): 189-192.

Schwandt, P., R. Kelishadi, R. Q. Ribeiro, G. M. Haas and P. Poursafa (2010). "A three-country study on the components of the metabolic syndrome in youths: the BIG Study." Int J Pediatr Obes 5(4): 334-341.

Sever, P. S., N. R. Poulter, B. Dahlof, H. Wedel, R. Collins, et al. (2005). "Reduction in cardiovascular events with atorvastatin in 2,532 patients with type 2 diabetes: Anglo-Scandinavian Cardiac Outcomes Trial--lipid-lowering arm (ASCOT-LLA)." Diabetes Care 28(5): 1151-1157.

Seviour, P. W., T. K. Teal, W. Richmond and R. S. Elkeles (1988). "Serum lipids, lipoproteins and macrovascular disease in non-insulin-dependent diabetics: a possible new approach to prevention." Diabet Med 5(2): 166-171.

Seyum, B., G. Mebrahtu, A. Usman, J. Mufunda, B. Tewolde, et al. (2010). "Profile of patients with diabetes in Eritrea: results of first phase registry analyses." Acta Diabetol 47(1): 23-27.

Shai, I., E. B. Rimm, M. B. Schulze, N. Rifai, M. J. Stampfer, et al. (2004). "Moderate alcohol intake and markers of inflammation and endothelial dysfunction among diabetic men." Diabetologia 47(10): 1760-1767.

Sharma, M. D. and V. N. Pavlik (2001). "Dyslipidaemia in African Americans, Hispanics and whites with type 2 diabetes mellitus and hypertension." Diabetes Obes Metab 3(1): 41-45.

Shepherd, J., P. Barter, R. Carmena, P. Deedwania, J. C. Fruchart, et al. (2006). "Effect of lowering LDL cholesterol substantially below currently recommended levels in patients with coronary heart disease and diabetes: the Treating to New Targets (TNT) study." Diabetes Care 29(6): 1220-1226.

Singh, I. M., M. H. Shishehbor and B. J. Ansell (2007). "High-density lipoprotein as a therapeutic target: a systematic review." Jama 298(7): 786-798.

Sisson, S. B., S. M. Camhi, T. S. Church, C. K. Martin, C. Tudor-Locke, et al. (2009). "Leisure time sedentary behavior, occupational/domestic physical activity, and metabolic syndrome in U.S. men and women." Metab Syndr Relat Disord 7(6): 529-536.

Smaoui, M., S. Hammami, R. Chaaba, N. Attia, K. B. Hamda, et al. (2004). "Lipids and lipoprotein(a) concentrations in Tunisian type 2 diabetic patients; Relationship to glycemic control and coronary heart disease." J Diabetes Complications 18(5): 258-263.

Snehalatha, C. and A. Ramachandran (2009). "Cardiovascular risk factors in the normoglycaemic Asian-Indian population--influence of urbanisation." Diabetologia 52(4): 596-599.

Sorrentino, S. A., C. Besler, L. Rohrer, M. Meyer, K. Heinrich, et al. (2010). "Endothelial-vasoprotective effects of high-density lipoprotein are impaired in patients with type 2 diabetes mellitus but are improved after extended-release niacin therapy." Circulation 121(1): 110-122.

Stamler, J., O. Vaccaro, J. D. Neaton and D. Wentworth (1993). "Diabetes, other risk factors, and 12-yr cardiovascular mortality for men screened in the Multiple Risk Factor Intervention Trial." Diabetes Care 16(2): 434-444.

Steinhagen-Thiessen, E., P. Bramlage, C. Losch, H. Hauner, H. Schunkert, et al. (2008). "Dyslipidemia in primary care--prevalence, recognition, treatment and control: data from the German Metabolic and Cardiovascular Risk Project (GEMCAS)." Cardiovasc Diabetol 7: 31.

Steven H, M. M., Helen H, Marc R, J.AVA K. (1986). "The role of behavioral variables and fat patterning in explaining ethnic differences in serum lipids and lipoproteins." Am. J. Epidemiol 123(5): 830-839.

Stone, N. J. (1994). "Secondary causes of hyperlipidemia." Med Clin North Am 78(1): 117-141.

Sumner AE, V. G., Genovese DJ, Finley KB, Bergman RN, Boston RC. (2005). "Normal triglyceride levels despite insulin resistance in African Americans: role of lipoprotein lipase." Metabolism 54(7): 902-909.

Sundquist J, W. M. (1999). "Cardiovascular risk factors in mexican american adults: a transcultural analysis of NHANES III, 1988-1994." Am. J. Public Health 89(5): 723-730.

Surana, S. P., D. B. Shah, K. Gala, S. Susheja, S. S. Hoskote, et al. (2008). "Prevalence of metabolic syndrome in an urban Indian diabetic population using the NCEP ATP III guidelines." J Assoc Physicians India 56: 865-868.

Tan, C. E., S. C. Emmanuel, B. Y. Tan and E. Jacob (1999). "Prevalence of diabetes and ethnic differences in cardiovascular risk factors. The 1992 Singapore National Health Survey." Diabetes Care 22(2): 241-247.

Tan, C. E., E. S. Tai, C. S. Tan, K. S. Chia, J. Lee, et al. (2003). "APOE polymorphism and lipid profile in three ethnic groups in the Singapore population." Atherosclerosis 170(2): 253-260.

Tanasescu, M., E. Cho, J. E. Manson and F. B. Hu (2004). "Dietary fat and cholesterol and the risk of cardiovascular disease among women with type 2 diabetes." Am J Clin Nutr 79(6): 999-1005.

Taylor, A. J., T. C. Villines, E. J. Stanek, P. J. Devine, L. Griffen, et al. (2009). "Extended-release niacin or ezetimibe and carotid intima-media thickness." N Engl J Med 361(22): 2113-2122.

Tekes-Manova, D., E. Israeli, T. Shochat, M. Swartzon, S. Gordon, et al. (2006). "The prevalence of reversible cardiovascular risk factors in Israelis aged 25-55 years." Isr Med Assoc J 8(8): 527-531.

Temelkova-Kurktschiev, T. S., D. P. Kurktschiev, L. G. Vladimirova-Kitova, I. Vaklinova and B. R. Todorova (2009). "Prevalence and type of dyslipidaemia in a population at risk for cardiovascular death in Bulgaria." Folia Med (Plovdiv) 51(2): 26-32.

Thavendiranathan, P., A. Bagai, M. A. Brookhart and N. K. Choudhry (2006). "Primary prevention of cardiovascular diseases with statin therapy: a meta-analysis of randomized controlled trials." Arch Intern Med 166(21): 2307-2313.

The DECODA Study Group (2007). "Prevalence of the metabolic syndrome in populations of Asian origin. Comparison of the IDF definition with the NCEP definition." Diabetes Res Clin Pract 76(1): 57-67.

The Emerging Risk Factors C (2009). "Lipoprotein(a) concentration and the risk of coronary heart disease, stroke, and nonvascular mortality." Jama 302(4): 412-423.

Tolonen, H., U. Keil, M. Ferrario and A. Evans (2005). "Prevalence, awareness and treatment of hypercholesterolaemia in 32 populations: results from the WHO MONICA Project." Int J Epidemiol 34(1): 181-192.

Tsimikas S, C. P., Brilakis ES. (2009). "Relationship of oxidized phospholipids on apolipoprotein B-100 particles to race/ethnicity, apolipoprotein(a) isoform size, and cardiovascular risk factors: results from the Dallas Heart Study." Circulation 119(13): 1711-1719.

Turner, R. C., H. Millns, H. A. Neil, I. M. Stratton, S. E. Manley, et al. (1998). "Risk factors for coronary artery disease in non-insulin dependent diabetes mellitus: United Kingdom Prospective Diabetes Study (UKPDS: 23)." Bmj 316(7134): 823-828.

U.K. Prospective Diabetes Study Investigators (1997). "U.K. Prospective Diabetes Study 27. Plasma lipids and lipoproteins at diagnosis of NIDDM by age and sex." Diabetes Care 20(11): 1683-1687.

Umeda, T., S. Kono, Y. Sakurai, K. Shinchi, K. Imanishi, et al. (1998). "Relationship of cigarette smoking, alcohol use, recreational exercise and obesity with serum lipid atherogenicity: a study of self-defense officials in Japan." J Epidemiol 8(4): 227-234.

Vega GL, C. L., Tang A, Marcovina S, Grundy SM, Cohen JC. (1998). "Hepatic lipase activity is lower in African-American men than in white American men: effects of 5' flanking polymorphism in the hepatic lipase gene (LIPC)." J Lipid Res 39(1): 228-232.

Venkatesan, A., A. Hemalatha, Z. Bobby, N. Selvaraj and V. Sathiyapriya (2006). "Effect of smoking on lipid profile and lipid peroxidation in normal subjects." Indian J Physiol Pharmacol 50(3): 273-278.

Villines, T. C., E. J. Stanek, P. J. Devine, M. Turco, M. Miller, et al. (2010). "The ARBITER 6-HALTS Trial (Arterial Biology for the Investigation of the Treatment Effects of Reducing Cholesterol 6-HDL and LDL Treatment Strategies in Atherosclerosis) Final Results and the Impact of Medication Adherence, Dose, and Treatment Duration." J Am Coll Cardiol: doi:10.1016/j.jacc.2010.1003.1017.

Vlajinac, H., M. Ilic and J. Marinkovic (1992). "Cardiovascular risk factors and prevalence of coronary heart disease in type 2 (non-insulin-dependent) diabetes." Eur J Epidemiol 8(6): 783-788.

Wang, J., S. Ruotsalainen, L. Moilanen, P. Lepisto, M. Laakso, et al. (2007). "The metabolic syndrome predicts cardiovascular mortality: a 13-year follow-up study in elderly non-diabetic Finns." Eur Heart J 28(7): 857-864.

Wang W, H. D., Lee ET. (2002). "Lipoprotein(a) in American Indians is low and not independently associated with cardiovascular disease: the Strong Heart Study." Ann. Epidemiol. 12(2): 107-114.

Werk, E. E., Jr., J. J. Gonzalez and J. E. Ranney (1993). "Lipid level differences and hypertension effect in blacks and whites with type II diabetes." Ethn Dis 3(3): 242-249.

Wilson, P. W., R. D. Abbott and W. P. Castelli (1988). "High density lipoprotein cholesterol and mortality. The Framingham Heart Study." Arteriosclerosis 8(6): 737-741.

Wood, P. D., M. P. Stern, A. Silvers, G. M. Reaven and J. von der Groeben (1972). "Prevalence of plasma lipoprotein abnormalities in a free-living population of the Central Valley, California." Circulation 45(1): 114-126.

World Health Organization (2007). "Prevention of cardiovascular disease: guideline for assessment and management of cardiovascular risk." WHO Press.

Wu, D. M., L. Pai, P. K. Sun, L. L. Hsu and C. A. Sun (2001). "Joint effects of alcohol consumption and cigarette smoking on atherogenic lipid and lipoprotein profiles: results from a study of Chinese male population in Taiwan." Eur J Epidemiol 17(7): 629-635.

Zaman, M. M., N. Yoshiike, M. A. Rouf, M. H. Syeed, M. R. Khan, et al. (2001). "Cardiovascular risk factors: distribution and prevalence in a rural population of Bangladesh." J Cardiovasc Risk 8(2): 103-108.

Zaninotto, P., J. Mindell and V. Hirani (2007). "Prevalence of cardiovascular risk factors among ethnic groups: results from the Health Surveys for England." Atherosclerosis 195(1): e48-57.

Zhang, X., Z. Sun, D. Zhang, L. Zheng, J. Li, et al. (2009). "Prevalence and association with diabetes and obesity of lipid phenotypes among the hypertensive Chinese rural adults." Heart Lung 38(1): 17-24.

Zhao, W. H., J. Zhang, Y. Zhai, Y. You, Q. Q. Man, et al. (2007). "Blood lipid profile and prevalence of dyslipidemia in Chinese adults." Biomed Environ Sci 20(4): 329-335.

4

Dyslipidemia and Type 2 Diabetes Mellitus: Implications and Role of Antiplatelet Agents in Primary Prevention of Cardiovascular Disease

Hasniza Zaman Huri

Department of Pharmacy, Faculty of Medicine,
University of Malaya, Kuala Lumpur,
Malaysia

1. Introduction

Dyslipidemia is the major risk factors for macrovascular complications leading to cardiovascular disease (CVD) in type 2 diabetes mellitus (T2DM). In addition to this, endothelial dysfunction, platelet hyperactivity, impaired fibrinolytic balance and abnormal blood flow may accelerate atherosclerosis and increased risk of thrombotic vascular events (Colwell & Nesto, 2003). Macrovascular disease is the most common cause of morbidity and mortality in T2DM (Koskinen, 1998). Macrovascular disease is defined as illnesses affecting the larger arteries supplying the heart, brain, and the legs, thereby causing ischemic heart disease, cerebrovascular disease, and peripheral vascular disease (Thompson, 1999). In patients with diabetes, alteration in distribution of lipid increased risk of atherosclerosis. Specifically, insulin resistance and insulin deficiency was identified as phenotype of dyslipidemia in diabetes mellitus (Taskinen, 2003; Krauss & Siri, 2004; Chahil & Ginsberg, 2006). This was characterized with high plasma triglyceride level, low HDL cholesterol level and increased level of small dense LDL-cholesterol (Mooradian, 2008). In these patient also, the increment of free fatty-acid release is due to insulin resistance. With the presence of adequate glycogen stores in the liver, this will promote triglyceride production, which stimulates the secretion of apolipoprotein B (Apo B) and VLDL cholesterol (Mooradian, 2008). Hepatic production of VLDL cholesterol is enhanced due to disability of insulin to inhibit the release of free fatty-acid. Low HDL cholesterol levels were also associated with hyperinsulinemia. There are several associations between dyslipidemia and the increased risk of cardiovascular disease in patients with type 2 diabetes mellitus. Low HDL cholesterol and increased triglyceride levels may contribute to the increased risk of cardiovascular disease. In conjunction with increased small dense LDL cholesterol and low HDL cholesterol levels, further evidence suggests that acceleration of atherosclerosis in diabetes mellitus and insulin-resistant conditions is regulated by hypertriglyceridemia. Nevertheless, the association between LDL cholesterol and CHD risk is stronger compared to the association between hypertriglyceridemia and CHD risk. Type 2 diabetes is also associated with insulin resistance and hyperinsulinemia or syndrome X comprises hypertension, dyslipidemia, decreased fibrinolysis and increased procoagulation factors (Serrano Rios, 1998). Besides dyslipidemia, platelet abnormalities contributed significantly to increased risk of CVD in these patients. In patients with type 2 diabetes, the platelet abnormalities are due to increased platelet aggregability and adhesiveness (Colwell & Nesto, 2003) and enhanced platelet aggregation activity may precede development of CVD (Halushka et al. 1981, Mandal et al. 1993). It has been well known that management of dyslipidemia in diabetes mellitus includes lifestyle changes such as increased physical activity and dietary modifications. Besides, various antihyperlipidemic agents have been utilized for this purpose. In contrast, antiplatelet agents are recommended mainly for primary and secondary prevention for cardiovascular disease in T2DM. Dyslipidemia is categorized as one of the cardiovascular risk factors besides others (family history CHD, hypertension, smoking, albuminuria) (American Diabetes Association, 2011). Patients with T2DM and having dyslipidemia are eligible for primary prevention of CVD with antiplatelet agents. This chapter will discuss on different types of antiplatelet agents used as primary prevention of cardiovascular disease in patients with T2DM. It will also emphasize appropriate selection of antiplatelet agents pertaining to clinical conditions of patients with T2DM and dyslipidemia.

2. Pathophysiology of dyslipidemia and platelet abnormalities in type 2 diabetes mellitus

Atherogenic dyslipidemia is characterized by three lipoprotein abnormalities: elevated VLDL, small LDL and decreased HDL cholesterol levels, named as atherogenic lipoprotein phenotype (Grundy, 1998). In patients with type 2 diabetes, the prothrombotic state is characterized by increased fibrinogen levels (Imperatore et al 1998), increased plasminogen activator inhibitor (PAI)-1 (Byberg et al., 1998) and abnormalities in platelet function (Trovati et al., 1988). The reason for three aforementioned phenotypes in athrogenic dyslipidemia is the increased free fatty-acid release from insulin-resistant fat cells (Taskinen, 2003; Krauss & Siri, 2004; Chahil & Ginsberg, 2006). The increased flux of free fatty acids into the liver in the presence of adequate glycogen stores promotes triglyceride production, which in turn stimulates the secretion of apolipoprotein B (ApoB) and VLDL cholesterol (Mooradian, 2008). The impaired ability of insulin to inhibit free fatty-acid release leads to enhanced hepatic VLDL cholesterol production (Frayn, 2001) which correlates with the degree of hepatic fat accumulation (Adiels et al., 2007). The increased number of plasma VLDL cholesterol and triglyceride levels decrease the level of HDL cholesterol and increase the concentration of small dense LDL cholesterol (Mooradian, 2008).

Platelet activation commenced with binding of thrombogenic substances (collagen, thrombin, components of atheromatous plaque) to receptors located on the platelet surface (Colwell & Nesto, 2003). Receptor binding triggers a series of events that include hydrolysis of membrane phospholipids, mobilization of intracellular calcium, and phosphorylation of important intracellular proteins (Colwell & Nesto, 2003). There are several platelet abnormalities seen in diabetes patients. Abnormalities of thromboxane A2 (TXA$_2$) production were among the earliest abnormalities in platelets of diabetes patients. TXA$_2$ is a potent activator and its synthesis is suppressed by aspirin (Natarajan et al., 2008). Platelets from patients with type 2 diabetes mellitus found to have increased expression of adhesion molecules CD31, CD36, CD49b, CD62P and CD63 (Eibl et al., 2004). Glycemic control improvement led to a significant decline in their expression (Eibl et al., 2004). In type 2 diabetes patients, platelets increased surface expressionof GP Ib and GP IIb/IIIa (Vinik et al., 2001). GP Ib mediates binding to von Willebrand factor (vWf) which is important in platelet-dependent thrombogenesis (Natarajan et al., 2008). Increased expression of GP IIb/IIIa on platelet surfaces leads to enhanced fibrinogen binding, platelet cross-linking and thrombogenesis (Colwell & Nesto, 2003). In patients with type 2 diabetes, decreased platelet insulin receptor number and affinity responsible for platelet hyperactivity (Vinik et al., 2001). Platelets have been shown to be targets of insulin action as they act as functional insulin receptor for insulin binding and autophosphorylation (Vinik et al., 2001). Insulin reduces platelet responses to the agonists' adenosine diphosphate (ADP), collagen, thrombin, arachidonate and platelet-activating factor. (Natarajan et al., 2008). In patients with type 2 diabetes also, platelets show disordered calcium homeostasis (Li et al., 2001). This may cause hyperactivity including platelet shape change, secretion, aggregation and thromboxane formation (Beckman et al., 2002). Furthermore, the deficiency of magnesium in diabetes has been associated with platelet hyperaggregability and adhesiveness (Gawaz et al., 1994). In type 2 diabetes patients, the reduced vascular synthesis of the anti-aggregants prostacyclin and nitric oxide by endothelium, shift the balance towards aggregation and vasoconstriction (Vinik et al., 2001; Ferroni et al., 2004). In type 2 diabetes patients with acute hyperglycaemia, shear stress-induced platelet activation and P-selection expression (Natarajan et al., 2008). Hyperglycaemia also causes non-enzymatic glycation of platelet membrane proteins resulting in changes in protein structure and conformation, as well as alterations of membrane lipid dynamics (Brownlee et al., 1988; Winocour et al., 1992). This could result in enhanced expression of certain crucial platelet receptors, for instance, P-selectin and GP IIb/IIIa, thus altering platelet activity (Ferroni et al., 2004). Glycated LDL causes an increase in intracellular calcium concentration and platelet nitric oxide (NO) production, as well as inhibition of the platelet membrane Na+/K+-adenosine triphosphatase (Na+/K+-ATPase) activity (Ferroni et al., 2004).

3. Implications of dyslipidemia and platelet abnormality in type 2 diabetes mellitus

In patients with type 2 diabetes mellitus, low HDL cholesterol and high triglyceride levels might contribute to the increased risk of cardiovascular disease (Mooradian, 2008). Based on the Expert panel on Detection, Evaluation and Treatment of High Blood Cholesterol in Adults (2011), hypertriglyceridemia, increased small dense LDL cholesterol and low HDL cholesterol found to be important in accelerating atherosclerosis in diabetes mellitus and insulin-resistant conditions. Abnormal platelet function is another important risk factors for cardiovascular disease in patients with diabetes (Colwell & Nesto, 2003). Atherosclerosis and thrombosis contribute significantly to the increased cardiovascular risk of diabetic patients (Colwell, 1997). The majority of ischemic coronary and cerebrovascular events are precipitated by vessel occlusion caused by atherosclerotic plaque disruption, platelet aggregation, platelet adhesion and thrombosis (Colwell & Nesto, 2003). Several systems that involved vasculature such as platelet, endothelial function, coagulation and fibrinolysis are impaired in patients with diabetes (Jokl & Colwell, 1997). Furthermore, increased platelet aggregability and adhesiveness are due to reduce membrane fluidity, increased intracellular Ca2+ and decreased intracellular Mg2+, increased arachidonic acid metabolism, increased

TXA$_2$ synthesis, decreased prostacyclin production, decreased NO production, decreased antioxidant levels and increased expression of activation-dependent adhesion molecules (Halushka et al., 1981; Mayfield et al., 1985; Watala et al., 1998; Martina et al., 1998; Trovati et al., 1997; Sarji et al., 1979; Tschoepe, et al., 1997; Leet et al., 1981). For patients with T2DM, the presence of dyslipidemia and platelet hyperactivity justifies the use of antiplatelet agents as primary prevention strategy of CVD.

4. Role of antiplatelet agents in primary prevention of CVD

Increased physical activity, dietary modifications and pharmacologic interventions are the key methods in management of dyslipidemia in type 2 diabetes mellitus (Mooradian, 2008). The Antithrombotic Trialists' Collaboration meta-analysis found that antiplatelet therapy reduces the relative risk of any serious vascular event by 25% in patients at high risk for a cardiovascular (CV) event (Antithrombotic Trialist' Collaboration, 2002). Antiplatelet agents are used for primary and secondary prevention of CVD in type 2 diabetes mellitus patients. Antiplatelet therapy is needed in the management of diabetes mellitus because there is an increase of platelet aggregability and adhesiveness due to platelet and endothelial dysfunction, impaired coagulation cascade, and fibrinolysis process among diabetic individuals compared to nondiabetic individuals (Colwell & Nesto, 2003). Consequently, the balance in normal hemostasis is shifted to favor thrombosis and accelerated atherosclerosis and results in increasing CVD (Colwell & Nesto, 2003). For primary prevention of cardiovascular diseases, type 2 diabetes mellitus patients with high risk acquiring cardiovascular events such as those with family history of cardiovascular disease, hypertension, obesity (BMI > 30 kg/m^2), smoking, dyslipidemia and albuminuria (Colwell, 2004). Several types of antiplatelet agents is being utilized for prevention of CVD which including aspirin, ticlopidine, clopidogrel and glycoprotein (Gp) IIb-IIIa antagonist such as abciximab, eptifibatide and tirofiban (Patrono et al., 2004; American Diabetes Association, 2006; Colwell & Nesto, 2003). Aspirin is one of the most common antiplatelet that been suggested in prevention of CVD in diabetes. Clopidogrel and ticlopidine are theinopyridine antiplatelet agents that generally suggested if patients are contraindicated to aspirin (American Diabetes Association, 2006). In contrast, Gp IIb-IIIa antagonist is usually given to diabetes patients who undergo precutaneous coronary intervention in order to intensify the antiplatelet therapy and to reduce the risk of procedure related thrombotic complication and reoccurrence of CV event (Patrono et al., 2004).

5. Types of antiplatelet

5.1 Aspirin

Aspirin selectively and irreversibly acetylates the COX-1 enzyme, thereby blocking the formation of thromboxane A2 in platelets and leads to inability of platelet to resynthesize COX-1 (Patrono et al., 2005). Aspirin has been used as a primary strategy to prevent CVD in type 2 diabetes due to its effectiveness in atherosclerosis prevention is well established. Various meta-analyses studies and large scale randomized controlled trials in T2DM support that low-dose aspirin therapy should be prescribed as prevention strategy in T2DM, if the contraindication is not exist (Colwell, 2004). Low dose of aspirin inhibits thromboxane production by platelets but has little or no effects on other sites of platelet activity (Colwell & Nesto, 2003). Several randomized controlled trials had been designed to assess the

efficacy of aspirin in primary prevention of CVD which included Primary Prevention Project
(PPP), US physicians' Health Study (USPHS), Early Treatment of Diabetes Retinopathy
Study (ETDRS), Hypertension Optimal Treatment Trial (HOT), British Male Doctors' Trial
(BMD) and the Thrombosis Prevention Trial (TPT) (Colwell & Nesto, 2003; Hayden et al.,
2002). In Primary Prevention Project (PPP), a low dose aspirin (100 mg/day) was evaluated
for the prevention of cardiovascular events in individuals with one or more of the following
conditions such as hypertension, hypercholesterolemia, diabetes, obese, family history of
premature myocardial infarction or being elderly. After a mean of 3.6 years follow-up,
aspirin was found to significantly lower the frequency of cardiovascular death (from 1.4 %
to 0.8 %); relative risk (RR) 0.56 [confidence interval (CI) 0.31-.99] and total cardiovascular
events (from 8.2 to 6.3% ; RR 0.77 [0.62-0.95]). This trial involved large sample size (n =
4495) with the largest proportion of patients with diabetes mellitus (17%) (Collaborative
Group of the Primary Prevention Project, 2001). Overall, PPP provides evidence to prove the
efficacy of aspirin in diabetes; though participants were not blinded and were not given
placebo pills. Additionally, a meta-analysis done by Hayden et al., (2002) also rated the
quality of PPP as "fair" if compared to the rest of studies. In addition to PPP, a 5 years
primary prevention trial in 22 701 healthy men; included 533 men with diabetes was
conducted in US Physicians' Health Study (USPHS) in which a low-dose aspirin regimen
(325 mg every other day) was given to treated group compared with placebo. A total of 44%
significant risk reduction in CVD treated group was noted and the subgroup analyses in the
diabetes reveals a reduction in myocardial infarction from 10.1 % (placebo) to 4.0 %
(aspirin), yield a relative risk reduction of 0.39 for the diabetes men on aspirin therapy
(Steering Committee of the Physicians' Health Study Research Group, 1989). Researcher and
participants were blinded in this trial. In contrast with PPP, women were included in the
study populations (2583 out of 4495 sample sizes). Hence, this study was more reliable
compared to previous ones even though only 2% of the study population was diagnosed
with diabetes. The Hypertension Optimal Treatment Trial (HOT) also examined the effects
of low dose of aspirin (75 mg/day) versus placebo in 18 790 hypertension patients and 8% of
them had diabetes. Results showed that aspirin significantly reduce cardiovascular event by
15% and myocardial infarction by 36% (Hansson et al., 1998). The HOT trial was another
primary prevention study that included women, which was 46.6 % from total study
population. Colwell (2004) commended that this study provided further evidence for the
efficacy and safety of aspirin therapy in diabetes with systolic blood pressure less than 160
mmHg. Hayden et al., (2002) was in agreement with Colwell (2004) and concluded that HOT
was a "good" quality of trial in their meta-analysis. Despite that, these findings were
mirrored by Early Treatment of Diabetes Retinopathy Study (ETDRS) where they reported
that although aspirin did not prevent progression of retinopathy but it did produce a
significant reduction in risk for myocardial infarction (28%) over 5 years (P=0.038). This
study may viewed as mixed primary and secondary prevention trials since those enrolled
had a history of myocardial infarction and less than 50% had elevated blood pressure and
history of CVD (ETDRS Investigators 1992). Conversely, the British Male Doctors' Trial
(BMD) had conflicting results regarding aspirin effects in reducing the risk for myocardial
infarction and adverse effects such as gastrointestinal bleeding and hemorrhagic stroke to
diabetes patients. A total of 39 % of participants were discontinued therapy during the study
due to adverse effect of aspirin (Hayden et al., 2002). Similar to PPP trial, participants in this
study were not blinded thus results may be varies. Following this, a meta-analysis of these

five randomized clinical trials (except ETDRS) was performed by Hayden et al., (2002) and systematic reviews on nine articles about the effect of aspirin on gastrointestinal bleeding and hemorrhagic stroke were conducted. They concluded that the net benefit of aspirin increase with CV risk. Nonetheless, this meta-analysis was found to have selection bias due to exclusion of 2 large trials that examined the effects of aspirin in patients with diabetes or stable angina. Sanmuganathan et al., (2001) also reached similar estimates of the beneficial effects of aspirin in primary prevention of CVD. The Japanese Primary Prevention of Atherosclerosis With Aspirin for Diabetes (JPAD) trial was the first prospectively designed trial to evaluate the use of aspirin (81 mg or 100 mg) in the primary prevention of cardiovascular events in patients with type 2 diabetes (n = 2539) aged 30–85 years in Japan (Ogawa et al., 2008). Among patients aged > 65 years (n =1363), aspirin was associated with a 32% reduction in the risk of the primary end point (6.3 vs. 9.2%; P = 0.047). Furthermore, in aspirin-treated patients, the incidence of fatal coronary and cerebrovascular events was significantly lower by 90% (0.08 vs. 0.8%; P = 0.0037). Paradoxically, there were no differences in nonfatal coronary and cerebrovascular events. Aspirin was well tolerated, with no significant increase in the composite of hemorrhagic stroke and severe gastrointestinal bleeding (Angiolillo, 2009). The outcome of this study was in opposite with the current recommendations on aspirin usage in primary prevention of CVD in diabetes patients (Angiolillo, 2009). However, the ASCEND and ACCEPT-D study are two ongoing trials will provide further insights to the appropriateness of aspirin usage in primary prevention of CVD in patients with diabetes. Another recent trial (POPADAD), failed to show any benefit with aspirin or antioxidants in primary prevention of cardiovascular events (Belch, 2008). The outcome of the study could be due to small number of patients with low event rates. A study on the utilization of antiplatelet therapy in type 2 diabetes patients revealed that many of the eligible patients did not receive the drugs as primary prevention strategy for CVD (Huri et al., 2008). Therefore, the recommendations on aspirin usage in primary prevention of CVD in type 2 diabetes patients must be fully justified after taking consideration against the benefit versus risk of its use. In another words, the recommendations should be base on individual patients' assessment and clinical judgment. Proper use of aspirin in primary prevention of CVD in type 2 diabetes patients may result in long-term benefits.

5.2 Clopidogrel

Clopidogrel is another type of antiplatelet agents used in primary prevention of CVD in type 2 diabetes when patients are intolerant to aspirin. It inhibits ADP-induced platelet aggregation by blocking the purinergic receptors and therefore prevents the activation of the GpIIb-IIIa receptor and subsequent binding to fibrinogen (Colwell & Nesto, 2003). Clopidogrel is preferable compared to ticlopidine because of its safety profile (Savi & Herbert, 2005; Bertrand et al., 2000). Nevertheless, the information regarding the usage of clopidogrel in primary prevention of CVD is limited than for secondary prevention of CVD in diabetes patients. Even though clopidogrel may be slightly more effective than aspirin, the size of any additional benefits is statistically uncertain and it has not been granted a claim of superiority against aspirin (Patrono et al., 2004). However, the publication of the Clopidogrel in Unstable Angina to Prevent Recurrent Events (CURE) recently had led to FDA approval of a new indication for clopidogrel in patients with acute coronary syndromes without ST-segment elevation (Patrono et al., 2004).The CURE trial examined CV outcomes with clopidogrel plus aspirin versus aspirin alone in patients with acute ischemic heart disease (IHD) (CURE Steering Committee, 2001). These findings demonstrated that clopidogrel has beneficial effects in patients with acute coronary syndromes without ST-segment elevation thus can be generalized as the study sample size (n =12,562) was large and patients were recruited from 482 centers in 28 countries. This trial also showed that 3.7% of patients in this combination therapy group had major bleeding and it was significant more compared with those solely on aspirin but there was no increase in life-threatening bleeds (CURE Steering Committee, 2001). Hence, a loading dose of 300mg clopidogrel should be used in this setting followed by 75 mg daily (Patrono et al., 2004). Bhatt et al., (2002) concluded that clopidogrel is an effective drug for secondary prevention in diabetes. Therefore, previous studies clearly justified the use of dual anti platelet therapy with aspirin and clopidogrel for secondary prevention of CVD in diabetes patients. Its role in primary prevention of CVD in diabetes patients is vague since no study has directly measure the outcome for this purpose.

5.3 Ticlopidine
Ticlopidine also inhibit ADP-induced platelet aggregation with no direct effects on the metabolism of arachidonic acid (Patrono, 1998). It has slower antiplatelet effect compared with clopidogrel (Patrono et al., 2004). Ticlopidine in Microangiopathy of Diabetes (TIMAD) study was conducted by involving 435 patients with nonproliferative diabetes retinopathy to evaluate for its effects on macrovascular disease in diabetes patients. Patients were randomized to receive ticlopidine, 250 mg twice daily and were followed up to 3 years. Ticlopidine was found significantly reduced annual microaneurysm progression by 67% and overall progression of retinopathy was significantly less severe with ticlopidine (TIMAD Study Group, 1990). However, this study was not designed to evaluate effect of ticlopidine on cardiovascular events. There are limited studies done on effect of ticlopidine in prevention of CVD in diabetes. In contrast to clopidogrel, ticlopidine does not have an approved indication for patients with a recent myocardial infarction (Patrono et al., 2004). Even though ticlopidine has lower cost compared to clopidogrel, (Drug Formulary University Malaya Medical Centre, 2005; Patrono et al., 2004), its role in primary prevention of CVD in type 2 diabetes patients have not been established.

5.4 Dipyridamole
Dipyridamole inhibits platelet cyclic-3′,5′-adenosine monophosphate and cyclic-3′, 5′-guanosine monophosphate phosphodiesterase (Natarajan et al. 2008). Overview of 25 trials among approximately 10000 high risks of CVD patients with the use of dipyridamole and aspirin, it was found that the addition of dipyridamole to aspirin has not been shown clearly to produce additional reductions in serious vascular events (Patrono et al., 2004). However, one of 25 trials suggested that there may be a worthwhile further reduction in stroke (Patrono *et al.* 2004). Patrono et al., (2004) also suggested that the combination of low dose aspirin and extended release dipyridamole (200 mg twice daily) is considered an acceptable option for initial therapy of patients with non-cardioembolic cerebral ischemic events and not in patients with ischemic heart attack. The benefits of dipyridamole in patients with diabetes have not been reported (Natarajan et al., 2008). Specifically, there are limited studies or trials conducted to examine the role of dipyridamole for primary and secondary prevention of CVD amongst T2DM patients.

5.5 GP IIb/IIIa inhibitors

The platelet glycoprotein (GP) IIb/IIIa complex receptor antagonists block activity at the fibrinogen binding site on platelet (Colwell & Nesto, 2003). These agents are useful in type 2 diabetes patients with acute coronary syndrome and in those undergoing percutaneous coronary interventions (Colwell & Nesto, 2003). These agents are administered intravenously with a rapid onset of action and short half-life (Natarajan et al., 2008). Numerous studies have been performed comparing various GP IIb/IIIa inhibitors. Currently, three different GP IIb/IIIa inhibitors (abciximab, eptifibatide, and tirofiban) are approved for clinical use. This group of drugs was mainly study for secondary prevention of CVD in diabetes patients. Evidence from three trials revealed that among 1,262 diabetes patients, use of these agents was associated with reduction in mortality from 4.5% to 2.5% (p=0.031) (Bhatt et al., 2000). In another meta-analysis of six large trials, with 6,458 patients with diabetes and acute coronary syndromes, GP IIb/IIIa inhibitor therapy was associated with a significant mortality reduction at 30 days, from 6.2% to 4.6% CI(0.59-0.92, p=0.007) (Roffi et al., 2001). Nonetheless, the role of GP IIb/IIIa inhibitors in primary prevention of CVD in type 2 diabetes mellitus has not been justified; therefore it is not recommended for this purpose.

6. Appropriate selection of antiplatelet agents for primary prevention of CVD in type 2 diabetes patients

Among all choices, there are considerations to be taken into account before types of antiplatelet agents chosen. According to American Diabetes Association (2011), aspirin (75-162mg/day) should be considered for primary prevention of cardiovascular disease in type 2 diabetes patients for men (>50 years) and women (>60 years) with at least one additional major risk factor (family history of cardiovascular disease, hypertension, smoking, dyslipidemia or albuminuria). The other types of antiplatelet agents either alone or combination with aspirin therapy has no established role in primary prevention of cardiovascular disease in type 2 diabetes patients. In contrast, aspirin should not be recommended for CVD prevention for diabetes patients with low CVD risk (10-year CVD risk <5%, such as in men <50 and women <60 years of age with no additional CVD risk factors, since the potential adverse effects from bleeding likely outweigh the potential benefits (ADA, 2011). A same recommendation goes to type 2 diabetes patients with multiple other risk factors (e.g. 10-year risk 5-10%), in which clinical judgment is required (American Diabetes Association, 2011).

7. Monitoring of aspirin efficacy and adverse effects

Aspirin once daily (75-100 mg) is recommended in primary prevention of CVD in type 2 diabetes patients when antiplatelet prophylaxis has a favorable benefit/risk profile (Patrono et al., 2004). For effectiveness of primary prevention strategy, patients should be followed on a regular basis and examined for signs and symptoms of any cardiovascular diseases. In consideration of dose-dependent GI toxicity and its potential impact on compliance, physicians are encouraged to use the lowest dose of aspirin that was shown to be effective in each clinical setting (Patrono et al., 2001). Aspirin should not be given to patients with gastrointestinal ulcerations; best tolerated after food. In conclusion, bleeding and gastrointestinal complications are the most common adverse effects of aspirin. Thus, the patients on aspirin should be monitored for stomach pain, heartburn, nausea and bleeding tendency.

8. Conclusion

Dyslipidemia is one of the risk factors for acquiring cardiovascular disease in patients with type 2 diabetes. In absent for contraindication, type 2 diabetes patients with dyslipidemia are eligible for primary prevention of cardiovascular disease although the routine use has not been documented. Aspirin plays a key role in primary prevention strategy of cardiovascular disease in type 2 diabetes patients. With limited studies and evidence for other antiplatelet agents, their role in primary prevention has not been established.

9. Summary

Dyslipidemia is one of the major risk factors for macrovascular disease leading to CVD in type 2 diabetes.

In type 2 diabetes patients with dyslipidemia, alteration in lipid distribution and platelet abnormalities increased risk of acquiring CVD.

Patients with type 2 diabetes with one of the following; dyslipidemia, family history of coronary heart disease, hypertension, smoking and albuminuria are at increased risk of CVD, thus eligible for primary prevention strategy of CVD.

With limited evidence, proper justification and clinical judgments of benefit versus risk, aspirin plays a key role as antiplatelet agent in primary prevention of CVD in patients with type 2 diabetes with dyslipidemia.

Patients with type 2 diabetes and dyslipidemia receiving aspirin for primary prevention strategy should be monitored for effectiveness of treatment (sign and symptoms of CVD) and adverse effects (stomach pain, heartburn, nausea and bleeding tendency).

10. References

Adiels, M., Westerbacka, J., Soro-Paavonen, A., Häkkinen, A.M., Vehkavaara, S., Caslake, M.J., Packard, C., Olofsson, S.O., Yki-Järvinen, H., Taskinen, M.R. & Borén, J. (2007). Acute suppression of VLDL1 secretion rate by insulin is associated with hepatic fat content and insulin resistance. *Diabetologia* Vol.50, No.11, (November 2007), pp. 2356-2365, ISSN 1432-0428

American Diabetes Association (2006). Standards of Medical Care in diabetes. *Diabetes Care* Vol.29, No.1, (January 2006), pp. 4-42, ISSN 1935-5548

American Diabetes Association (2011). Standard of Medical Care in Diabetes 2011. *Diabetes Care* Vol.34, No.1, (January 2011), pp. S11-S61, ISSN 1935-5548

Angiolillo, D.J. (2009). Antiplatelet therapy in diabetes: efficacy and limitations of current treatment strategies and future directions. *Diabetes Care* Vol.32, No.4, (April 2009), pp. 531-540, ISSN 1935-5548

Antithrombotic Trialists' Collaboration (2002): Collaboration meta-analysis of randomized trials of antiplatelet therapy for prevention of death, myocardial infarction, and stroke in high risk patients. *BMJ Vol.*324, No.7329, (January 2002), pp. 71–86, ISSN 1468-5833

Beckman, J.A., Creager, M.A. & Libby, P. (2002). Diabetes and atherosclerosis: epidemiology, pathophysiology, and management. *JAMA* Vol.287, No.19, (May 2002), pp. 2570-81, ISSN 1538-3598

Belch, J., MacCuish, A., Campbell, I., et al. (2008). The prevention of progression of arterial disease and diabetes (POPADAD) trial: factorial randomised placebo controlled trial of aspirin and antioxidants in patients with diabetes and asymptomatic peripheral arterial disease. *BMJ Vol.337*, (October 2008), pp. a1840, ISSN 1468-5833

Bertrand, M.E., Rupprecht, H.J., Urban, P. et al. (2000). Double-blind study of the safety of clopidogrel with and without a loading dose in combination with aspirin compared with ticlopidine in combination with aspirin after coronary stenting. The clopidogrel aspirin stent international cooperative study (CLASSICS). *Circulation* Vol.102, No.6, (August 2000), pp. 624–629, ISSN 1524-4539

Bhatt, D.L., Marso, S.P., Lincoff, A.M., Wolski, K.E., Ellis, S.G. & Topol, E.J. (2000). Abciximab reduces mortality in diabetics following percutaneous coronary intervention. *J Am Coll Cardiol* Vol.35, No.4, (March 2000), pp. 922-928, ISSN 1558-3597

Bhatt, D.L., Marso, S.P., Hirsch, A.T., et al. (2002). Amplified benefit of clopidogrel versus aspirin in patients with diabetes mellitus. *Am J Cardiol Vol.90*, No.6, (September 2002), pp. 625– 628, ISSN 0735-1097

Brownlee, M., Cerami, A. & Vlassara, H. (1988). Advanced products of nonenzymatic glycosylation and the pathogenesis of diabetic vascular disease. *Diabetes Metab Rev* Vol.4, No.5, (August 1988), pp. 437-51, ISSN 1520- 7560

Byberg, L., Siegbahn, A., Berglund, L., Mc-Keigue, P., Reneland, R. & Lithell, H. (1998). Plasminogen activator inhibitor-1 activity is independently related to both insulin sensitivity and serum triglycerides in 70-year-old men. *Arterioscler Thromb Vasc Biol* Vol.18, No.2, (February 1998), pp. 258 –264, ISSN 1079-5642

Chahil, T.J. & Ginsberg, H.N. (2006). Diabetic dyslipidemia. *Endocrinol Metab Clin North Am* Vol.35, No.3, pp. 491–510, ISSN 1558-4410

Collaborative Group of the Primary Prevention Project (2001). Low-dose aspirin and vitamin E in people at cardiovascular risk: a randomized trial in general practice. *Lancet Vol.357*, No.9250, (January 2001), 89–95, ISSN 1474-4465

Colwell, J.A. (1997). Multifactorial aspects of the treatment of the type II diabetic patient. *Metabolism* Vol.46, No.12, (December 1997), pp.1–4, ISSN 1532-8600

Colwell, J.A. & Nesto, R.W. (2003). The platelet in diabetes: focus on prevention of ischemic events. *Diabetes Care,* Vol.26, No.7, pp. 2181–2188, ISSN 1935-5548

Colwell, J.A. (2004). Aspirin therapy in diabetes. *Diabetes Care* Vol.27, No.1, (January 2004), pp. S72-S73, ISSN 1935-5548

CURE Steering Committee (2001). Effects of clopidogrel in addition to aspirin in patients with acute coronary syndromes without ST-segment elevation. *N Engl J Med* Vol.345, No.7, (August 2001), pp. 494–502, ISSN 1533-4406

Drug Formulary University Malaya Medical Centre (2005). Senarai Ubat-Ubatan. Malaysia: University Malaya Medical Centre; 2005.

ETDRS Investigators (1992). Aspirin effects on mortality and morbidity in patients with diabetes mellitus. *JAMA* Vol.268, No.10, (September 1992), pp. 1292–1300, ISSN 1538-3598

Eibl, N., Krugluger, W., Streit, G., Schrattbauer, K., Hopmeier, P. & Schernthaner, G. (2004). Improved metabolic control decreases platelet activation markers in patients with type-2 diabetes. *Eur J Clin Invest* Vol.34, No.3, (March 2004), pp. 205-209, ISSN 1365-2362

Ferroni, P., Basili, S., Falco, A. & Davi, G. (2004). Platelet activation in type 2 diabetes mellitus. *J Thromb Haemost* Vol.2, No.8, (August 2004), pp. 1282-1291, ISSN 1538-7836

Frayn, K.N. (2001) Adipose tissue and the insulin resistance syndrome. *Proc Nutr Soc* Vol.60, No.3, (August 2001), pp. 375–380, ISSN 1475- 2719

Gawaz, M., Ott, I., Reininger, A.J. & Neumann, F.J. (1994). Effects of magnesium on platelet aggregation and adhesion. Magnesium modulates surface expression of glycoproteins on platelets in vitro and ex vivo. *Thromb Haemost* Vol.72, No.6, (December 1994), pp. 912-918, ISSN 0340-6245

Grundy, S.M. (1998). Hypertriglyceridemia, atherogenic dyslipidemia, and the metabolic syndrome. *Am J Cardiol* Vol.81, No. 4A, (February 1998), pp. 18B–25B, ISSN 0002-9149

Halushka, P.V., Rogers, R.C., Loadholt, C.B. & Colwell, J.A. (1981). Increased platelet thromboxane synthesis in diabetes mellitus. *J Lab Clin Med* Vol.97, No.1, (January 1981), pp. 87–96, ISSN 1532-6543

Hansson, L., Zanchetti, A., Carruthers, S.G., Dahlof, B., Elmfeldt, D., Julius, S., Menard, J., Rahn, K.H., Wedel, H., Westerling, S., for the HOT Study Group (1998). Effects of intensive blood-pressure lowering and low-dose aspirin in patients with hypertension: principal results of the Hypertension Optimal Treatment (HOT) randomised trial. *Lancet* Vol.351, No.9118, (June 1998), pp. 1755–1762, ISSN 1474-547X

Hayden, M., Pignone, M., Phillips, C. & Mulrow, C. (2002). Aspirin for the primary prevention of cardiovascular events: a summary of the evidence for the U.S. Preventive Services Task Force. *Ann Intern Med* Vol.136, No.2, (January 2002), pp. 161-172, ISSN 1539-3704

Huri, H.Z., Yi, L.Q., Pendek, R. & Sulaiman, C.Z. 2008. Use of antiplatelet agents for primary and secondary prevention of cardiovascular disease amongst type 2 diabetic patients. *Journal of Pharmacy Practice*, Vol.21, No.4, (August 2008), pp. 287-301, ISSN 1531-1937

Imperatore, G., Riccardi, G., Iovine, C., Rivellese, A.A. & Vaccaro, O. (1998). Plasma fibrinogen: a new factor of the metabolic syndrome: a population-based study. *Diabetes Care* Vol.21, No.4, (April 1998), pp. 649–654, ISSN 1935-5548

Koskinen, S.V., Reunanen, A.R., Martelin, T.P. & Valkonen, T. (1998). Mortality in a large population-based cohort of patients with drug-treated diabetes mellitus. *Am J Publ Health* Vol.88, No.5, (May 1998), pp. 765-770, ISSN 1541-0048

Krauss, R.M. & Siri, P.W. (2004). Dyslipidemia in type 2 diabetes. *Med Clin North Am* Vol.88, No.4, pp. 897–909, ISSN 1557-9859

Jokl, R. & Colwell, J.A. (1997). Arterial thrombosis and atherosclerosis in diabetes. *Diabetes Metab Rev Vol.5*, pp. 1–15, ISSN 1520- 7560

Leet, H., Paton, R.C., Passa, P. & Caen, J.P. (1981). Fibrinogen binding and ADP-induced aggregation in platelets from diabetic subjects. *Thromb Res* Vol.24, No.1-2, (October 1981), pp. 143–150, ISSN 0049-3848

Li, Y., Woo, V. & Bose, R. (2001). Platelet hyperactivity and abnormal Ca(2+) homeostasis in diabetes mellitus. *Am J Physiol Heart Circ Physiol* Vol.280, No.4, (April 2001), pp. H1480-H1489, ISSN 1522-1539

Mandal, S., Sarode, R., Dash, S. & Dash, R.J. (1993) Hyperaggregation of platelets detected by whole blood platelet aggregometry in newly diagnosed noninsulindependent diabetes mellitus. *American Journal of Clinical Pathology*, Vol.100, No.2, (August 1993), pp. 103-107, ISSN 0002-9173

Martina, V., Bruno, G.A., Trucco, F., Zumpano, E., Tagliabue, M. & Di Bisceglie, C. (1998). Platelet cNOS activity is reduced in patients with IDDM and NIDDM. *Thromb Haemost* Vol.79, No. 3, (March 1998), pp. 520–522, ISSN 0340-6245

Mayfield, R.K., Halushka, P.V., Wohltmann, H.J., Lopes-Virella, M. & Chambers, J.K. (1985). Platelet function during continuous insulin infusion treatment in insulin-dependent diabetic patients. *Diabetes* Vol.34, No.11, (November 1985), pp. 1127–1133, ISSN 1939-327X

Mooradian, A.D (2008). Dsylipidemia in type 2 diabetes mellitus. Nature Clinical Practice *Endocrinology & Metabolism*, Vol.5, No.3, (March 2009), pp. 150-159, ISSN 1759-5029

Natarajan, A., Zaman, A.G. & Marshall, S.M. (2008). Platelet hyperactivity in type 2 diabetes: role of antiplatelet agents. *Diab Vasc Dis Res* Vol.5, No.2, (June 2008), pp. 138-144, ISSN 1752-8984

Ogawa H, Nakayama M, Morimoto T, et al. (2008). Low-dose aspirin for primary prevention of atherosclerotic events in patients with type 2 diabetes: a randomized controlled trial. *JAMA* Vol. 300, No.18, (November 2008), pp. 2134-2141, ISSN 1538-3598

Patrono, C., Coller, B., Dalen, J.E., Fuster, V., Gent, M., Harker, L.A., Hirsh, J. & Roth, G. (1998). Platetet-active drugs: the relationship among dose, effectiveness and side-effects. *Chest* Vol.114, No.5, (November 1998), pp. 470s-488s, ISSN 1931- 3543

Patrono, C., Coller, B. & Dalen, J.E. et al. (2001). Platelet-Active Drugs: The relationships among dose, effectiveness, and side effects. *Chest* Vol.119, No.1, (January 2001), pp. 39S–63S, ISSN 1931- 3543

Patrono, C., Bachmann, F., Baigent, C., Bode, C., Caterina, R.D., Charbonnier, B., Fitzgerald, D., Hirsh, J., Husted, S., Kvasnicka, J., Montalescot, G., Garcia Rodriguez, L.A., Verhueght, F., Vermylen, J., Wallentin, L. et al. (2004). Expert Consensus Document on the Use of Antiplatelet Agents. *European Heart Journal* Vol.25, No.2, (January 2004), pp. 166-181, ISSN 1522-9645

Patrono, C., Garcia Rodriguez, L.A., Landolfi, R. & Baigent, C. (2005). Low-dose aspirin for the prevention of atherothrombosis. *N Engl J Med* Vol.353, No.22, (December 2005), 2373–2383, ISSN 1533-4406

Roffi, M., Chew, D.P., Mukherjee, D., Bhatt, D.L., White, J.A., Heeschen, C., Hamm, C.W.,
  Moliterno, D.J., Califf, R.M., White, H.D., Kleiman, N.S., Theroux, P. & Topol, E.J.
  (2001). Platelet glycoprotein IIb/IIIa inhibitors reduce mortality in diabetic patients
  with non-ST-segment-elevation acute coronary syndromes. *Circulation* Vol.104, No.
  23, (December 2001), pp. 2767–2771, ISSN 0009-7322

Sanmuganathan, P.S., Ghahramani, P., Jackson, P.R., Wallis, E.J. & Ramsay, L.E. (2001).
  Aspirin for primary prevention of coronary heart disease: safety and absolute
  benefit related to coronary risk derived from meta-analysis of randomised trials.
  Heart Vol.85, No.3, (March 2001), pp. 265-271, ISSN 1468-201X

Sarji, K.E., Kleinfelder, J., Brewington, P., Gonzalez, J., Hempling, H. & Colwell, J.A. (1979).
  Decreased platelet vitamin C in diabetes mellitus: possible role in
  hyperaggregation. *Thromb Res* Vol.15, No.5-6, pp. 639–650, ISSN 0049-3848

Savi, P. & Herbert, J.M. (2005). Clopidogrel and ticlopidine: P2Y12 adenosine diphosphate-
  receptor antagonists for the prevention of atherothrombosis. *Semin Thromb Hemost*
  Vol.31, No.2, (April 2005), pp. 174 –183, ISSN 0094-6176

Serrano Rios, M. (1998). Relationship between obesity and the increased risk of major
  complications in non-insulin-dependent diabetes mellitus. *Eur J Clin Invest* Vol.28,
  No.2, (September 1998), pp. 14–18, ISSN 1365-2362

Steering Committee of the Physicians' Health Study Research Group (1989). Final report on
  the aspirin component of the ongoing Physicians' Health Study. *N Engl J Med*
  Vol.321, No.3, (July 1989), pp. 129–135, ISSN 1533-4406

Taskinen, M.R. (2003) Diabetic dyslipidaemia: from basic research to clinical practice.
  Diabetologia Vol. 46, No.6, pp. 733–749, ISSN 1432-0428

Thompson, D.M. (1999). Cardiovascular disease and diabetes. *BC Endocrine Research
  Foundation Newsletter* 1: 3, ISSN 1755-3245

TIMAD Study Group (1990). Ticlopidine treatment reduces the progression of
  nonproliferative diabetic retinopathy. *Arch Ophthalmol* Vol.108, pp. 1577–1583, ISSN
  1538-3601

Trovati, M., Anfossi, G., Cavalot, F., Massucco, P., Mularoni, E. & Emanuelli, G. (1988).
  Insulin directly reduces platelet sensitivity to aggregating agents: studies in vitro
  and in vivo. *Diabetes* Vol.37, No.6, (June 1988), pp. 780–786, ISSN 1939-327X

Trovati, M., Anfossi, G., Massucco, P., Mattiello, L., Costamagna, C., Piretto, V., Mularoni,
  E., Cavalot, F., Bosia, A. & Ghigo, D. (1997). Insulin stimulates nitric oxide synthesis
  in human platelets and, through nitric oxide, increases platelet concentrations of
  both guanosine-3ˏ, 5ˏ-cyclic monophosphate and adenosine-3ˏ, 5ˏ-cyclic
  monophosphate. *Diabetes* Vol.46, No.5, (May 1997), pp. 742–749, ISSN 1939-327X

Tschoepe, D., Rauch, U. & Schwippert, B. (1997). Platelet-leukocyte-cross-talk in diabetes
  mellitus. *Horm Metab Res* Vol.29, No.12, (December 1997), pp. 631–635, ISSN 1439-
  4286

Vinik, A.I., Erbas, T., Park. T.S., Nolan, R. & Pittenger, G.L. (2001). Platelet dysfunction in
  type 2 diabetes. Diabetes Care Vol.24, No.8, (August 2001), pp. 1476-85, ISSN 1935-
  5548

Watala C, Boncer M, Golanski J, Koziolkiewcz W, Trojanowski Z, Walkowiak B: Platelet
      membrane lipid fluidity and intraplatelet calcium mobilization in type 2 diabetes.
      Eur J Haematol Vol.61, No.5, (November 1998), pp. 319–326, ISSN 1600-0609
Winocour, P.D., Watala, C. & Kinlough-Rathbone, R.L. (1992). Reduced membrane fluidity
      and increased glycation of membrane proteins of platelets from diabetic subjects
      are not associated with increased platelet adherence to glycated collagen. *J Lab Clin
      Med* Vol.120, No.6, (December 1992), pp. 921-928, ISSN 1532-6543

5

Dyslipidemia: Genetics and Role in the Metabolic Syndrome

Nora L. Nock and Aiswarya L.P. Chandran Pillai
Case Western Reserve University
USA

1. Introduction

Dyslipidemia is characterized by an aggregation of lipoprotein abnormalities including low high density lipoprotein cholesterol (HDL-C), high serum triglycerides (TG) and increased small low density lipoprotein cholesterol (LDL-C). Lipoproteins, which contain lipids and proteins (apolipoproteins, APO) are responsible, primarily, for transporting water insoluble lipids (cholesterol, TG) in plasma from the intestines and liver, where they are absorbed and synthesized, respectively, to peripheral tissues (muscle, adipose) for utilization, processing and/or storage (Kwan et al., 2007). There are several subtypes of lipoproteins with specific functions including, from smallest to largest: 1) chylomicrons, which transport dietary TG from the intestines to the peripheral tissue and liver; 2) very LDL (VLDL) particles, which transport TG from the liver to peripheral tissues; 3) intermediate density lipoproteins (IDL), which are produced from VLDL particle metabolism and may be taken up by the liver or further hydrolyzed to LDL; and, 4) HDL, which is key in 'reverse cholesterol transport' or shuttling cholesterol from peripheral cells to the liver (Kwan et al., 2007).

The Metabolic Syndrome (MetSyn) is a clustering of traits including dyslipidemia as well as hypertension (raised systolic and/or diastolic blood pressure), dysglycemia (high fasting glucose) and obesity (high body mass index (BMI) and/or waist circumference). Dyslipidemia is formally defined within the context of MetSyn. Various diagnostic definitions have been proposed for MetSyn by several organizations including the World Health Organization (WHO) (Alberti and Zimmet, 1998), European Group Insulin Resistance (EGIR) (Balkau and Charles, 1999), National Cholesterol Education Program Adult Treatment Panel III (NCEP ATP III, (2001), International Diabetes Federation (IDF, (Alberti et al., 2005), American Heart Association/National Heart, Lung, and Blood Institute (AHA/NHLBI) (Grundy et al., 2006) and, with the most recent joint interim statement proposed by the AHA/NHLBI, IDF and other organizations (Alberti et al., 2009). Although the recommendations differ widely on the obesity component, the dyslipidemia component has been fairly consistently defined as having TG ≥ 150 mg/l, HDL-C <40 mg/dL (1.03 mmol/l, in males) or <50 mg/dL (1.29 mmol/l in females) or drug treatment for elevated TG or low HDL-C (NCEP ATP III: (2001), IDF: (Alberti et al., 2005), Joint Statement: (Alberti et al., 2009)). However, the WHO (Alberti and Zimmet, 1998) proposed slightly lower limits for HDL-C (male: < 0.9 mmol/l (35 mg/dl); female: < 1.0 mmol/l (39 mg/dl)) and the EGIR (Balkau and Charles, 1999) recommended dyslipidemia be defined by HDL-C < 1.0 mmol/l (39 mg/dl) or TG > 2.0 mmol/l (177 mg/dl). There is currently no recommended value for

LDL-C levels in the context of MetSyn yet LDL-C remains the primary target of therapy for the management of high blood cholesterol per the most recent guidelines from the NCEP ATPIII, which recommended drug therapy for LDL-C values ranging from ≥100 mg/dl to ≥190 mg/dl depending on the presence/absence of other coronary heart disease (CHD) risk factors (Grundy et al., 2004). When LDL becomes lipid depleted, small dense LDL (sdLDL) particles are formed, which have a lower affinity for the LDL receptor (LDLR), more susceptibility to oxidation and a higher affinity for macrophages; and, thus, sdLDL particles contribute to the atherosclerotic process (Austin et al., 1990; Littlewood and Bennett, 2003) and likely MetSyn (Kruit et al., 2010).

Dyslipidemia and MetSyn are common in developed nations and the prevalence of both are rising worldwide, which may be attributed, in part, to the rising rates of overweight and obesity (Alberti et al., 2009; Halpern et al., 2010). According to the National Health and Nutrition Examination Survey (NHANES) III (1988-1994) in the United States (U.S.), which used the NCEP ATP III criteria, the age-adjusted prevalence of dyslipidemia defined by high TG or low HDL-C, was approximately 30.0% and 37.1%, respectively; and, the prevalence of MetSyn was approximately 23.7% (Ford et al., 2002). The prevalence of dyslipidemia and MetSyn generally increase with increasing age (Ford et al., 2002). However, in a more recent study that used the Health Survey for England (HSE) (2003-2006) survey data and NHANES (1999-2006) data with exclusion of persons over 80 years old, the prevalence of low HDL-C (defined in both males and females as <40 mg/dL) was 10.0% in England and 19.2% in the U.S. (Martinson et al., 2010). Thus, the prevalence can vary markedly depending on how these traits are defined (Cook et al., 2008). Interestingly, trends in the U.S. and England indicate during the past two decades an increase in the proportion of individuals diagnosed with high cholesterol (≥240 mg/dL) but who achieved therapeutic control (Roth et al., 2010). For example, in the U.S. in 2006, 54.0% of men (95% CI: 47.6–60.4) and 49.7% of women (95% CI: 44.3–55.0) with high total serum cholesterol were on cholesterol-lowering medication, as opposed to 10.8% of men (95% CI: 8.0–13.6) and 8.6% (95% CI: 6.7–10.6) of women in 1993 (Roth et al., 2010). In England, in 2006, 35.5% of men (95% CI: 32.8–38.3) and 25.7% of women (95% CI: 23.4–28.1) were on cholesterol-lowering medication as opposed to 0.6% of men (95% CI: 0.3–1.3) and 0.4% of women (95% CI: 0.1–0.7%) in 1993 (Roth et al., 2010). Thus, prevalence rates will also vary by whether or not relevant drug treatments have been considered and, perhaps, the list of relevant drugs should include cholesterol lowering therapies (e.g., statins) as well as other drugs (e.g., tamoxifen, glucocorticoids) known to alter TG and cholesterol levels (Garg and Simha, 2007).

Both dyslipidemia and MetSyn increase the risk of Type II diabetes mellitus (T2DM) (Adiels et al., 2006; Kruit et al., 2010) and cardiovascular disease (CVD) morbidity (Alberti et al., 2009; Linsel-Nitschke and Tall, 2005) and CVD mortality (Lewington et al., 2007). Patients with MetSyn have a five-fold increase in the risk of developing T2DM and are at twice the risk of developing CVD over the next 5 to 10 years compared to individuals without the syndrome (Alberti et al., 2009). In the presence of both MetSyn and T2DM, the prevalence of CVD is markedly increased with an odds ratio (OR) of 3.04 [95% confidence interval (CI) of OR: 1.98-4.11] in comparison to those with none of these conditions (Athyros et al., 2004). The importance of MetSyn is exemplified by its ICD-9 code (277.7), which was initially established as a diagnosis of "Dysmetabolic Syndrome X" (Einhorn et al., 2003; Kahn et al., 2005). In summary, both dyslipidemia and MetSyn are substantial public health problems, which require a better understanding of their respective etiologies to develop more effective lifestyle and therapeutic interventions.

Heritability estimates suggest there is a strong genetic component to dyslipidemia and MetSyn. Heritability estimates for dyslipidemia range from 0.20 to 0.60 (Edwards et al., 1997; Goode et al., 2007; Herbeth et al., 2010; Kronenberg et al., 2002; Wang and Paigen, 2005) and from 0.24 to 0.63 for MetSyn (Lin et al., 2005; Sung et al., 2009).

Multiple genetic variants in the form of single nucleotide polymorphisms (SNPs) (i.e., single DNA base changes) have been associated with manifestation of dyslipidemia and MetSyn. In this chapter, we review and summarize associations between common SNPs (i.e., those with a minor allele frequency (MAF) ≥0.05) in the most biologically plausible candidate genes and HDL-C, LDL-C and TG levels as well as MetSyn as a single, unifying trait. Previous estimates suggest all common variants together explain less than 10 percent of HDL-C levels in the general population (Kronenberg et al., 2002); however, more elegant statistical modeling methods that combine SNPs in a more biologically meaningful way may be needed to better understand the collective role of genetic variants in manifestation of dyslipidemia, MetSyn and other complex metabolic traits. As a result, at the end of this chapter, we review studies that have undertaken more complex modeling strategies to understand the aggregate effects of SNPs in manifestation of dyslipidemia and MetSyn and provide our insights for future directions in this field.

2. Genetic variants in lipid metabolism and HDL-C levels

As mentioned above, HDL-C is important for "reverse cholesterol transport" or the shuttling of cholesterol from peripheral cells to the liver. Many of the genetic variants associated with HDL-C levels have been summarized nicely in a recent comprehensive review by Boes et al. (Boes et al., 2009). In Table 1, we include common SNPs tabulated in Boes et al. (2009) review of large studies (ethnic group sample sizes ≥500) as well as common SNPs in large studies that have been identified since their review.

Gene	Polym.	rs Number	MAF	Ethn.	Sample Size	Results (Effect Size, p-value)	Reference
ABCA1	C (-297)T	rs2246298	0.25 (T)	A	1625 (GP)	p=0.0455	(Shioji et al. 2004b)
ABCA1	G (-273)C	rs1800976	0.40 (C)	A	1626 (GP) 735 (HBP)	+1.9/+2.7 mg/dl (1/2copies); p=0.03 +1.9 /+5.0 mg/dl (1/2 copies); p=0.03	(Shioji et al. 2004b)
ABCA1	G (-273)C	rs1800976	0.38 (T)	Tu	2332 (GP)	+0.7/+1.9 mg/dl (1/2 copies); p<0.02	(Hodoglugil et al. 2005)
ABCA1	G378C	rs1800978	0.13 (C)	W	5040 (GP)	-1.2/- 2.7 mg/dl (1/2 copies); p=0.03	(Porchay et al. 2006)
ABCA1		rs3890182	0.13 (A)	W	5287 (GP)	-1/-3 mg/dl (1/2 copies) ; p=0.003	(Kathiresan et al. 2008)
ABCA1		rs2275542		A	<1880 (GP)	p=0.006	(Shioji et al. 2004b)

ABCA1		rs2515602	0.27	B	1943 (P)	M; p=0.034; F; p<0.001	(Klos et al. 2006a)
ABCA1	G596A	rs2853578	0.28 (A)	W	2468 CVD 834 (Co)	0.2 / +2.8 mg/dl (1/2 copies); p=0.02	(Whiting et al. 2005)
ABCA1	2310G>A	rs2066718	0.03 (A)	W	9123 (P)	F: higher levels in carriers; p=0.02	(Frikke-Schmidt et al. 2004)
ABCA1	G2706A	rs2066718	0.05 (A)	Tu	2458 (GP)	M: +2.0 mg/dl for heterozygotes; p<0.01	(Hodoglugil et al. 2005)
ABCA1	2472G>A G2868A	rs2066718	0.06 (A)	Tu	2105 (GP)	F: +3.1 mg/dl for carriers; p=0.0005	(Hodoglugil et al. 2005)
ABCA1	1883M	rs4149313	0.12 (G)	W	9123 (P)	F: + heterozygotes; p=0.05	(Frikke-Schmidt et al. 2004)
ABCA1	32b.+30, ABC32			W	1543 (P)	-2.2 mg/dl for carriers ; p=0.0040	(Costanza et al. 2005)
ABCA1	R1587K	rs2230808	0.24 (A)	W	9123 (P)	M: - 1.5 mg/dl for heterozygotes; p=0.008	(Frikke-Schmidt et al. 2004)
ABCA1	4759G > A	rs2230808	0.26 (K)	W	779 (CVD)	-1.5 mg/dl for carriers; p=0.03	(Clee et al. 2001)
ABCA1	50b.3038, ABC50	rs41474449	.	W	1543 (P)	+1.6 mg/dl for carriers; p=0.043	(Costanza et al. 2005)
ABCA1		rs3890182	0.12 (A)	EA	25,167	p= 4.53E-07	(Dumitrescu et al. 2011)
APOA1	T84C (HaeIII)	rs5070	0.23 (C)	A	1637 (GP)	+1.9 / +5.4 mg/dl (1/2copies); p=0.0005	(Shioji et al. 2004a)
APOA1	MspI RFLP	rs5069	0.31 (C)	B	3831 (P)	M/F; p=n.s/0.022	(Brown et al. 2006)
APOA1		rs28927680	0.93 (G)	EA	25,167	p= 8.61E-09	(Dumitrescu et al. 2011)
APOA1		rs964184	0.86 (C)	EA	25,167	p= 6.08E-10	(Dumitrescu et al. 2011)
APOA5	- 1131T > C	rs662799	0.06 (C)	UK	1696 (P)	-1.5 mg/dl /-5.4 mg/dl (1/2 copies) ; p=0.04	(Talmud et al. 2002a)
APOA5	- 1131T > C	rs662799	0.07 (C)	W	1596(SA PHIR)	-3.5 mg/dl per copy; p=0.00038	(Grallert et al. 2007)
APOA5	- 1131T > C	rs662799	0.23– 0.30 (C)	C, Ma	2711 (C) 707 (M)	-2.3/- 5.4 mg/dl 1/2 copies; p<0.0001 - 1.2 /- 8.1 mg/dl 1/2 copies; p<0.0001	(Lai et al. 2003)

APOA5	- 1131T > C	rs662799	0.34 (C)	A	521 HoCo	-3.3 mg/dl per copy; p<0.001	(Yamada et al. 2007)
APOA5	-3A > G	rs651821	0.07	W	2056 (P)	M; p=0.30; F; p=0.26	(Klos et al. 2006a)
APOA5	-3A > G	rs651821	0.18 (G)	C	2711 (GP)	-2.3/-5.8 mg/dl 1/2 copies ; p<0.0001	(Lai et al. 2003)
APOA5	-3A > G	rs651821	0.34 (C)	A	5207 (Ho Co, P)	-2.7 mg/dl per copy; p<0.001	(Yamada et al. 2007)
APOA5	-3A > G	rs651821	0.36 (G)	A	2417 (Ho Co)	-3.9 /- 7.0 mg/dl 1/2 copies ; p<0.001	(Yamada et al. 2008)
APOA5	S19W	rs3135506	0.06 (W)	UK	1660 (P)	-1.9 /+1.2 mg/dl (1/2 copies); p=0.02	(Talmud et al. 2002a)
APOA5	56C>G	rs3135506	0.06 (G)	W	2347 (P)	-2.0 mg/dl for carriers; p=0.008	(Lai et al. 2004)
APOA5		rs2072560	0.16 (A)	C	2711 (GP)	-1.9 /-3.9 mg/dl (1/2 copies) ; p=0.003	(Lai et al. 2003)
APOA5	IVS3+476 G>A	rs2072560		Ma	707 (P)	-0.4 /9.3 mg/dl (1/2 copies) ; p=0.004	(Qi et al. 2007)
APOA5	V153M	rs3135507		W	2557	F:- 3.5 mg/dl for carriers; p<0.01	(Hubacek 2005)
APOA5	+553	rs2075291	0.07 (T)	A	5206 HoCo	-4.6 mg/dl per copy; p<0.001	(Yamada et al. 2007)
APOA5	Gly185Cys	rs2075291	0.08 (T)	A	2417 HoCo	-5.0 /-11.2 mg/dl (1/2 copies); p<0.001	(Yamada et al. 2008)
APOA5	1259T>C	rs2266788	0.18 (C)	C	2711 (GP)	-2.3 /-3.1 mg/dl 1/2 copies; p<0.0001	(Lai et al. 2003)
APOB		rs11902417	0.78 (G)	E	17723	p= 3.7×10^{-7}	(Waterworth et al. 2010)
APOC3	C455T	rs2854116	0.41 (C)	In	1308 (P)	-3.1/-5.4 mg/dl (1/2 copies) ; p<0.05	(Lahiry et al. 2007)
APOC3	PvuII	rs618354	0.49	A	F:291 (GP)	F: +0.1/-4.2 mg/dl 1/2 copies;p=0.029	(Kamboh et al. 1999)
APOC3	Sst1 RFLP	rs5128	0.09 (S2)	W	M:1219 (P)	M: -1.8 mg/dl for carriers; p=0.04.	(Russo et al. 2001)
APOC3	3'-utr/Sac I	rs5128	0.09 (+)	Hu	713 (P)	-5.0 mg/dl for heteroz.; p=0.0014	(Hegele et al. 1995)

APOC3	3238C > G	rs5128	0.07 (S2)	W	906 (GP)	+1.9 mg/dl for carriers; p=0.079	(Corella et al. 2002)
APOE	Cys112Arg	rs429358	0.16 (A)	N	3575	p=0.001	(Povel et al. 2011)
CETP	G2708A	rs12149545	0.30 (A)	W	2683 GP 556 Cvd	+1.9 mg/dl per copy; p<0.001	(McCaskie et al. 2007)
CETP	G2708A	rs12149545	0.31 (A)	W	709 (CVD)	+1.5 /+3.5 mg/dl (1/2 copies) ;p=0.0016	(Klerkx et al. 2003)
CETP		rs3764261	0.14 (T)	C	4192	+0.07 mg/dl; p=4.3x10⁻¹⁴	(Liu et al. 2011)
CETP	G971A	rs4783961	0.49 (A)	W	709 (CVD)	+1.2/+1.9 mg/dl (1/2 copies) ; p=0.09	(Klerkx et al. 2003)
CETP	C629A	rs1800775	0.48 (A)	W	7083 (P)	+2.7 /+5.4 mg/dl (1/2 copies); p<0.001	(Borggreve et al. 2005a)
CETP	C629A	rs1800775	0.51 (A)	W	847 M, 873 F (P)	+4.2 mg/dl for homoz.; p<0.002	(Bernstein et al. 2003)
CETP	C629A	rs1800775	0.49 (A)	W	5287 (GP)	+3 /+5 mg/dl (1/2 copies) ; p= 2x10-29	(Kathiresan et al. 2008)
CETP	C629A	rs1800775	0.42 A	A	4050 (GP)	+2.2/+3.4 mg/dl 1/2 copies; p=3.28x10-9	(Tai et al. 2003b)
CETP	C629A	rs1800775	0.48 (A)	W	2683 GP 556 Cvd	+2.7 mg/dl per copy; p<0.001	(McCaskie et al. 2007)
CETP	C629A	rs1800775	0.40 (A)	W	1214 (CVD) 574 (Co)	CVD: +2.0/3.5mg/dl (1/2 copies) ; p=0.02 Co: +3.3/6.1 mg/dl (1/2 copies) ; p=0.05	(Blankenberg et al. 2004)
CETP	C629A	rs1800775	0.44 (A)	W	709 (CVD)	+0.8/3.9 mg/dl (1/2 copies) ; p<0.0001	(Klerkx et al. 2003)
CETP	C629A	rs1800775	0.50 (A)	W	309 (MI) 757 (Co)	+1.9/6.1 mg/dl (1/2 copies) ; p<0.0001	(Eiriksdottir et al. 2001)
CETP	C629A	rs1800775	0.48 (A)	W	498 (cvd) 1107(Co)	+2.9/4.4 mg/dl (1/2 copies) ; p<0.001	(Freeman et al. 2003)
CETP	Taq1B	rs708272	0.40 (B2)		13,677 (Meta)	+1.2 /+3.8 mg/dl 1/2 copies; p<0.0001	(Boekholdt et al. 2005)

CETP	Taq1B	rs708272			>10,000 (Meta)	+4.6 mg/dl for homoz.; p<0.00001	(Boekholdt & Thompson 2003)
CETP	Taq1B	rs708272	0.42 (B2)	W	7083 (P)	+2.7/5.0 mg/dl (1/2 copies) ; p<0.001	(Borggreve et al. 2005b)
CETP	Taq1B	rs708272	0.44 (B2)	W	2916 (P)	+2.5/4.7 mg/dl (1/2 copies) ; p<0.001	(Ordovas et al. 2000)
CETP	Taq1B	rs708272	0.43 0.26 (A)	W B	2056 1943 (P)	p<0.01; p<0.02	(Klos et al. 2006b)
CETP	Taq1B	rs708272	0.44 0.27 (A)	W B	8764 (P)	+2.3/5.8 mg/dl (1/2 copies) ; p<0.001 +3.8/9.8 mg/dl (1/2 copies) ; p<0.001	(Nettleton et al. 2007)
CETP	Taq1B	rs708272	0.41 (A)	W	1503 (P)	+2 /+5 mg/dl (1/2 copies) ; p<0.001	(Sandhofer et al. 2008)
CETP	Taq1B	rs708272	0.33 (A)	A	4207 (GP)	+2.5/4.4 mg/dl (1/2 copies ; p=1.25x10-10	(Tai et al. 2003b)
CETP	Taq1B	rs708272	0.40 (A)	A	1729 (GP)	M: +1.2/3.5 mg/dl (1/2 copies); p=0.096 F: +1.9/6.2 mg/dl (1/2 copies); p<0.001	(Tsujita et al. 2007)
CETP	Taq1B	rs708272	0.42 (A)	W	2683 GP 556 CVd	+2.7 mg/dl per copy; p<0.001	(McCaskie et al. 2007)
CETP	Taq1B	rs708272	0.42 (A)	W	2392 cvd 827 Co	+1.7/3.6 mg/dl (1/2 copies) ; p<0.001	(Whiting et al. 2005)
CETP	Taq1B	rs708272	0.40 (A)	W	1464 CVD	+2.1/3.0 mg/dl (1/2 copies) ; p=0.003	(Carlquist & Anderson 2007)
CETP	Taq1B	rs708272	0.41 (A)	W	1200 CV 571 (Co)	+2.6 /+4.3 mg/dl (1/2 copies) ; p<0.02	(Blankenberg et al. 2004)
CETP	Taq1B	rs708272	0.44 (A)	W	499 CVD 1105 Co	+2.1/3.6 mg/dl (1/2 copies) ; p<0.001	(Freeman et al. 2003)
CETP	+784CCC	rs34145065	0.39 (A)	W	709 (CVD)	+1.2/3.5 mg/dl (1/2 copies) ; p=0.0009	(Klerkx et al. 2003)

CETP	A373P	rs5880	0.05 (A)	W	8467 P 1636 CV	5.4 mg/dl for heteroz.; p<0.0001	(Agerholm-Larsen et al. 2000)
CETP	Ile405Val	rs5882			>10,000 (Meta)	+1.9 mg/dl for homoz. ; p<0.00001	(Boekholdt & Thompson 2003)
CETP	A + 16G/Ex.14	rs61212082	0.32 (A)	W	6421 (P)	M: +1.5/2.3 mg/dl (1/2 copies); p=0.002 F: +0.0/+2.3 mg/dl (1/2 copies); p=0.007	(Isaacs et al. 2007)
CETP		rs61212082	0.30 (A)	W	1208 (CVD) 572 (Co)	+1.4 /+3.1 mg/dl (1/2 copies) ; p=0.08 +0.3 /+8.4 mg/dl (1/2 copies); p=0.003	(Blankenberg et al. 2004)
CETP		rs61212082	0.30 (A)	W	498 (CVD) 1108 (Co)	+1.2 /+3.5 mg/dl (1/2 copies); p<0.05 +1.5 /+1.5 mg/dl (1/2 copies); p<0.05	(Freeman et al. 2003)
CETP	D442G	rs2303790b	0.03 (A)	A	3469 (He Ex)	+4.9 mg/dl for heteroz.; p<0.001	(Zhong et al. 1996)
CETP	R451Q	rs1800777	0.04 (A)	W	8467 (P) 1636 (CVD)	5.4 mg/dl for heterozygotes ; p<0.001	(Agerholm-Larsen et al. 2000)
CETP	G + 82A/Ex15	rs1800777	0.03 (A)	W	1071 CV 532 Co	3.6 /5.2 mg/dl for heteroz.; p=0.06/0.07	(Blankenberg et al. 2004)
CETP		rs12596776	0.90 (C)	EA	25,167	p=1.18E-05	(Dumitrescu et al. 2011)
CETP		rs9989419	0.39 (A)	EA	25,167	p=1.71E-53	(Dumitrescu et al. 2011)
LCAT	Gly230Arg			W	156 low 160 high	Variant sig. only in low HDL group	(Miettinen et al. 1998)
LCAT	608C/T	rs5922	.	A	203 (CVD)	Increase in HDL; p=0.015	(Zhang et al. 2003)
LCAT		rs5922		A	150 Str 122 Co	Lower HDL-C in heteroz.; p<0.05	(Zhu et al. 2006)
LCAT	P143L +511C>T			A	190 CVD 209 (Co)	Association with low HDLC; p<0.01	(Zhang et al. 2004)
LCAT		rs2292318	0.12 (A)	W	1442 CVD,Co	Increases HDLC; p=2 x 10 -5	(Pare et al. 2007)

LDLR	Exon 2	rs2228671		W	1543 (P)	+3.8 mg/dl for carriers; p=0.0056	(Costanza et al. 2005)
LDLR	1866C > T Asn591Asn	rs688 = rs57911429	0.12 (T)	A	2417 (Ho Co)	+1.5 /+8.5 mg/dl (1/2 copies) ; p=0.0155	(Yamada et al. 2008)
LDLR	Exon 12/HincII	rs688 = rs57911429	0.39 (+)	Hu	713 (P)	2.3 / 4.3 mg/dl (1/2 copies) ; p=0.047	(Hegele et al. 1995)
LDLR	2052T >C	rs5925 = rs57369606	0.17 (C)	A	2417 HoCo	+1.2/+5.4 (1/2 copies) ; p=0.043	(Yamada et al. 2008)
LIPC	T-710C	rs1077834	0.22 (C)	W	9121 (P)	+3–4% per copy; p<0.001	(Andersen et al. 2003)
LIPC	C-514Ta	rs1800588	0.25 (T)	Va	>24,000 (Meta)	+1.5 /+3.5 mg/dl (1/2 copies); p<0.001	(Isaacs et al. 2004)
LIPC	Pos.-480T	rs1800588	0.21 (T) 0.53 (T)	W B	8897 (P) 2909 (P)	W: +2.2/+3.8 mg/dl (1/2 copies); p<0.001 B: +1.6/+4.0 mg/dl (1/2 copies); p<0.001	(Nettleton et al. 2007)
LIPC		rs1800588	0.21 (T)	W	6239 (P)	+1.3/+4.3 mg/dl (1/2 copies); p<0.001	(Isaacs et al. 2007)
LIPC		rs1800588	0.38 (T)	A	2170 (P)	+2.3 /+2.7 mg/dl (1/2 copies); p=0.001	(Tai et al. 2003a)
LIPC		rs1800588	0.21 (T)	W	5287 (GP)	+1 /+4 mg/dl (1/2 copies) ; p=4x 10 -10	(Kathiresan et al. 2008)
LIPC		rs1800588	0.25 (T)	W	2773 (GP)	+1.5 mg/dl per copy; p=0.04	(Talmud et al. 2002b)
LIPC		rs1800588	0.24 (T)	W	3319 CV 1385 Co	+1.0 /+3.8 mg/dl (1/2 copies); p=0.001	(Whiting et al. 2005)
LIPC		rs1800588	0.51 (T)	A	5207 Ho Co	+2.5 mg/dl per copy; p<0.001	(Yamada et al. 2007)
LIPC		rs1800588	0.21 (T)	W	6412 (CVD)	+2.0–2.5 mg/dl per copy; p<0.001	(McCaskie et al. 2006)
LIPC	G -250A	rs2070895	0.22 (A)	W	9121 (P)	+3–4% per copy; p<0.001	(Andersen et al. 2003)
LIPC		rs2070895		W	1543 (P)	+1.5 mg/dl for carriers; p=0.020	(Costanza et al. 2005)
LIPC		rs2070895	0.32 (A)	W	514 (P)	M; p=0.001	(de Andrade et al. 2004)

Gene	Variant	rs number	MAF	Pop	N	Effect	Reference
LIPC		rs2070895	0.23 (A)	W	5585 (P)	+3.9/3.9 mg/dl (1/2 copies); p=8x10-10	(Grarup et al. 2008)
LIPC		rs2070895	0.51 (A)	A	5213 HoCo	+2.7 mg/dl per copy; p<0.001	(Yamada et al. 2007)
LIPC		rs2070895	0.39 (A)	A	716 HeEx	+2.1 mg/dl for carriers; p=0.026	(Ko et al. 2004)
LIPC		rs12594375	0.37 (A)	A	2970 (GP)	p=0.00003	(Iijima et al. 2008)
LIPC		rs8023503	0.38 (T)	A	2970 (GP)	p=0.0001	(Iijima et al. 2008)
LIPC	+1075C	rs3829462	0.05 (C)	A	823	+8.0 mg/dl for heterozygotes; p<0.05	(Fang & Liu 2002)
LIPC		rs4775041	0.29C	EA	25,167	p=1.03E-16	(Dumitrescu et al. 2011)
LIPC		rs261332	0.20 (A)	EA	25,167	p=1.99E-13	(Dumitrescu et al. 2011)
LPC		rs261334	0.20 (T)	E	17723	p= 4.9×10^{-22}	(Waterworth et al. 2010)
LIPG	-384A > C	rs3813082	0.12 (C)	A	541 (Co)	+1.3/+10.2 mg/dl (1/2 copies) ; p=0.021	(Hutter et al. 2006)
LIPG		rs3813082	0.12 (C)	A	340 (Kids)	+0.7/+9.8 (1/2 copies) ; p=0.0086	(Yamakawa-Kobayashi et al. 2003)
LIPG	584 C/T T111l	rs2000813	0.32 (I)	W	495 (GP)	M: 1.2 /+2.7 mg/dl (1/2 copies) ; p=0.82 F: 0.4 /+1.9 mg/dl (1/2 copies) ; p=0.09	(Paradis et al. 2003)
LIPG		rs2000813	0.24 (T)	A	541 (Co)	+0.5/+6.1 mg/dl (1/2 copies) ; p=0.048	(Hutter et al. 2006)
LIPG		rs2000813	0.30 (T)	A	265 CVD 265 Co	+3.7 for carries; p=<0.02	(Tang et al. 2008)
LIPG		rs2000813	0.29 (T)	W 90%	372 (CVD)	+1.6 /+6.0 mg/dl (1/2 copies) ; p=0.035	(Ma et al. 2003)
LIPG	C+42T/ln 5	rs2276269	0.44 (T)	W	594 (HDL)	Decreases HDLC; p=0.007	(Mank-Seymour et al. 2004)

LIPG	T+2864C/In8	rs6507931	0.42 (C)	W	594 (HDL)	Decreases HDLC; p=0.004	(Mank-Seymour et al. 2004)
LIPG	2237G > A	rs3744841	0.36 (A)	A	340 (Kids)	4.0 mg/dl /-4.3 mg/dl (1/2 copies) ; p=0.011	(Yamakawa-Kobayashi et al. 2003)
LPL	D9N; Asp9Asn	rs1801177		–	5067 (Meta)	-3.1 mg/dl for heteroz.; p=0.002	(Wittrup et al. 1999)
LPL	Gly188Glu			–	10,434 (Meta)	- 9.7 mg/dl for heteroz.; p<0.001	(Wittrup et al. 1999)
LPL	N291S	rs268		–	14,912 (Meta)	-4.6 mg/dl for heteroz.; p<0.001	(Wittrup et al. 1999)
LPL	HindIll; Int8	rs320	0.30 (H)	W	520 (P)	+5.5 mg/dl in H – H- vs. H+H+; p=0.025	(Senti et al. 2001)
LPL	HindIll; Int8	rs320	0.26 (H1)	W	1361 (P)	M: +3.5 mg/dl for heteroz. ; p=0.0018 F : +4.2 mg/dl for heteroz. ; p=0.0212	(Holmer et al. 2000)
LPL	HindIll; Int8	rs320	0.32 (H)	W	906 (GP)	+1.9 mg/dl; p=0.003	(Corella et al. 2002)
LPL	HindIll; Int8	rs320		A	550 (NGT) 465 (DM)	NGT: +3.0 mg/dl for carriers; p<0.05 DM: +1.0 mg/dl for carriers; p<0.05	(Radha et al. 2006)
LPL	HindIll; Int8	rs320	0.27-0.31	NHW, H	615(W); 579(H)	p=0.005	(Ahn et al. 1993)
LPL		rs326	0.44	B	1943 (P)	M; p=0.013; F; p=0.004	(Klos et al. 2006a)
LPL	S447X Ser447Ter	rs328			4388 (Meta)	+1.5 mg/dl for heteroz.; p<0.001	(Wittrup et al. 1999)
LPL	S447X Ser447Ter	rs328	0.10 (G)	W	8968 (P)	+2.8 /+4.0 mg/dl (1/2 copies); p<0.001	(Nettleton et al. 2007)
LPL	S447X Ser447Ter	rs328	0.07 (G)	B	2677 (P)	+3.1 /+12.6 mg/dl (1/2 copies); p<0.001	
LPL	S447X	rs328	0.11 (X)	A	4058 (P)	+3.1 mg/dl; p<0.001	(Lee et al. 2004)
LPL		rs328		W	1543 (P)	+2.7 mg/dl; p=0.0017	(Costanza et al. 2005)
LPL		rs328			25,167	P=5.6E-22	(Dumitrescu et al. 2011)
LPL		rs328	0.09 (G)	W	5287 (GP)	+3 /+5 mg/dl (1/2 copies); p=3 x 10-12	(Kathiresan et al. 2008)

LPL		rs325	0.89 (T)	E	17723	p= 7.8×10-25	(Waterworth et al. 2010)
MLXIPL		rs17145738	0.12 (T)	EA	25,167	p=1.64E-05	(Dumitrescu et al. 2011)
PON1	Q192R	rs662 = rs60480675	0.30 (G)	W	1232 (P)	W: +0.1 /+2.3 mg/dl (1/2 copies) ; p=0.041	(Srinivasan et al. 2004)
PON1	Gln192Arg	rs662 = rs60480675	0.67	B	554	-5.4 /- 6.7 mg/dl (1/2 copies) ; p=0.008	"
PON1		rs662 = rs60480675	0.29 (R)	Hu	738 (P)	-3.1 mg/dl /- 3.1 mg/dl (1/2 copies) ; p=0.001	(Hegele et al. 1995)
PON1		rs662 = rs60480675	0.36 (R)	W-Bra	261 CVD, Co	M: +1.5 /+2.7 mg/dl (1/2 copies) ; p=0.035	(Rios et al. 2007)
PON1	C -107T	rs705379	0.48 (C)	W	710 (CVD)	-3.1/- 2.3 mg/dl (1/2 copies) ; p=0.006	(Blatter Garin et al. 2006)
PON1	Leu55M	rs85456	0.20 (T)	MA	741	p=0.02	(Chang et al. 2010)
SCARB 1	Exon 8 C>T	rs5888	0.44 (T)	W	865 (P)	+1.9/2.7 mg/dl 1/2 copies;p=0.006	(Morabia et al. 2004)
SCARB 1	C1050T	rs5888	0.49 (T)	W	546 (CVD)	+2.3 /+1.9 mg/dl (1/2 copies); p=0.03	(Boekholdt et al. 2006)

Table 1. Genetic Polymorphisms Associated With HDL-C. MAF=Minor Allele Frequency; Ethn.: A=Asians; AA=African Americans; Am=Amish; A-I=Asian Indian; B=Blacks; C=Chinese; CH=Caribbean Hispanics; In=Inuit; Ma= Malays; N=Netherlands; NHW=Non-Hispanic Whites; H=Hispanics; Hu=Hutteries; Tu=Turks; UK=United Kingdom; W-Bra=Caucasian Brazilians; W= Whites; Va=Various; Non-DM C0=Non diabetic control subjects; MI=Myocardial infarction; NGT=Normal glucose tolerance; DM= Diabetes mellitus; Ho Sta= Hospital staff; HBP= Hypertensive patients; He Ex=Health examination; Cor Ang=coronary angiography; hyperCH=hypercholesterolemia patients; CVD= Cardiovascular Disease; Co=Controls; Ho Co=Hospital based controls; GP=General Population; Meta= Meta Analysis; P=Population based; M= Males; F= females; + =increase; - = decrease; n.s.=not significant; see text for full gene names. Adapted from Boes et al. (2009) with permission from Elsevier.

2.1 Genetic variation in enzymes involved in lipid metabolism and HDL-C levels

Perhaps, the most notable gene in the HDL-C synthesis and metabolism pathways, whose variants have been consistently associated with HDL-C, is the cholesterol ester transfer protein (CETP), which is a key plasma protein that mediates the transfer of esterfied cholesterol from HDL to APOB containing particles in exchange for TG. Although complete loss of CETP function is rare and can yield HDL-C levels up to five times higher than normal (Klos and Kullo, 2007), three common polymorphisms (Table 1: TaqIB (rs708272); -

629C>A (rs1800775); Ile405Val (rs5882)) can all modestly inhibit CETP activity and have been consistently associated with higher HDL-C levels (Bernstein et al., 2003; Blankenberg et al., 2004; Boekholdt et al., 2005; Boekholdt and Thompson, 2003; Borggreve et al., 2005; Eiriksdottir et al., 2001; Freeman et al., 2003; Kathiresan et al., 2008a; Klerkx et al., 2003; Tai et al., 2003b; Thompson et al., 2008). The CETP gene is located on chromosome 16 (16q21).

Lipoprotein lipase (LPL) is an enzyme involved in lipolysis of TG-containing lipoproteins such as VLDL and chlyomicrons (Miller and Zhan, 2004), which generate free fatty acids (FFA) that can be taken up by the liver, muscle and adipose tissues (Kwan et al., 2007). Thus, LPL affects LDL levels directly (see Section 3.2) may only affect HDL-C levels indirectly (Lewis and Rader, 2005). The human LPL gene is located on chromosome 8 (8p22). Several LPL SNPs have been associated with HDL-C (Table 1) (Ahn et al., 1993; Corella et al., 2002; Holmer et al., 2000; Klos and Kullo, 2007; Klos et al., 2006; Komurcu-Bayrak et al., 2007; Lee et al., 2004; Nettleton et al., 2007; Senti et al., 2001; Wittrup et al., 1999); however, many of them are in strong linkage disequilibrium with each other (e.g., rs320, rs326, rs13702, rs10105606) (Boes et al., 2009; Heid et al., 2008).

Hepatic lipase (HL; LIPC) is a glycoprotein that is synthesized by liver cells (hepatocytes) and catalyzes the hydrolysis of TG and phospholipids (Miller et al., 2003). For example, after hydrolysis of TG by LPL, VLDL particles are reduced to IDL particles and can be further hydrolyzed by HL/LIPC to LDL or taken up by the liver (Kwan et al., 2007). The human HL/LIPC gene is located on chromosome 15 (15q21). Several HL/LIPC SNPs have been associated with HDL-C levels (Table 1) (Andersen et al., 2003; Costanza et al., 2005; de Andrade et al., 2004; Fang and Liu, 2002; Grarup et al., 2008; Iijima et al., 2008; Isaacs et al., 2007; Kathiresan et al., 2008b; Ko et al., 2004; McCaskie et al., 2006; Nettleton et al., 2007; Tai et al., 2003a; Talmud et al., 2002b; Whiting et al., 2005; Yamada et al., 2007). However, the most consistent associations have been observed for rs1800588 and rs2070895 and, several SNPs in the promoter region are in strong LD (Boes et al., 2009).

Endothelial lipase (EL; LIPG) is an enzyme expressed in endothelial cells that, in the presence of HL/LIPC, metabolizes larger (HDL$_3$) to smaller (HDL$_2$) HDL-C particles and increases the catabolism of APOA-I (see Section 2.3) (Jaye and Krawiec, 2004). EL/LIPG plays a role in the dyslipidemia component and, possibly, the yet to be established, proinflammatrory component of MetSyn (Lamarche and Paradis, 2007) (see Section 5.0). The human EL/LIPG gene is located on chromosome 18 (18q21.1). Several polymorphisms in EL/LPIG have been associated with HDL-C levels (Table 1) (Hutter et al., 2006; Ma et al., 2003; Mank-Seymour et al., 2004; Paradis et al., 2003; Tang et al., 2008; Yamakawa-Kobayashi et al., 2003). However, most of these SNPs have not been as well studied as those in CETP, LPL and EL; and, only the nonsynonymous SNP, rs2000813, has been consistently associated with HDL-C levels in African-American populations (Hutter et al., 2006; Tang et al., 2008; Yamakawa-Kobayashi et al., 2003).

In the presence of cofactor, APOA-I (see Section 2.3), lecithin-cholesteryl acyltransferase (LCAT), catalyzes the esterification of free cholesterol and, can metabolize larger HDL-C particles to smaller HDL-C particles (Klos and Kullo, 2007; Miller and Zhan, 2004). The human LCAT is located on chromosome 16 (16q22.1). Although mutations leading to complete loss of LCAT and marked (5-10%) reduction in HDL-C levels are rare and can cause cornea opacifications (fish eye disease) and renal disease (Garg and Simha, 2007), several common polymorphisms in LCAT have been associated, albeit inconsistently, with much more modest changes in HDL-C levels (Table 1) (Boekholdt et al., 2006; Miettinen et al., 1998; Pare et al., 2007; Zhang et al., 2004; Zhu et al., 2006).

Parroxanonase 1 (PON1), inhibits the oxidation of LDL (Mackness et al., 1991) and, therefore, may only indirectly affect antioxidant properties of HDL-C. The human PON1 gene is located on chromosome 7 (7q21.3). Several SNPs in PON1 have been associated with HDL-C levels, most notably, two nonsynonymous SNPs, rs662 and rs3202100, which are in strong LD, but results are inconsistent across studies (Table 1) (Blatter Garin et al., 2006; Hegele et al., 1995; Manresa et al., 2006; Rios et al., 2007; van Aalst-Cohen et al., 2005).

2.2 Genetic variation in receptors and transporters and HDL-C levels

Scavenger receptor class B, type 1 (SCARB1; SR-B1), which is highly expressed in liver and steroidogenic tissues (testes, ovaries, adrenal) (Cao et al., 1997), has been shown to participate in the uptake of HDL in animals by transferring cholesterol from the HDL-C particle and releasing the lipid-depleted HDL particle into the circulation (Acton et al., 1996; Miller et al., 2003). The human SCARB1 gene is located on chromosome 12 (12q24.31). Only a few studies have examined potential associations between SCARB1 polymorphisms and HDL-C levels (Table 1) (Boekholdt et al., 2006; Costanza et al., 2005; Hsu et al., 2003; Morabia et al., 2004; Osgood et al., 2003; Roberts et al., 2007). The most well studied polymorphism has been rs5888; however, the association with rs5888 and HDL-C levels was only significant among Caucasian (White, W) males in one study (Morabia et al., 2004), Amish females (Roberts et al., 2007) and Caucasian CVD patients (Boekholdt et al., 2006).

The LDL receptor (LDLR) and LDLR-related protein participate in the uptake of LDL and chylomicron remnants by hepatocytes (Kwan et al., 2007) and, therefore, may only indirectly affect HDL-C levels. The human LDLR is located on chromosome 19 (19p13.2). Although some common polymorphisms in LDLR have been associated with HDL-C levels (Table 1: (Costanza et al., 2005; Hegele et al., 1995; Yamada et al., 2008), their impact is likely greater on LDL-C levels (see Section 3.1).

The ATP-binding cassette transporter A1 (ABCA1), which is highly expressed in the liver, steroidogenic tissues and macrophages, plays a key role in 'reverse cholesterol transport' by mediating the efflux of cholesterol and phospholipids from macrophages to the nascent lipid-free, APOA-1 HDL particle (Cavelier et al., 2006; Miller et al., 2003). The human ABCA1 gene is located on chromosome 9 (9q31.1). Due to its functional importance, genetic variants in this gene have been well investigated but many of them are quite rare including the homozygous deletion that leads to Tangier's disease that is characterized by very low HDL-C levels (~5 mg/dl), orange colored tonsils, peripheral neuropathy and, sometimes, premature CHD (Garg and Simha, 2007). Several common polymorphisms have been fairly consistently associated with more modest changes in HDL-C levels but different variants appear to drive this association in different ethnic groups (Table 1) (Clee et al., 2001; Costanza et al., 2005; Frikke-Schmidt et al., 2004; Hodoglugil et al., 2005; Kathiresan et al., 2008b; Klos et al., 2006; Porchay et al., 2006; Shioji et al., 2004b; Whiting et al., 2005).

2.3 Genetic variation in apolipoproteins and HDL-C levels

Apolipoprotein A-1 (APOA1; APOA-I) is a ligand required for HDL-C binding to its receptors including SCARB1 and ABCA1 and, is an important cofactor in 'reverse cholesterol transport' (Miller et al., 2003; Remaley et al., 2001; Rigotti et al., 1997). The human APOA1 gene is located on chromosome 11 (11q23-24). APOA-I is a major constituent of HDL particles and deletions leading to complete APOA-I deficiency are rare but lead to HDL deficiency (HDL-C <10 mg/dl) and sometimes CHD (Garg and Simha, 2007). Several common polymorphisms in APOA-I have been associated with more modest reductions in HDL-C but results across studies are inconsistent (Table 1) (Brown et al., 2006; Kamboh et al., 1999b; Larson et al., 2002; Shioji et al., 2004a).

Apolipoprotein A-4 (APOA4; APOA-IV) is a potent activator of LCAT and modulates the activation of LPL and transfer of cholestryl esters from HDL to LDL (Kwan et al., 2007). The human APOA4 gene is located on chromosome 11 near APOA1 (11q23) and is part of what is known as the APOA1/C3/A4/A5 gene cluster. Polymorphisms in APOA4 have not been as well studied; however, the nonsynonymous SNP, rs5110 (Gln360His), has recently been associated with reduced HDL-C levels in Brazilian elderly (Ota et al., 2011) and coronary artery calcification (CAC) progression, a marker of subclinical atherosclerosis, in patients with Type I Diabetes Mellitus (T1DM) (Kretowski et al., 2006). The rs675 polymorphism has been associated with reduced HDL-C levels in females with T2DM (Qi et al., 2007).

Apolipoprotein A-5 (APOA5; APOA-V) is located predominantly on TG-rich chylomicrons and VLDL and activates LPL (Hubacek, 2005). The human APOA5 gene is located on chromosome 11 (11q23) in the APOA1/C3/A4/A5 gene cluster. Several APOA5 SNPs have been associated with reduced HDL-C levels; and, perhaps, the most well studied and consistent associations have been observed for rs651821 and rs662799 (Table 1) (Grallert et al., 2007; Hubacek, 2005; Klos et al., 2006; Lai et al., 2003; Qi et al., 2007; Talmud et al., 2002a; Yamada et al., 2008; Yamada et al., 2007).

Apolipoprotein C-3 (APOC3; APOC-III) is an inhibitor of LPL and is transferred to HDL during the hydrolysis of TG-rich lipoproteins (Kwan et al., 2007; Miller and Zhan, 2004). The human APOC3 gene is located on chromosome 11 (11q23) in the APOA1/C3/A4/A5 gene cluster. Although several APOC3 SNPs have been identified and investigated, associations between these SNPs and HDL-C levels have been quite inconsistent (Table 1) (Arai and Hirose, 2004; Brown et al., 2006; Corella et al., 2002; Hegele et al., 1995; Kamboh et al., 1999a; Lahiry et al., 2007; Pallaud et al., 2001; Qi et al., 2007; Russo et al., 2001).

Chylomicron remnants, VLDL and IDL particles are rich in apolipoprotein E (APOE) and APOE is a critical ligand for binding to hepatic receptors that remove these particles from the circulation (Kwan et al., 2007). Mutations in APOE are well known to modify LDL-C levels; however, their independent influence on HDL-C levels remains controversial (Sviridov and Nestel, 2007). Nevertheless, associations between APOE SNPs and HDL-C levels in large scale studies have been fairly consistent (Costanza et al., 2005; Frikke-Schmidt et al., 2000; Gronroos et al., 2008; Kataoka et al., 1996; Srinivasan et al., 1999; Volcik et al., 2006; Wilson et al., 1994; Wu et al., 2007).

2.4 GWAS and HDL-C Levels

Results from genomewide association studies (GWAS) have confirmed associations between polymorphisms in viable candidate genes including CETP, LPL, HL/LIPIC, EL/LIPG, ABCA1, LCAT and the APOA1/C3/A4/A5 gene cluster and HDL-C levels (Boes et al., 2009). GWAS have also identified several novel putative loci, which are discussed in detail in a recent review (Teslovich et al., 2010).

3. Genetic variants in lipid metabolism and LDL-C levels

3.1 Genetic variation in enzymes, receptors and transporters and LDL-C levels

LDL-C is a widely accepted risk factor for atherosclerotic cardiovascular diseases. The most marketed drugs for lowering LDL-C are statins, which inhibit hydroxy-3-methylglutaryl coenzyme A reductase (HMGCR), the rate limiting enzyme in cholesterol synthesis that is normally suppressed (Endo, 1992). The human HMGCR gene is located on chromosome 5 (5q13.3-14). Only a few common HMGCR polymorphisms have been associated with LDL-C levels including rs3846662, which was identified through GWAS (Table 2) (Burkhardt et al., 2008; Hiura et al., 2010; Polisecki et al., 2008; Teslovich et al., 2010).

As mentioned above, the LDL receptor (LDLR) regulates the uptake of LDL and chylomicron remnants by hepatocytes (Kwan et al., 2007) and, the human LDLR gene is located on chromosome 19 (19p13.2). Familial (or monogenic) hypercholesterolemia (FH: OMIM No. 143890), which is due to mutations in LDLR occurring at a frequency of approximately 1 in 500 (heterozygotes) to 1 in 1,000,000 (homozygotes), is one of the most common inherited metabolic diseases and results in a reduced number of LDL receptors and, in heterozygotes, a 2- to 3-fold increase in LDL–C levels and, in homozygotes, complete loss of LDLR function and a greater than 5-fold increase in LDL-C (Garg and Simha, 2007). A few common polymorphisms in LDLR have been identified and associated with more modest changes in LDL-C levels, most notably, rs6511720, which was highly significantly associated with LDL-C in a recent meta analysis (Table 2) (Teslovich et al., 2010; Willer et al., 2008).

ATP-binding cassette transporters G5 and G8 (ABCG5/8) regulate the efflux of cholesterol back into the intestinal lumen and, in hepatocytes, the efflux of cholesterol into bile (Graf et al., 2003). The human ABCG5/8 gene cluster is located on chromosome 2 (2p21). A rare autosomal recessive mutation in ABCG5/8 leads to sitosterolemia characterized by xanthomas, premature atherosclerosis and other features (Berge et al., 2000). Only a couple of common variants in ABCG5/8 have been associated with LDL-C levels and a recent meta-analysis failed to find associations between ABCG5/G8 polymorphisms including, ABCG8 rs6544718, and plasma lipid levels (Table 2) (Jakulj et al., 2010; Teslovich et al., 2010)

3.2 Genetic variation in lipoproteins and LDL-C levels

Apolipoprotein B (APOB; main isoform: ApoB-100) is responsible for the recognition and uptake of LDL by LDLR, which clears approximately 60-80% of the LDL in 'normal' individuals with the remaining taken up by LRP or SCARB1 (Kwan et al., 2007). The human APOB gene is located on chromosome 2 (2p23-24). Familial defective APOB (FDB: OMIM No. 144010) is an autosomal codominant disorder due to mutations in APOB that are a bit more rare than FH mutations at approximately 1 in 500 to 1 in 700 resulting in lower LDL-C levels than in FH patients (Garg and Simha, 2007). Common polymorphisms have also been identified and associated with more modest changes in LDL-C (Table 2) (Haas et al., 2011; Teslovich et al., 2010; Waterworth et al., 2010; Willer et al., 2008).

As mentioned above, APOE is a critical ligand for binding chylomicron remnants, VLDL and IDL particles to hepatic receptors to remove these particles from the circulation (Kwan et al., 2007). The human APOE gene is located on chromosome 19 (19q13.2). The structural APOE gene is polymorphic with three common alleles, designated as ε2, ε3 and ε4 which encode for E2, E3 and E4 proteins, respectively. Although several APOE polymorphisms have been identified, the APOE ε4 allele has been the most consistently associated with CHD and LDL-C levels (Table 2) (Anoop et al., 2010; Chang et al., 2010; Eichner et al., 2002; Teslovich et al., 2010; Willer et al., 2008).

Gene	Polym.	rs Number	MAF	Ethn.	Sample Size	Results (Effect Size, p-value)	Reference
ABCG8		rs4299376	0.30 (G)	E	95,454 (Meta)	+2.75 mg/dl; $p=2 \times 10^{-8}$	(Teslovich et al. 2010)
ABCG8	A632V	rs6544718		Va	982	p=0.02	(Jakuljl et al. 2010)
APOB		rs562338	0.18 (A)	Va	10,849	+4.89 mg/dl; $p=3.6 \times 10^{-12}$	(Willer et al. 2008)
APOB		rs754523	0.28 (A)	Va	6,542	+2.78 mg/dl; $p=1.3 \times 10^{-6}$	(Willer et al. 2008)
APOB		rs693	0.42 (G)	Va	3,222	+2.44 mg/dl; p=0.0034	(Willer et al. 2008)
APOB	Thr98Ile	rs1367117	0.30 (A)	E	95,454 (Meta)	+4.05 mg/dl; $p=4 \times 10^{-114}$	(Teslovich et al. 2010)
APOB		rs7575840	0.28 (T)	F	5054	0.131 $p= 3.88 \times 10^{-9}$	(Haas et al. 2011)
APOB		rs515135	0.19 (A)	Va	982	$p=2.4 \times 10^{-20}$	Waterworth et al. (2010)
APOE		rs4420638	0.17 (G)	E	95,454 (Meta)	+7.14 mg/dl; $p=9 \times 10^{-147}$	(Teslovich et al. 2010)
APOE	Arg176 Cys	rs7412	0.06 (T)	N-HB	683	-22.52mg/dl; p< 0.0001	(Chang et al. 2010)
APOE	Cys130 Arg	rs429358	0.076 (T)	M-A	739	10.54mg/dl; p< 0.0001	(Chang et al. 2010)
APOC1		rs4420638	0.82 (A)	Va	10,806	+6.61 mg/dl; $p = 4.9 \times 10^{-24}$	(Willer et al. 2008)
APOE/ C1/C4		rs10402271	0.67 (T)	Va	6,519	+2.62 mg/dl; $p =1.5 \times 10^{-5}$	(Willer et al. 2008)
LDLR		rs6511720	0.11 (T)	E	95,454 (Meta)	-6.99 mg/dl; $p=4 \times 10^{-117}$	(Teslovich et al. 2010)
LDLR		rs6511720	0.90 (T)	Va	7,442	+9.17 mg/dl; $p =3.3 \times 10^{-19}$	(Willer et al. 2008)
PCSK9		rs11206510	0.81 (C)	Va	10,805	+3.04 mg/dl; $p=5.4 \times 10^{-7}$	(Willer et al. 2008)
PCSK9		rs2479409	0.30 (G)	E	95,454 (Meta)	+2.01mg/dl; $p= 2 \times 10^{-28}$	(Teslovich et al. 2010)
PCSK9	A443T Ala443Thr	rs28362263	0.06 (A)	B	1750	95.5 vs. 106.9 mg/dl;p<0.001	(Huang et al. 2009)
PCSK9	C679X	rs28362286		B	1750	81.5 vs. 106.9 mg/dl;p<0.001	(Huang et al. 2009)
PCSK9	E670G	rs505151	0.11 (G)	W	691	P=0.001	(Chen et al. 2005)
PCSK9		rs11206510	0.81 (T)	EA	21,986 (Meta)	p=1.44E-05	(Dumitrescu et al. 2011)
SORT1		rs629301	0.22 (G)	E	95,454 (Meta)	-5.65 mg/dl; $p=1 \times 10^{-170}$	(Teslovich et al. 2010)

Table 2. Genetic Polymorphisms Associated with LDL-C. See Table 1 legend.

3.3 Genetic variation in proteases and LDL-C levels
Proprotein convertase subtilisin-like kexin type 9 (PCSK9) is a serine protease that degrades hepatic LDLR in endosomes (Maxwell et al., 2005). The human PCSK9 gene is located on chromosome 1 (1p32.3). A mutation in PCSK9 results in an autosomal dominant form of hypercholesterolemia (OMIM No. 607786) with clinical features similar to FH patients (Garg and Simha, 2007). Over 50 variants in PCSK9 have been shown to affect circulating levels of cholesterol; however, most of these are relatively rare (see Davignon et al., 2010) for a complete list). The number of common polymorphisms in PCSK9 is substantially less with only a few SNPs having been associated with changes in LDL-C levels (Table 2) (Chen et al., 2005; Evans and Beil, 2006; Huang et al., 2009; Teslovich et al., 2010; Willer et al., 2008).

3.4 GWAS and LDL-C Levels
GWAS have confirmed associations between polymorphisms in viable candidate genes including APOB, APOE, LDLR and PCSK9, and have identified novel SNPs associated with LDL-C levels with strong biological plausibility including an inhibitor of lipase (ANGPTL3), see Section 4.1 and a transcription factor activating triglyceride synthesis (MLXIPL) see Section 4.2 (Teslovich et al., 2010).

4. Genetic variants in lipid metabolism and TG levels

Plasma triglycerides (TG) integrate multiple TG-rich lipoprotein particles, predominantly, intestinally synthesized chylomicrons in the postprandial state and hepatically synthesized VLDL in the fasted state. Therefore, not surprisingly, there is considerable overlap between genetic variants associated with HDL-C and LDL-C levels as well as TG levels. For example, the Global Lipids Genetics Consortium (GLGC) found that 15 of the 32 loci associated with TG levels were also jointly associated with HDL-C levels, explaining 9.6% of the total variation in plasma TG, which corresponded to 25–30% of the total genetic contribution to TG variability (Teslovich et al., 2010). However, the joint associations reported do not appear additionally adjusted for the other lipid phenotype. Furthermore, certain loci appear to be more strongly associated with one lipid phenotype over the other while others have similar effect sizes; and, genetic heterogeneity between loci clearly exists between major ethnic groups.

4.1 Genetic variation in aolipoproteins and TG levels
As mentioned above (see Section 3.2), APOB is the backbone of atherogenic lipoproteins and is located on chromosome 2 (2p23-24). A rare monogenic autosomal recessive disorder called homozygous hypobetalipoproteinemia and rare autosomal codominant disorder called familial hypobetalipoproteinaemia (HHBL and FHBL, respectively: OMIM No. 107730), characterized by very low (<5th percentile of age- and sex-specific values) of plasma TG (and LDL-C) levels, which are caused by rare mutations in APOB (Burnett and Hooper, 2008; Di et al., 2009). Although common APOB polymorphisms have primarily been associated with LDL-C levels (Benn, 2009), GWAS has revealed that a common SNP in APOB, rs1042034, is associated with TG (Johansen and Hegele, 2011; Teslovich et al., 2010).
Common polymorphisms in the APOA1/C3/A4/A5 gene cluster, located on chromosome 11 (11q23), have been associated with HDL-C levels (see Section 2.3) as well as TG levels (Teslovich et al., 2010; Willer et al., 2008). A SNP in the APOE gene, rs439401, has also been shown to be strongly associated with TG levels in a recent GWAS meta analyses (Johansen and Hegele, 2011; Teslovich et al., 2010).

z	Polym.	rs Number	MAF	Ethn.	Sample Size	Results (Effect Size, p-value)	Reference
ANGPTL3		rs2131925	0.32 (G)	E	96,598 (Meta)	-4.94mg/dl; $p=9\times10^{-43}$	(Teslovich et al. 2010)
ANGPTL3		rs1748195	0.70 (G)	Va	9,559	7.12 mg/dl; $p=5.4\times10^{-8}$	(Willer et al. 2008)
APOA5		rs964184	0.13 (G)	E	96,598 (Meta)	+16.95mg/dl; $p=7\times10^{-240}$	(Teslovich et al. 2010)
APOA5/A4/C3/A1		rs12286037	0.94 (C)	Va	9,738	25.82 mg/dl; $p=1.6\times10^{-22}$	(Willer et al. 2008)
APOA5		rs662799	0.05 (A)	Va	3,248	16.88 mg/dl $p=2.7\times10^{-10}$	(Willer et al. 2008)
APOA5/A4/C3/A1		rs2000571	0.17 (G)	Va	3,209	6.93 mg/dl; $p=8.7\times10^{-5}$	(Willer et al. 2008)
APOA5/A4/C3/A1		rs486394	0.28 (A)	Va	3,597	1.50 mg/dl; p=0.0073	(Willer et al. 2008)
APOE		rs439401	0.40 (C)	C	4.192	$p=2.2\times10^{-5}$	(Liu et al. 2011)
APOE		rs439401	0.64 (C)	Va	Meta	$p=5.5\times10^{-30}$	Johansen et al. (2010)
LIPC/HL		rs4775041	0.67 (G)	Va	8,462	3.62 mg/dl; $p=2.9\times10^{-5}$	(Willer et al. 2008)
LIPC/HL		rs261342	0.22 (G)	Va	Meta	$p=2.0\times10^{-13}$	Johansen et al. (2010)
LPL		rs12678919	0.12 (G)	E	96,598 (Meta)	-13.64 mg/dl $p=2\times10^{-115}$	(Teslovich et al. 2010)
LPL		rs10503669	0.90 (A)	Va	9,711	11.57 mg/dl; $p=1.6\times10^{-14}$	(Willer et al. 2008)
LPL		rs2197089	0.58 (A)	Va	3,202	3.38 mg/dl; p=0.0029	(Willer et al. 2008)
LPL		rs6586891	0.66 (A)	Va	3,622	4.60 mg/dl; $p=5\times10^{-4}$	(Willer et al. 2008)
LPL	S447X	rs328	0.90 (C)	EA	24,258	p=4.16E-30	(Dumitrescu et al. 2011)
LPL	S447X	rs328	0.10 (X)	Va	43,242	-0.15 (-0.12- -0.19) mmol/l	(Sagoo et al. 2008)
LPL	D9N	rs1801177	0.03 (N)	Va	21,040	0.14 (0.08-0.20) mmol/l	(Sagoo et al. 2008)
LPL	N291S	rs368	0.03 (S)	Va	27,204	0.19 (0.12-0.26) mmol/l	(Sagoo et al. 2008)
LPL		rs326	0.18 (G)	C	4,192	$p=2.3\times10^{-6}$	(Liu et al. 2011)
LRP1		rs11613352	0.23 (T)	E	96,598 (Meta)	-2.70 mg/dl $p=4\times10^{-10}$	(Teslovich et al. 2010)
MLXIPL		rs17145738	0.12 (T)	E	96,598 (Meta)	-9.32 mg/dl $p=6\times10^{-58}$	(Teslovich et al. 2010)
MLXIPL		rs17145738	0.84 (T)	Va	9,741	8.21 mg/dl; $p=5\times10^{-8}$	(Willer et al. 2008)
MLXIPL		rs7811265	0.81 (A)	Va	Meta	7.91 mg/dl $p=9.0\times10^{-59}$	(Johansen et al. 2011)

Table 3. Genetic Polymorphisms Associated With TG Levels. See Table 1 legend.

Angiopoietin-like 3 protein (ANGPTL3) inhibits LPL catalytic activity but this process is reversible (Shan et al., 2009; Shimizugawa et al., 2002). A monogenic autosomal recessive disorder called familial combined hypolipidemia (FCH: OMIM No. 605019), characterized by very low TG levels, is genetically complex and poorly understood; however, mutations in ANGPTL3 are believed to play a role. Common polymorphisms in ANGPTL3, most notably, rs2131925, have been associated with more modest changes in TG levels (Johansen and Hegele, 2011; Keebler et al., 2009; Lanktree et al., 2009; Teslovich et al., 2010; Willer et al., 2008). Sequencing individuals in the Dallas Heart Study has identified several additional nonsynonymous ANGPTL3 variants affecting TG levels (Musunuru et al., 2010); however, these SNPs require further investigation in other populations.

4.2 Genetic variation in enzymes and transcription factors and TG levels

As mentioned above (see Section 2.1), LPL is an enzyme that hydrolyzes TG-rich particles in peripheral tissues (muscle, macrophages, adipose) generating FFA and glycerol for energy metabolism and storage (Goldberg, 1996). More than 100 mutations in LPL have been identified (Murthy et al., 1996); however, only a few common nonsynonymous SNPs have been consistently associated with TG levels including rs1801177, rs328 and rs268 (Mailly et al., 1995; Rip et al., 2006; Sagoo et al., 2008; Teslovich et al., 2010; Willer et al., 2008). Two SNPs, rs1801177 and rs328, have also been consistently associated with CHD; however, there is fairly strong LD between these SNPs, at least in Caucasians (Sagoo et al., 2008).

MLX interacting protein like (MLXIPL) locus encodes a transcription factor of the Myc/Max/Mad superfamily which activates, in a glucose-dependent manner, carbohydrate response element binding protein (CREBP) that is expressed in lipogenic tissues coordinating the subsequent activation of lipogenic enzymes such as fatty acid synthase (FAS) to convert dietary carbohydrate to TG (Iizuka and Horikawa, 2008). The human MLXIPL gene is located on chromosome 7 (7q11.23). Although initially identified through GWAS, the rs1745738 polymorphism has been replicated in other studies (Johansen and Hegele, 2011; Teslovich et al., 2010; Wang et al., 2008; Willer et al., 2008).

5. Genetic variants in dyslipidemia and the Metabolic Syndrome (MetSyn)

As mentioned in the Introduction (see Section 1.0), MetSyn is a clustering of traits including dyslipidemia as well as obesity, hypertension and insulin resistance/dysglycemia. Undoubtedly, there is complex interplay between genetic determinants of each of these traits and 'environmental' factors including those related to lifestyle (diet, exercise, sleep) and those related to toxin exposure. Due to space limitations, we focus only on the genetic determinants of dyslipidemia that overlap with MetSyn defined as a single, unifying trait and refer the reader to other reviews for genetic determinants of the other traits involved in MetSyn (Joy et al., 2008; Monda et al., 2010; Pollex and Hegele, 2006; Sharma and McNeill, 2006) and their interactions with lifestyle factors (Adamo and Tesson, 2008; Garaulet et al., 2009; Ordovas and Shen, 2008; Phillips et al., 2008) and toxins (Andreassi, 2009).

Lipoprotein related genes with common SNPs associated with MetSyn (as defined by NCEP ATP III and AHA/NHLBI criteria) and HDL-C, LDL-C or TG levels include APOA5 and APOC3 (Table 4) (Grallert et al., 2007; Joy et al., 2008; Miller et al., 2007; Pollex et al., 2006; Pollex and Hegele, 2006; Yamada et al., 2008). Enzymes involved in lipid metabolism with genetic polymorphisms that have also been associated with MetSyn (using the NCEP ATPIII criteria) appear limited to the nonsynonymous SNP in LPL, rs328 (Table 4) (Joy et al., 2008;

Komurcu-Bayrak et al., 2007). Several SNPs in the LDLR have been associated with MetSyn (using AHA/NHLBI criteria) and LDL-C or HDL-C (Joy et al., 2008; Yamada et al., 2008).

Gene	Polymorphism	rs Number	Ethn.	Sample Size	Results (p-value)	Reference	Comments (definition)
APOA5	-1131T→C		J	1788	p< 0.0009	(Yamada et al. 2007)	NCEP ATP III
APOA5	c.56C→G		C	3124	p=0.026	(Grallert et al. 2007)	NCEP ATP III
APOA5	-3A→G		J	2417	p< 0.0001	(Yamada et al. 2008)	AHA/NHLBI
APOC3	-455T→C		O-C	515	p=0.029*	(Miller et al. 2007) (Pollex et al. 2006)	*Women only NCEP ATP III
LDLR	2052TmC		J	2417	p=0.0005	(Yamada et al. 2008)	AHA/NHLBI
LPL	S447X		Tu	1586	p=0.04	(Komurcu-Bayrak et al. 2007)	NCEP ATP III
LPL		rs295	Va	1407	OR= 0.7; p=2.1 x 10⁻³	(Grassi et al. 2011)	NCEP ATPIII

Table 4. Genetic Polymorphisms in Lipid Metabolism Associated with MetSyn. See Table 1 legend. WHO= World Health Organization; NCEP ATP III=National Cholesterol Education Program Adult Treatment Panel III, IDF=International Diabetes Federation; AHA=American Heart Association; NHLBI=National Heart, Lung, and Blood institute.

6. Genetic variants in dyslipidemia and MetSyn: Future directions

Given the polygenic nature and multi-level complexity of Dyslipidemia and MetSyn, a better understanding of the genetic determinants of each intermediate (lower level) phenotype as well as the collective integration of these traits as unifying syndromes (higher/hierarchical level) is needed, which will require more elegant statistical modeling methods and, perhaps, a paradigm shift in the way in which we think about dissecting genetic and environmental factors in complex traits. As stated throughout this chapter, there is considerable overlap between genetic variants associated with HDL-C, LDL-C and TG levels as well MetSyn as a unifying trait. As a result, there is great need to understand not only the aggregate effects of multiple variants in each of these genes but to also understand how the effects of variation in one gene are modified in the presence of other genes.

Aggregate effects of multiple variants in genes affecting dyslipidemia and MetSyn related traits have included calculation of 'risk scores', which simply add the number of 'risk alleles' in a weighted or unweighted manner. For example, unweighted risk scores were constructed by summing the number of 'TG-raising' alleles at 32 loci and placed in 'risk bins' (categories) to show that higher risk scores were significantly associated with patients with hypertriglyceridemia (HTG) compared to controls (Johansen and Hegele, 2011; Teslovich et al., 2010). Increasing genotype risk scores comprised by summing risk alleles in 9 common SNPs were associated with decreasing HDL-C levels (Kathiresan et al., 2008a).

We have used the multivariate statistical framework of structural equation modeling (SEM) to evaluate multiple genetic determinants of MetSyn and aggregate effects of individual genes by modeling MetSyn as a second-order factor together with multiple putative candidate genes represented by latent constructs, which we mathematically defined by multiple SNPs in each gene (Nock et al., 2009b). Using this approach with the Framingham Heart Study (Offspring Cohort, Exam 7; Affymetrix 50k Human Gene Panel) data, we found that the CETP gene had a very strong association with the Dyslipidemia factor but little effect on MetSyn directly. Furthermore, we found that the effects of the CSMD1 gene diminished when modeled simultaneously with six other candidate genes, most notably CETP and STARD13. Work to identify the genetic determinants of 'Syndrome Z', modeled as a higher-order, unifying syndrome defined by 5 first-order factors (dyslipidemia, insulin resistance, obesity, hypertension, sleep disturbance) (Nock et al., 2009a) using the latent gene construct SEM approach is underway.

The use of other forms of 'causal modeling' (edge/node; integrative genetics) has been proposed (Lusis et al., 2008), particularly, to improve our understanding of differential effects by gender as well as to better understand how maternal nutrition and epigenetics affect MetSyn. Furthermore, a complex model for the genetic determinants of MetSyn associated phenotypes was recently proposed and, using gene enrichment analysis and protein-protein interaction network approaches, the retinoid X receptor and farnesoid X receptor (FXR) were identified as key players in MetSyn given their multiple interactions with metabolism, cell proliferation and oxidative stress (Sookoian and Pirola, 2011). However, more elegant kinetic models may be required to understand the true influence of genetic variants on Dsylipidemia and MetSyn given the presence of multiple feedback loops and reversible reactions (Bakker et al., 2010; Gutierrez-Cirlos et al., 2011).

7. Acknowledgement

This work was supported, in part, by the National Institutes of Health/National Cancer Institute Grant [K07CA129162] awarded to NLN.

8. References

2001. Executive Summary of The Third Report of The National Cholesterol Education Program (NCEP) Expert Panel on Detection, Evaluation, And Treatment of High Blood Cholesterol In Adults (Adult Treatment Panel III). JAMA 285: 2486-2497.

Acton S, Rigotti A, Landschulz KT, Xu S, Hobbs HH, Krieger M. 1996. Identification of scavenger receptor SR-BI as a high density lipoprotein receptor. Science 271: 518-520.

Adamo KB, Tesson F. 2008. Gene-environment interaction and the metabolic syndrome. Novartis. Found. Symp. 293: 103-119.

Adiels M, Olofsson SO, Taskinen MR, Boren J. 2006. Diabetic dyslipidaemia. Curr. Opin. Lipidol. 17: 238-246.

Ahn YI, Kamboh MI, Hamman RF, Cole SA, Ferrell RE. 1993. Two DNA polymorphisms in the lipoprotein lipase gene and their associations with factors related to cardiovascular disease. J. Lipid Res. 34: 421-428.

Alberti KG, Eckel RH, Grundy SM, et al. 2009. Harmonizing the metabolic syndrome: a joint interim statement of the International Diabetes Federation Task Force on Epidemiology and Prevention; National Heart, Lung, and Blood Institute; American Heart Association; World Heart Federation; International Atherosclerosis Society; and International Association for the Study of Obesity. Circulation 120: 1640-1645.

Alberti KG, Zimmet P, Shaw J. 2005. The metabolic syndrome--a new worldwide definition. Lancet 366: 1059-1062.

Alberti KG, Zimmet PZ. 1998. Definition, diagnosis and classification of diabetes mellitus and its complications. Part 1: diagnosis and classification of diabetes mellitus provisional report of a WHO consultation. Diabet. Med. 15: 539-553.

Andersen RV, Wittrup HH, Tybjaerg-Hansen A, Steffensen R, Schnohr P, Nordestgaard BG. 2003. Hepatic lipase mutations,elevated high-density lipoprotein cholesterol, and increased risk of ischemic heart disease: the Copenhagen City Heart Study. J. Am. Coll. Cardiol. 41: 1972-1982.

Andreassi MG. 2009. Metabolic syndrome, diabetes and atherosclerosis: influence of gene-environment interaction. Mutat. Res. 667: 35-43.

Anoop S, Misra A, Meena K, Luthra K. 2010. Apolipoprotein E polymorphism in cerebrovascular & coronary heart diseases. Indian J. Med. Res. 132: 363-378.

Arai Y, Hirose N. 2004. Aging and HDL metabolism in elderly people more than 100 years old. J. Atheroscler. Thromb. 11: 246-252.

Athyros VG, Mikhailidis DP, Papageorgiou AA, et al. 2004. Prevalence of atherosclerotic vascular disease among subjects with the metabolic syndrome with or without diabetes mellitus: the METS-GREECE Multicentre Study. Curr. Med. Res. Opin. 20: 1691-1701.

Austin MA, King MC, Vranizan KM, Krauss RM. 1990. Atherogenic lipoprotein phenotype. A proposed genetic marker for coronary heart disease risk. Circulation 82: 495-506.

Bakker BM, van EK, Jeneson JA, van Riel NA, Bruggeman FJ, Teusink B. 2010. Systems biology from micro-organisms to human metabolic diseases: the role of detailed kinetic models. Biochem. Soc. Trans. 38: 1294-1301.

Balkau B, Charles MA. 1999. Comment on the provisional report from the WHO consultation. European Group for the Study of Insulin Resistance (EGIR). Diabet. Med. 16: 442-443.

Benn M. 2009. Apolipoprotein B levels, APOB alleles, and risk of ischemic cardiovascular disease in the general population, a review. Atherosclerosis 206: 17-30.

Berge KE, Tian H, Graf GA, Yu L, Grishin NV, Schultz J, Kwiterovich P, Shan B, Barnes R, Hobbs HH. 2000. Accumulation of dietary cholesterol in sitosterolemia caused by mutations in adjacent ABC transporters. Science 290: 1771-1775.

Bernstein MS, Costanza MC, James RW, Morris MA, Cambien F, Raoux S, Morabia A. 2003. No physical activity x CETP 1b.-629 interaction effects on lipid profile. Med. Sci. Sports Exerc. 35: 1124-1129.

Blankenberg S, Tiret L, Bickel C, et al. 2004. [Genetic variation of the cholesterol ester transfer protein gene and the prevalence of coronary artery disease. The AtheroGene case control study]. Z. Kardiol. 93 Suppl 4: IV16-IV23.

Blatter Garin MC, Moren X, James RW. 2006. Paraoxonase-1 and serum concentrations of HDL-cholesterol and apoA-I. J. Lipid Res. 47: 515-520.

Boekholdt SM, Sacks FM, Jukema JW, et al. 2005. Cholesteryl ester transfer protein TaqIB variant, high-density lipoprotein cholesterol levels, cardiovascular risk, and efficacy of pravastatin treatment: individual patient meta-analysis of 13,677 subjects. Circulation 111: 278-287.

Boekholdt SM, Souverein OW, Tanck MW, et al. 2006. Common variants of multiple genes that control reverse cholesterol transport together explain only a minor part of the variation of HDL cholesterol levels. Clin. Genet. 69: 263-270.

Boekholdt SM, Thompson JF. 2003. Natural genetic variation as a tool in understanding the role of CETP in lipid levels and disease. J. Lipid Res. 44: 1080-1093.

Boes E, Coassin S, Kollerits B, Heid IM, Kronenberg F. 2009. Genetic-epidemiological evidence on genes associated with HDL cholesterol levels: a systematic in-depth review. Exp Gerontol. 44: 136-160.

Borggreve SE, Hillege HL, Wolffenbuttel BH, de Jong PE, Bakker SJ, van der Steege G, van TA, Dullaart RP. 2005. The effect of cholesteryl ester transfer protein -629C->A promoter polymorphism on high-density lipoprotein cholesterol is dependent on serum triglycerides. J. Clin. Endocrinol. Metab 90: 4198-4204.

Brown CM, Rea TJ, Hamon SC, Hixson JE, Boerwinkle E, Clark AG, Sing CF. 2006. The contribution of individual and pairwise combinations of SNPs in the APOA1 and APOC3 genes to interindividual HDL-C variability. J. Mol. Med. (Berl) 84: 561-572.

Burkhardt R, Kenny EE, Lowe JK, et al.. 2008. Common SNPs in HMGCR in micronesians and whites associated with LDL-cholesterol levels affect alternative splicing of exon13. Arterioscler. Thromb. Vasc. Biol. 28: 2078-2084.

Burnett JR, Hooper AJ. 2008. Common and rare gene variants affecting plasma LDL cholesterol. Clin Biochem. Rev. 29: 11-26.

Cao G, Garcia CK, Wyne KL, Schultz RA, Parker KL, Hobbs HH. 1997. Structure and localization of the human gene encoding SR-BI/CLA-1. Evidence for transcriptional control by steroidogenic factor 1. J. Biol. Chem. 272: 33068-33076.

Cavelier C, Rohrer L, von EA. 2006. ATP-Binding cassette transporter A1 modulates apolipoprotein A-I transcytosis through aortic endothelial cells. Circ. Res. 99: 1060-1066.

Chang MH, Yesupriya A, Ned RM, Mueller PW, Dowling NF. 2010. Genetic variants associated with fasting blood lipids in the U.S. population: Third National Health and Nutrition Examination Survey. BMC. Med. Genet. 11: 62.

Chen SN, Ballantyne CM, Gotto AM, Jr., Tan Y, Willerson JT, Marian AJ. 2005. A common PCSK9 haplotype, encompassing the E670G coding single nucleotide polymorphism, is a novel genetic marker for plasma low-density lipoprotein cholesterol levels and severity of coronary atherosclerosis. J. Am. Coll. Cardiol. 45: 1611-1619.

Clee SM, Zwinderman AH, Engert JC, et al. 2001. Common genetic variation in ABCA1 is associated with altered lipoprotein levels and a modified risk for coronary artery disease. Circulation 103: 1198-1205.

Corella D, Guillen M, Saiz C, Portoles O, Sabater A, Folch J, Ordovas JM. 2002. Associations of LPL and APOC3 gene polymorphisms on plasma lipids in a Mediterranean population: interaction with tobacco smoking and the APOE locus. J. Lipid Res. 43: 416-427.

Costanza MC, Cayanis E, Ross BM, Flaherty MS, Alvin GB, Das K, Morabia A. 2005. Relative contributions of genes, environment, and interactions to blood lipid concentrations in a general adult population. Am. J. Epidemiol. 161: 714-724.

Davignon J, Dubuc G, Seidah NG. 2010. The influence of PCSK9 polymorphisms on serum low-density lipoprotein cholesterol and risk of atherosclerosis. Curr. Atheroscler. Rep. 12: 308-315.

de Andrade FM, Silveira FR, Arsand M, et al. 2004. Association between -250G/A polymorphism of the hepatic lipase gene promoter and coronary artery disease and HDL-C levels in a Southern Brazilian population. Clin. Genet. 65: 390-395.

Di LE, Magnolo L, Pinotti E, et al. 2009. Functional analysis of two novel splice site mutations of APOB gene in familial hypobetalipoproteinemia. Mol. Genet. Metab 96: 66-72.

Edwards KL, Newman B, Mayer E, Selby JV, Krauss RM, Austin MA. 1997. Heritability of factors of the insulin resistance syndrome in women twins. Genet. Epidemiol. 14: 241-253.

Eichner JE, Dunn ST, Perveen G, Thompson DM, Stewart KE, Stroehla BC. 2002. Apolipoprotein E polymorphism and cardiovascular disease: a HuGE review. Am. J. Epidemiol. 155: 487-495.

Einhorn D, Reaven GM, Cobin RH, et al. 2003. American College of Endocrinology position statement on the insulin resistance syndrome. Endocr. Pract. 9: 237-252.

Eiriksdottir G, Bolla MK, Thorsson B, Sigurdsson G, Humphries SE, Gudnason V. 2001. The -629C>A polymorphism in the CETP gene does not explain the association of TaqIB polymorphism with risk and age of myocardial infarction in Icelandic men. Atherosclerosis 159: 187-192.

Endo A. 1992. The discovery and development of HMG-CoA reductase inhibitors. J. Lipid Res. 33: 1569-1582.

Evans D, Beil FU. 2006. The E670G SNP in the PCSK9 gene is associated with polygenic hypercholesterolemia in men but not in women. BMC. Med. Genet. 7: 66.

Fang DZ, Liu BW. 2002. Polymorphism of HL +1075C, but not -480T, is associated with plasma high density lipoprotein cholesterol and apolipoprotein AI in men of a Chinese population. Atherosclerosis 161: 417-424.

Ford ES, Giles WH, Dietz WH. 2002. Prevalence of the metabolic syndrome among US adults: findings from the third National Health and Nutrition Examination Survey. JAMA 287: 356-359.

Freeman DJ, Samani NJ, Wilson V, et al. 2003. A polymorphism of the cholesteryl ester transfer protein gene predicts cardiovascular events in non-smokers in the West of Scotland Coronary Prevention Study. Eur. Heart J. 24: 1833-1842.

Frikke-Schmidt R, Nordestgaard BG, Jensen GB, Tybjaerg-Hansen A. 2004. Genetic variation in ABC transporter A1 contributes to HDL cholesterol in the general population. J. Clin. Invest 114: 1343-1353.

Frikke-Schmidt R, Tybjaerg-Hansen A, Steffensen R, Jensen G, Nordestgaard BG. 2000. Apolipoprotein E genotype: epsilon32 women are protected while epsilon43 and epsilon44 men are susceptible to ischemic heart disease: the Copenhagen City Heart Study. J. Am. Coll. Cardiol. 35: 1192-1199.

Garaulet M, Lee YC, Shen J, Parnell LD, Arnett DK, Tsai MY, Lai CQ, Ordovas JM. 2009. CLOCK genetic variation and metabolic syndrome risk: modulation by monounsaturated fatty acids. Am. J. Clin Nutr. 90: 1466-1475.

Garg A, Simha V. 2007. Update on dyslipidemia. J. Clin Endocrinol. Metab 92: 1581-1589.

Goldberg IJ. 1996. Lipoprotein lipase and lipolysis: central roles in lipoprotein metabolism and atherogenesis. J. Lipid Res. 37: 693-707.

Goode EL, Cherny SS, Christian JC, Jarvik GP, de AM. 2007. Heritability of longitudinal measures of body mass index and lipid and lipoprotein levels in aging twins. Twin. Res. Hum. Genet. 10: 703-711.

Graf GA, Yu L, Li WP, Gerard R, Tuma PL, Cohen JC, Hobbs HH. 2003. ABCG5 and ABCG8 are obligate heterodimers for protein trafficking and biliary cholesterol excretion. J. Biol. Chem. 278: 48275-48282.

Grallert H, Sedlmeier EM, Huth C, Kolz M, Heid IM, Meisinger C, Herder C, Strassburger K, Gehringer A, Haak M, Giani G, Kronenberg F, Wichmann HE, Adamski J, Paulweber B, Illig T, Rathmann W. 2007. APOA5 variants and metabolic syndrome in Caucasians. J. Lipid Res. 48: 2614-2621.

Grarup N, Andreasen CH, Andersen MK, et al. 2008. The -250G>A promoter variant in hepatic lipase associates with elevated fasting serum high-density lipoprotein cholesterol modulated by interaction with physical activity in a study of 16,156 Danish subjects. J. Clin. Endocrinol. Metab 93: 2294-2299.

Gronroos P, Raitakari OT, Kahonen M, et al.. 2008. Relation of apolipoprotein E polymorphism to markers of early atherosclerotic changes in young adults--the Cardiovascular Risk in Young Finns Study. Circ. J. 72: 29-34.

Grundy SM, Cleeman JI, Daniels SR, et al. 2006. Diagnosis and management of the metabolic syndrome: an American Heart Association/National Heart, Lung, and Blood Institute scientific statement. Curr. Opin. Cardiol. 21: 1-6.

Grundy SM, Cleeman JI, Merz CN, et al. 2004. Implications of recent clinical trials for the National Cholesterol Education Program Adult Treatment Panel III Guidelines. J. Am. Coll. Cardiol. 44: 720-732.

Gutierrez-Cirlos C, Ordonez-Sanchez ML, Tusie-Luna MT, Patterson BW, Schonfeld G, Aguilar-Salinas CA. 2011. Familial hypobetalipoproteinemia in a hospital survey: genetics, metabolism and non-alcoholic fatty liver disease. Ann. Hepatol. 10: 155-164.

Haas BE, Weissglas-Volkov D, Aguilar-Salinas CA, et al. 2011. Evidence of how rs7575840 influences apolipoprotein B-containing lipid particles. Arterioscler. Thromb. Vasc. Biol. 31: 1201-1207.

Halpern A, Mancini MC, Magalhaes ME, et al. 2010. Metabolic syndrome, dyslipidemia, hypertension and type 2 diabetes in youth: from diagnosis to treatment. Diabetol. Metab Syndr. 2: 55.

Hegele RA, Brunt JH, Connelly PW. 1995. Multiple genetic determinants of variation of plasma lipoproteins in Alberta Hutterites. Arterioscler. Thromb. Vasc. Biol. 15: 861-871.

Heid IM, Boes E, Muller M, Kollerits B, et al. 2008. Genome-wide association analysis of high-density lipoprotein cholesterol in the population-based KORA study sheds new light on intergenic regions. Circ. Cardiovasc. Genet. 1: 10-20.

Herbeth B, Samara A, Ndiaye C, Marteau JB, Berrahmoune H, Siest G, Visvikis-Siest S. 2010. Metabolic syndrome-related composite factors over 5 years in the STANISLAS family study: genetic heritability and common environmental influences. Clin Chim. Acta 411: 833-839.

Hiura Y, Tabara Y, Kokubo Y, Okamura T, Goto Y, Nonogi H, Miki T, Tomoike H, Iwai N. 2010. Association of the functional variant in the 3-hydroxy-3-methylglutaryl-coenzyme a reductase gene with low-density lipoprotein-cholesterol in Japanese. Circ. J. 74: 518-522.

Hodoglugil U, Williamson DW, Huang Y, Mahley RW. 2005. Common polymorphisms of ATP binding cassette transporter A1, including a functional promoter polymorphism, associated with plasma high density lipoprotein cholesterol levels in Turks. Atherosclerosis 183: 199-212.

Holmer SR, Hengstenberg C, Mayer B, Doring A, Lowel H, Engel S, Hense HW, Wolf M, Klein G, Riegger GA, Schunkert H. 2000. Lipoprotein lipase gene polymorphism, cholesterol subfractions and myocardial infarction in large samples of the general population. Cardiovasc. Res. 47: 806-812.

Hsu LA, Ko YL, Wu S, Teng MS, Peng TY, Chen CF, Chen CF, Lee YS. 2003. Association between a novel 11-base pair deletion mutation in the promoter region of the scavenger receptor class B type I gene and plasma HDL cholesterol levels in Taiwanese Chinese. Arterioscler. Thromb. Vasc. Biol. 23: 1869-1874.

Huang CC, Fornage M, Lloyd-Jones DM, Wei GS, Boerwinkle E, Liu K. 2009. Longitudinal association of PCSK9 sequence variations with low-density lipoprotein cholesterol levels: the Coronary Artery Risk Development in Young Adults Study. Circ. Cardiovasc. Genet. 2: 354-361.

Hubacek JA. 2005. Apolipoprotein A5 and triglyceridemia. Focus on the effects of the common variants. Clin. Chem. Lab Med. 43: 897-902.

Hutter CM, Austin MA, Farin FM, Viernes HM, Edwards KL, Leonetti DL, McNeely MJ, Fujimoto WY. 2006. Association of endothelial lipase gene (LIPG) haplotypes with high-density lipoprotein cholesterol subfractions and apolipoprotein AI plasma levels in Japanese Americans. Atherosclerosis 185: 78-86.

Iijima H, Emi M, Wada M, Daimon M, Toriyama S, Koyano S, Sato H, Hopkins PN, Hunt SC, Kubota I, Kawata S, Kato T. 2008. Association of an intronic haplotype of the LIPC gene with hyperalphalipoproteinemia in two independent populations. J. Hum. Genet. 53: 193-200.

Iizuka K, Horikawa Y. 2008. ChREBP: a glucose-activated transcription factor involved in the development of metabolic syndrome. Endocr. J. 55: 617-624.

Isaacs A, Aulchenko YS, Hofman A, et al. 2007. Epistatic effect of cholesteryl ester transfer protein and hepatic lipase on serum high-density lipoprotein cholesterol levels. J. Clin. Endocrinol. Metab 92: 2680-2687.

Jakulj L, Vissers MN, Tanck MW, Hutten BA, Stellaard F, Kastelein JJ, Dallinga-Thie GM. 2010. ABCG5/G8 polymorphisms and markers of cholesterol metabolism: systematic review and meta-analysis. J. Lipid Res. 51: 3016-3023.

Jaye M, Krawiec J. 2004. Endothelial lipase and HDL metabolism. Curr. Opin. Lipidol. 15: 183-189.

Johansen CT, Hegele RA. 2011. Genetic bases of hypertriglyceridemic phenotypes. Curr. Opin. Lipidol. 22: 247-253.

Joy T, Lahiry P, Pollex RL, Hegele RA. 2008. Genetics of metabolic syndrome. Curr. Diab. Rep. 8: 141-148.

Kahn R, Buse J, Ferrannini E, Stern M. 2005. The metabolic syndrome: time for a critical appraisal: joint statement from the American Diabetes Association and the European Association for the Study of Diabetes. Diabetes Care 28: 2289-2304.

Kamboh MI, Bunker CH, Aston CE, Nestlerode CS, McAllister AE, Ukoli FA. 1999a. Genetic association of five apolipoprotein polymorphisms with serum lipoprotein-lipid levels in African blacks. Genet. Epidemiol. 16: 205-222.

Kamboh MI, Manzi S, Mehdi H, Fitzgerald S, Sanghera DK, Kuller LH, Atson CE. 1999b. Genetic variation in apolipoprotein H (beta2-glycoprotein I) affects the occurrence of antiphospholipid antibodies and apolipoprotein H concentrations in systemic lupus erythematosus. Lupus 8: 742-750.

Kataoka S, Robbins DC, Cowan LD, Go O, Yeh JL, Devereux RB, Fabsitz RR, Lee ET, Welty TK, Howard BV. 1996. Apolipoprotein E polymorphism in American Indians and its relation to plasma lipoproteins and diabetes. The Strong Heart Study. Arterioscler. Thromb. Vasc. Biol. 16: 918-925.

Kathiresan S, Melander O, Anevski D, et al. 2008a. Polymorphisms associated with cholesterol and risk of cardiovascular events. N. Engl. J. Med. 358: 1240-1249.

Kathiresan S, Melander O, Guiducci C, et al. 2008b. Six new loci associated with blood low-density lipoprotein cholesterol, high-density lipoprotein cholesterol or triglycerides in humans. Nat. Genet. 40: 189-197.

Keebler ME, Sanders CL, Surti A, Guiducci C, Burtt NP, Kathiresan S. 2009. Association of blood lipids with common DNA sequence variants at 19 genetic loci in the multiethnic United States National Health and Nutrition Examination Survey III. Circ. Cardiovasc. Genet. 2: 238-243.

Klerkx AH, Tanck MW, Kastelein JJ, Molhuizen HO, Jukema JW, Zwinderman AH, Kuivenhoven JA. 2003. Haplotype analysis of the CETP gene: not TaqIB, but the closely linked -629C-->A polymorphism and a novel promoter variant are independently associated with CETP concentration. Hum. Mol. Genet. 12: 111-123.

Klos KL, Kullo IJ. 2007. Genetic determinants of HDL: monogenic disorders and contributions to variation. Curr. Opin. Cardiol. 22: 344-351.

Klos KL, Sing CF, Boerwinkle E, Hamon SC, Rea TJ, Clark A, Fornage M, Hixson JE. 2006. Consistent effects of genes involved in reverse cholesterol transport on plasma lipid and apolipoprotein levels in CARDIA participants. Arterioscler. Thromb. Vasc. Biol. 26: 1828-1836.

Ko YL, Hsu LA, Hsu KH, Ko YH, Lee YS. 2004. The interactive effects of hepatic lipase gene promoter polymorphisms with sex and obesity on high-density-lipoprotein cholesterol levels in Taiwanese-Chinese. Atherosclerosis 172: 135-142.

Komurcu-Bayrak E, Onat A, Poda M, Humphries SE, Acharya J, Hergenc G, Coban N, Can G, Erginel-Unaltuna N. 2007. The S447X variant of lipoprotein lipase gene is associated with metabolic syndrome and lipid levels among Turks. Clin. Chim. Acta 383: 110-115.

Kretowski A, Hokanson JE, McFann K, Kinney GL, Snell-Bergeon JK, Maahs DM, Wadwa RP, Eckel RH, Ogden LG, Garg SK, Li J, Cheng S, Erlich HA, Rewers M. 2006. The apolipoprotein A-IV Gln360His polymorphism predicts progression of coronary artery calcification in patients with type 1 diabetes. Diabetologia 49: 1946-1954.

Kronenberg F, Coon H, Ellison RC, Borecki I, Arnett DK, Province MA, Eckfeldt JH, Hopkins PN, Hunt SC. 2002. Segregation analysis of HDL cholesterol in the NHLBI Family Heart Study and in Utah pedigrees. Eur. J. Hum. Genet. 10: 367-374.

Kruit JK, Brunham LR, Verchere CB, Hayden MR. 2010. HDL and LDL cholesterol significantly influence beta-cell function in type 2 diabetes mellitus. Curr. Opin. Lipidol. 21: 178-185.

Kwan BC, Kronenberg F, Beddhu S, Cheung AK. 2007. Lipoprotein metabolism and lipid management in chronic kidney disease. J. Am. Soc. Nephrol. 18: 1246-1261.

Lahiry P, Ban MR, Pollex RL, et al. 2007. Common variants APOC3, APOA5, APOE and PON1 are associated with variation in plasma lipoprotein traits in Greenlanders. Int. J. Circumpolar. Health 66: 390-400.

Lai CQ, Tai ES, Tan CE, Cutter J, Chew SK, Zhu YP, Adiconis X, Ordovas JM. 2003. The APOA5 locus is a strong determinant of plasma triglyceride concentrations across ethnic groups in Singapore. J. Lipid Res. 44: 2365-2373.

Lamarche B, Paradis ME. 2007. Endothelial lipase and the metabolic syndrome. Curr. Opin. Lipidol. 18: 298-303.

Lanktree MB, Anand SS, Yusuf S, Hegele RA. 2009. Replication of genetic associations with plasma lipoprotein traits in a multiethnic sample. J. Lipid Res. 50: 1487-1496.

Larson IA, Ordovas JM, Barnard JR, Hoffmann MM, Feussner G, Lamon-Fava S, Schaefer EJ. 2002. Effects of apolipoprotein A-I genetic variations on plasma apolipoprotein, serum lipoprotein and glucose levels. Clin Genet. 61: 176-184.

Lee J, Tan CS, Chia KS, Tan CE, Chew SK, Ordovas JM, Tai ES. 2004. The lipoprotein lipase S447X polymorphism and plasma lipids: interactions with APOE polymorphisms, smoking, and alcohol consumption. J. Lipid Res. 45: 1132-1139.

Lewington S, Whitlock G, Clarke R, Sherliker P, Emberson J, Halsey J, Qizilbash N, Peto R, Collins R. 2007. Blood cholesterol and vascular mortality by age, sex, and blood pressure: a meta-analysis of individual data from 61 prospective studies with 55,000 vascular deaths. Lancet 370: 1829-1839.

Lewis GF, Rader DJ. 2005. New insights into the regulation of HDL metabolism and reverse cholesterol transport. Circ. Res. 96: 1221-1232.

Lin HF, Boden-Albala B, Juo SH, Park N, Rundek T, Sacco RL. 2005. Heritabilities of the metabolic syndrome and its components in the Northern Manhattan Family Study. Diabetologia 48: 2006-2012.

Linsel-Nitschke P, Tall AR. 2005. HDL as a target in the treatment of atherosclerotic cardiovascular disease. Nat. Rev. Drug Discov. 4: 193-205.

Littlewood TD, Bennett MR. 2003. Apoptotic cell death in atherosclerosis. Curr. Opin. Lipidol. 14: 469-475.

Lusis AJ, Attie AD, Reue K. 2008. Metabolic syndrome: from epidemiology to systems biology. Nat. Rev. Genet. 9: 819-830.

Ma K, Cilingiroglu M, Otvos JD, Ballantyne CM, Marian AJ, Chan L. 2003. Endothelial lipase is a major genetic determinant for high-density lipoprotein concentration, structure, and metabolism. Proc. Natl. Acad. Sci. U. S. A 100: 2748-2753.

Mackness MI, Arrol S, Durrington PN. 1991. Paraoxonase prevents accumulation of lipoperoxides in low-density lipoprotein. FEBS Lett. 286: 152-154.

Mailly F, Tugrul Y, Reymer PW, et al. 1995. A common variant in the gene for lipoprotein lipase (Asp9-->Asn). Functional implications and prevalence in normal and hyperlipidemic subjects. Arterioscler. Thromb. Vasc. Biol. 15: 468-478.

Mank-Seymour AR, Durham KL, Thompson JF, Seymour AB, Milos PM. 2004. Association between single-nucleotide polymorphisms in the endothelial lipase (LIPG) gene and high-density lipoprotein cholesterol levels. Biochim. Biophys. Acta 1636: 40-46.

Manresa JM, Zamora A, Tomas M, et al. 2006. Relationship of classical and non-classical risk factors with genetic variants relevant to coronary heart disease. Eur. J. Cardiovasc. Prev. Rehabil. 13: 738-744.

Maxwell KN, Fisher EA, Breslow JL. 2005. Overexpression of PCSK9 accelerates the degradation of the LDLR in a post-endoplasmic reticulum compartment. Proc. Natl. Acad. Sci. U. S. A 102: 2069-2074.

McCaskie PA, Cadby G, Hung J, McQuillan BM, Chapman CM, Carter KW, Thompson PL, Palmer LJ, Beilby JP. 2006. The C-480T hepatic lipase polymorphism is associated with HDL-C but not with risk of coronary heart disease. Clin. Genet. 70: 114-121.

Miettinen HE, Gylling H, Tenhunen J, et al. 1998. Molecular genetic study of Finns with hypoalphalipoproteinemia and hyperalphalipoproteinemia: a novel Gly230 Arg mutation (LCAT[Fin]) of lecithin:cholesterol acyltransferase (LCAT) accounts for 5% of cases with very low serum HDL cholesterol levels. Arterioscler. Thromb. Vasc. Biol. 18: 591-598.

Miller M, Rhyne J, Chen H, Beach V, Ericson R, Luthra K, Dwivedi M, Misra A. 2007. APOC3 promoter polymorphisms C-482T and T-455C are associated with the metabolic syndrome. Arch. Med. Res. 38: 444-451.

Miller M, Rhyne J, Hamlette S, Birnbaum J, Rodriguez A. 2003. Genetics of HDL regulation in humans. Curr. Opin. Lipidol. 14: 273-279.

Miller M, Zhan M. 2004. Genetic determinants of low high-density lipoprotein cholesterol. Curr. Opin. Cardiol. 19: 380-384.

Monda KL, North KE, Hunt SC, Rao DC, Province MA, Kraja AT. 2010. The genetics of obesity and the metabolic syndrome. Endocr. Metab Immune. Disord. Drug Targets. 10: 86-108.

Morabia A, Ross BM, Costanza MC, Cayanis E, Flaherty MS, Alvin GB, Das K, James R, Yang AS, Evagrafov O, Gilliam TC. 2004. Population-based study of SR-BI genetic variation and lipid profile. Atherosclerosis 175: 159-168.

Murthy V, Julien P, Gagne C. 1996. Molecular pathobiology of the human lipoprotein lipase gene. Pharmacol Ther. 70: 101-135.

Musunuru K, Pirruccello JP, Do R, et al. 2010. Exome sequencing, ANGPTL3 mutations, and familial combined hypolipidemia. N. Engl. J. Med. 363: 2220-2227.

Nettleton JA, Steffen LM, Ballantyne CM, Boerwinkle E, Folsom AR. 2007. Associations between HDL-cholesterol and polymorphisms in hepatic lipase and lipoprotein lipase genes are modified by dietary fat intake in African American and White adults. Atherosclerosis 194: e131-e140.

Nock NL, Li L, Larkin EK, Patel SR, Redline S. 2009a. Empirical evidence for "syndrome Z": a hierarchical 5-factor model of the metabolic syndrome incorporating sleep disturbance measures. Sleep 32: 615-622.

Nock NL, Wang X, Thompson CL, Song Y, Baechle D, Raska P, Stein CM, Gray-McGuire C. 2009b. Defining genetic determinants of the Metabolic Syndrome in the Framingham Heart Study using association and structural equation modeling methods. BMC. Proc. 3 Suppl 7: S50.

Ordovas JM, Shen J. 2008. Gene-environment interactions and susceptibility to metabolic syndrome and other chronic diseases. J. Periodontol. 79: 1508-1513.

Osgood D, Corella D, Demissie S, et al. 2003. Genetic variation at the scavenger receptor class B type I gene locus determines plasma lipoprotein concentrations and particle size and interacts with type 2 diabetes: the framingham study. J. Clin Endocrinol. Metab 88: 2869-2879.

Ota VK, Chen ES, Ejchel TF, Furuya TK, Mazzotti DR, Cendoroglo MS, Ramos LR, Araujo LQ, Burbano RR, Smith MD. 2011. APOA4 Polymorphism as a Risk Factor for Unfavorable Lipid Serum Profile and Depression: A Cross-Sectional Study. J. Investig. Med.

Pallaud C, Sass C, Zannad F, Siest G, Visvikis S. 2001. APOC3, CETP, fibrinogen, and MTHFR are genetic determinants of carotid intima-media thickness in healthy men (the Stanislas cohort). Clin Genet. 59: 316-324.

Paradis ME, Couture P, Bosse Y, Despres JP, Perusse L, Bouchard C, Vohl MC, Lamarche B. 2003. The T111I mutation in the EL gene modulates the impact of dietary fat on the HDL profile in women. J. Lipid Res. 44: 1902-1908.

Pare G, Serre D, Brisson D, Anand SS, Montpetit A, Tremblay G, Engert JC, Hudson TJ, Gaudet D. 2007. Genetic analysis of 103 candidate genes for coronary artery disease and associated phenotypes in a founder population reveals a new association between endothelin-1 and high-density lipoprotein cholesterol. Am. J. Hum. Genet. 80: 673-682.

Phillips CM, Tierney AC, Roche HM. 2008. Gene-nutrient interactions in the metabolic syndrome. J. Nutrigenet. Nutrigenomics. 1: 136-151.

Polisecki E, Muallem H, Maeda N, et al. 2008. Genetic variation at the LDL receptor and HMG-CoA reductase gene loci, lipid levels, statin response, and cardiovascular disease incidence in PROSPER. Atherosclerosis 200: 109-114.

Pollex RL, Hanley AJ, Zinman B, Harris SB, Khan HM, Hegele RA. 2006. Metabolic syndrome in aboriginal Canadians: prevalence and genetic associations. Atherosclerosis 184: 121-129.

Pollex RL, Hegele RA. 2006. Genetic determinants of the metabolic syndrome. Nat. Clin Pract. Cardiovasc. Med. 3: 482-489.

Porchay I, Pean F, Bellili N, et al. 2006. ABCA1 single nucleotide polymorphisms on high-density lipoprotein-cholesterol and overweight: the D.E.S.I.R. study. Obesity. (Silver. Spring) 14: 1874-1879.

Qi L, Liu S, Rifai N, Hunter D, Hu FB. 2007. Associations of the apolipoprotein A1/C3/A4/A5 gene cluster with triglyceride and HDL cholesterol levels in women with type 2 diabetes. Atherosclerosis 192: 204-210.

Remaley AT, Stonik JA, Demosky SJ, et al. 2001. Apolipoprotein specificity for lipid efflux by the human ABCAI transporter. Biochem. Biophys. Res. Commun. 280: 818-823.

Rigotti A, Trigatti B, Babitt J, Penman M, Xu S, Krieger M. 1997. Scavenger receptor BI--a cell surface receptor for high density lipoprotein. Curr. Opin. Lipidol. 8: 181-188.

Rios DL, D'Onofrio LO, Cerqueira CC, et al. 2007. Paraoxonase 1 gene polymorphisms in angiographically assessed coronary artery disease: evidence for gender interaction among Brazilians. Clin. Chem. Lab Med. 45: 874-878.

Rip J, Nierman MC, Ross CJ, Jukema JW, Hayden MR, Kastelein JJ, Stroes ES, Kuivenhoven JA. 2006. Lipoprotein lipase S447X: a naturally occurring gain-of-function mutation. Arterioscler. Thromb. Vasc. Biol. 26: 1236-1245.

Roberts CG, Shen H, Mitchell BD, Damcott CM, Shuldiner AR, Rodriguez A. 2007. Variants in scavenger receptor class B type I gene are associated with HDL cholesterol levels in younger women. Hum. Hered. 64: 107-113.

Roth GA, Fihn SD, Mokdad AH. 2010. High total serum cholesterol, medication coverage and therapeutic control: an analysis of national health examination survey data from eight countries. In: pp. 92-101.

Russo GT, Meigs JB, Cupples LA, et al. 2001. Association of the Sst-I polymorphism at the APOC3 gene locus with variations in lipid levels, lipoprotein subclass profiles and coronary heart disease risk: the Framingham offspring study. Atherosclerosis 158: 173-181.

Sagoo GS, Tatt I, Salanti G, Butterworth AS, Sarwar N, van MM, Jukema JW, Wiman B, Kastelein JJ, Bennet AM, de FU, Danesh J, Higgins JP. 2008. Seven lipoprotein lipase gene polymorphisms, lipid fractions, and coronary disease: a HuGE association review and meta-analysis. Am. J. Epidemiol. 168: 1233-1246.

Senti M, Elosua R, Tomas M, Sala J, Masia R, Ordovas JM, Shen H, Marrugat J. 2001. Physical activity modulates the combined effect of a common variant of the lipoprotein lipase gene and smoking on serum triglyceride levels and high-density lipoprotein cholesterol in men. Hum. Genet. 109: 385-392.

Shan L, Yu XC, Liu Z, Hu Y, Sturgis LT, Miranda ML, Liu Q. 2009. The angiopoietin-like proteins ANGPTL3 and ANGPTL4 inhibit lipoprotein lipase activity through distinct mechanisms. J. Biol. Chem. 284: 1419-1424.

Sharma V, McNeill JH. 2006. The etiology of hypertension in the metabolic syndrome part one: an introduction to the history, the concept and the models. Curr. Vasc. Pharmacol 4: 293-304.

Shimizugawa T, Ono M, Shimamura M, Yoshida K, Ando Y, Koishi R, Ueda K, Inaba T, Minekura H, Kohama T, Furukawa H. 2002. ANGPTL3 decreases very low density lipoprotein triglyceride clearance by inhibition of lipoprotein lipase. J. Biol. Chem. 277: 33742-33748.

Shioji K, Mannami T, Kokubo Y, Goto Y, Nonogi H, Iwai N. 2004a. An association analysis between ApoA1 polymorphisms and the high-density lipoprotein (HDL) cholesterol level and myocardial infarction (MI) in Japanese. J. Hum. Genet. 49: 433-439.

Shioji K, Nishioka J, Naraba H, et al. 2004b. A promoter variant of the ATP-binding cassette transporter A1 gene alters the HDL cholesterol level in the general Japanese population. J. Hum. Genet. 49: 141-147.

Sookoian S, Pirola CJ. 2011. Metabolic syndrome: from the genetics to the pathophysiology. Curr. Hypertens. Rep. 13: 149-157.

Srinivasan SR, Ehnholm C, Elkasabany A, Berenson G. 1999. Influence of apolipoprotein E polymorphism on serum lipids and lipoprotein changes from childhood to adulthood: the Bogalusa Heart Study. Atherosclerosis 143: 435-443.

Sung J, Lee K, Song YM. 2009. Heritabilities of the metabolic syndrome phenotypes and related factors in Korean twins. J. Clin Endocrinol. Metab 94: 4946-4952.

Sviridov D, Nestel PJ. 2007. Genetic factors affecting HDL levels, structure, metabolism and function. Curr. Opin. Lipidol. 18: 157-163.

Tai ES, Corella D, Deurenberg-Yap M, Cutter J, Chew SK, Tan CE, Ordovas JM. 2003a. Dietary fat interacts with the -514C>T polymorphism in the hepatic lipase gene promoter on plasma lipid profiles in a multiethnic Asian population: the 1998 Singapore National Health Survey. J. Nutr. 133: 3399-3408.

Tai ES, Ordovas JM, Corella D, Deurenberg-Yap M, Chan E, Adiconis X, Chew SK, Loh LM, Tan CE. 2003b. The TaqIB and -629C>A polymorphisms at the cholesteryl ester transfer protein locus: associations with lipid levels in a multiethnic population. The 1998 Singapore National Health Survey. Clin. Genet. 63: 19-30.

Talmud PJ, Hawe E, Martin S, Olivier M, Miller GJ, Rubin EM, Pennacchio LA, Humphries SE. 2002a. Relative contribution of variation within the APOC3/A4/A5 gene cluster in determining plasma triglycerides. Hum. Mol. Genet. 11: 3039-3046.

Talmud PJ, Hawe E, Robertson K, Miller GJ, Miller NE, Humphries SE. 2002b. Genetic and environmental determinants of plasma high density lipoprotein cholesterol and apolipoprotein AI concentrations in healthy middle-aged men. Ann. Hum. Genet. 66: 111-124.

Tang NP, Wang LS, Yang L, Zhou B, Gu HJ, Sun QM, Cong RH, Zhu HJ, Wang B. 2008. Protective effect of an endothelial lipase gene variant on coronary artery disease in a Chinese population. J. Lipid Res. 49: 369-375.

Teslovich TM, Musunuru K, Smith AV, Edmondson AC, et al. 2010. Biological, clinical and population relevance of 95 loci for blood lipids. Nature 466: 707-713.

Thompson A, Di AE, Sarwar N, Erqou S, Saleheen D, Dullaart RP, Keavney B, Ye Z, Danesh J. 2008. Association of cholesteryl ester transfer protein genotypes with CETP mass and activity, lipid levels, and coronary risk. JAMA 299: 2777-2788.

van Aalst-Cohen ES, Jansen AC, Boekholdt SM, Tanck MW, Fontecha MR, Cheng S, Li J, Defesche JC, Kuivenhoven JA, Kastelein JJ. 2005. Genetic determinants of plasma HDL-cholesterol levels in familial hypercholesterolemia. Eur. J. Hum. Genet. 13: 1137-1142.

Volcik KA, Barkley RA, Hutchinson RG, Mosley TH, Heiss G, Sharrett AR, Ballantyne CM, Boerwinkle E. 2006. Apolipoprotein E polymorphisms predict low density lipoprotein cholesterol levels and carotid artery wall thickness but not incident coronary heart disease in 12,491 ARIC study participants. Am. J. Epidemiol. 164: 342-348.

Wang J, Ban MR, Zou GY, Cao H, Lin T, Kennedy BA, Anand S, Yusuf S, Huff MW, Pollex RL, Hegele RA. 2008. Polygenic determinants of severe hypertriglyceridemia. Hum. Mol. Genet. 17: 2894-2899.

Wang X, Paigen B. 2005. Genetics of variation in HDL cholesterol in humans and mice. Circ. Res. 96: 27-42.

Waterworth DM, Ricketts SL, Song K, et al. 2010. Genetic variants influencing circulating lipid levels and risk of coronary artery disease. Arterioscler. Thromb. Vasc. Biol. 30: 2264-2276.

Whiting BM, Anderson JL, Muhlestein JB, Horne BD, Bair TL, Pearson RR, Carlquist JF. 2005. Candidate gene susceptibility variants predict intermediate end points but not angiographic coronary artery disease. Am. Heart J. 150: 243-250.

Willer CJ, Sanna S, Jackson AU, et al. 2008. Newly identified loci that influence lipid concentrations and risk of coronary artery disease. Nat. Genet. 40: 161-169.

Wilson PW, Myers RH, Larson MG, Ordovas JM, Wolf PA, Schaefer EJ. 1994. Apolipoprotein E alleles, dyslipidemia, and coronary heart disease. The Framingham Offspring Study. JAMA 272: 1666-1671.

Wittrup HH, Tybjaerg-Hansen A, Nordestgaard BG. 1999. Lipoprotein lipase mutations, plasma lipids and lipoproteins, and risk of ischemic heart disease. A meta-analysis. Circulation 99: 2901-2907.

Wu K, Bowman R, Welch AA, Luben RN, Wareham N, Khaw KT, Bingham SA. 2007. Apolipoprotein E polymorphisms, dietary fat and fibre, and serum lipids: the EPIC Norfolk study. Eur. Heart J. 28: 2930-2936.

Yamada Y, Ichihara S, Kato K, et al. 2008. Genetic risk for metabolic syndrome: examination of candidate gene polymorphisms related to lipid metabolism in Japanese people. J. Med. Genet. 45: 22-28.

Yamada Y, Matsuo H, Warita S, et al. 2007. Prediction of genetic risk for dyslipidemia. Genomics 90: 551-558.

Yamakawa-Kobayashi K, Yanagi H, Endo K, Arinami T, Hamaguchi H. 2003. Relationship between serum HDL-C levels and common genetic variants of the endothelial lipase gene in Japanese school-aged children. Hum. Genet. 113: 311-315.

Zhang K, Zhang S, Zheng K, Hou Y, Liao L, He Y, Zhang L, Nebert DW, Shi J, Su Z, Xiao C. 2004. Novel P143L polymorphism of the LCAT gene is associated with dyslipidemia in Chinese patients who have coronary atherosclerotic heart disease. Biochem. Biophys. Res. Commun. 318: 4-10.

Zhu XY, Xu HW, Hou RY, Liu HF, Xiao B, Yang XS, Yang QD, Tang BS. 2006. [Lecithin-cholesterol acyltransferase gene 608C/T polymorphism associated with atherosclerotic cerebral infarction]. Zhonghua Yi. Xue. Yi. Chuan Xue. Za Zhi. 23: 419-422.

6

Impact of Climate Change and Air Pollution on Dyslipidemia and the Components of Metabolic Syndrome

Roya Kelishadi[1] and Parinaz Poursafa[2]
[1]Faculty of Medicine & Child Health Promotion Research Center,
Isfahan University of Medical Sciences, Isfahan,
[2]Environment Research Center,
Isfahan University of Medical Sciences, Isfahan,
Iran

1. Introduction

Environmental factors, notably climate change and air pollution influence health before conception, and continue during pregnancy, childhood, and adolescence. Experts have suggested that such health hazards may represent the greatest public health challenge humanity has faced. The accumulation of greenhouse gases such as carbon dioxide, primarily from burning fossil fuels results in warming, which has an impact on air pollution, particularly on levels of ozone and particulates. Heat-related health effects include increased rates of pregnancy complications, pre-eclampsia, eclampsia, low birth weight, renal effects, vector-borne diseases as malaria and dengue; increased diarrheal and respiratory disease, food insecurity, decreased quality of foods (notably grains), malnutrition, water scarcity, exposures to toxic chemicals, worsened poverty, natural disasters, and population displacement. Air pollution has many adverse health effects, which would have long-term impact on the components of the metabolic syndrome. In addition to short-term effects as premature labor, intrauterine growth retardation, neonatal and infant mortality rate, malignancies (notably leukemia and Hodgkin lymphoma), respiratory diseases, allergic disorders and anemia, exposure to criteria air pollutants from early life might be associated with dyslipidemia, increase in stress oxidative, inflammation and endothelial dysfunction which in turn might have long-term effects on chronic non-communicable diseases.

2. Environmental factors: Climate change and air pollution

2.1 Air pollutants

Air pollution is a mixture of solid particles and gases in the air. The six common and hazardous air pollutants consist of particulate matter, ground-level ozone, carbon monoxide, sulfur oxides, nitrogen oxides, and lead; of which, particle pollution and ground-level ozone are the most widespread health hazards (Samet & Krewski, 2007; Chen & Kan, 2008).

Particulate matter or PM consists of a diverse mixture of very small particles and liquid droplets suspended in air. The PM size is directly related to their potential for affecting health. Particles with diameter < 10 micrometers are the particles that usually pass through the throat and nose to enter the lungs. Then, they can affect different body organs especially the heart and lungs, and may cause serious health effects. According to the size, the particle pollution is grouped into: "inhalable coarse particles" which have a diameter of 2.5 to 10 micrometers, and are found near roadways and industries, and "fine particles" < 2.5 micrometers in diameter such as those found in smoke and haze; they can form when gases emitted from power plants, industries and automobiles react in the air. Ozone (O_3) is a gas composed of three oxygen atoms. In the presence of sunlight, it is created at ground-level by a chemical reaction between oxides of nitrogen and volatile organic compounds. Ozone might have harmful effects when formed in the earth's lower atmosphere, i.e. at ground-level. Hot weather and sunlight cause ground-level ozone to form in harmful concentrations in the air. Carbon monoxide (CO) is an odorless and colorless gas formed by incomplete carbon combustion. It is mainly emitted from the motor vehicle exhaust followed by non-road engines as construction equipment, industrial processes and wood burning. The increasing number of cars has an important role in the increase in CO emission worldwide. Sulfur Dioxide (SO_2) is a gas formed when fuel containing sulfur, such as coal and oil, is burned, and when gasoline is extracted from oil or metals are extracted from ore. Nitrogen oxides (Nox) are a group of highly reactive gases containing various levels of nitrogen and oxygen. Lead is usually emitted from motor vehicles and industrial sources (Chen & Kan, 2008; Brook et al., 2004). Other stationary sources are waste incinerators, utilities, and lead-acid battery manufacturers. In addition to exposure to lead in air, other major exposure pathways include ingestion of lead in drinking water and lead-contaminated food as well as incidental ingestion of lead-contaminated soil and dust. Lead-based paint remains a major exposure pathway in older homes. Some toys might contain considerable amounts of lead that would be harmful for children's health (Samet & Krewski, 2007; Han & Naeher, 2006).

2.2 Climate change

Climate change and global warming have various health hazards (Poursafa & Kelishadi 2011).

Climate change has an impact on levels of ozone and particulate matters, which are both associated with various health hazards. The accumulation of greenhouse gases such as carbon dioxide, primarily from burning fossil fuels results in warming. Heat increases ground level ozone production, which in turn augments morbidity and mortality (Bell et al., 2007). Moreover, warming increases water vapor and ground-level ozone formation, and will result in harmful ozone levels (Jacob & Winner, 2009). Warming modify the risk of forest fires, and may generate massive amounts of carcinogens, as formaldehyde and benzene, potent lung irritants, as acrolein and other aldehydes, carbon monoxide, and particulates (Wegesser et al., 2009).

3. Association of environmental factors and dyslipidemia

Environmental factors are associated with many chronic diseases. Air pollution and climate change are associated with risk factors of non-communicable diseases in children and adolescents (Kelishadi et al., 2009; Sheffield & Landrigan, 2011; Kelishadi & Poursafa, 2010; Mansourian et al., 2010; Poursafa et al., 2011; Kargarfard et al., 2011).

The effects of environmental factors on intrauterine growth retardation and preterm labor are well documented. In turn, low birth weight (Sinclair et al., 2007) and prematurity (Evensen et al., 2008) would increase the risk of chronic non-communicable diseases and their risk factors. Exposure to air pollutants is reported to be associated with stress oxidative and markers of insulin resistance (Kelishadi et al., 2010) as well as with diabetes mellitus (Brook et al., 2008). These systemic responses to environmental factors can potentially increase the risk for dyslipidemia, development of the metabolic syndrome, hypertension, and other chronic diseases.Moreover, it is documented that some environmental factors as increased humidity are associated with preeclampsia and eclampsia, and their related consequences (Subramaniam, 2007).

Several reports exist on the association of environmental factors with dyslipidemia and the components of metabolic syndrome. By applying generalized additive models, Secondary analyses of a Taiwanese survey in 2002 demonstrated that increased particulate matter with aerodynamic diameters <10 microm was associated with elevated systolic blood pressure, triglycerides, apolipoprotein B, hemoglobin A1c, and reduced high-density lipoprotein (HDL) cholesterol. Elevated ozone was associated with increased diastolic blood pressure, apolipoprotein B, and hemoglobin A1c (Chuang et al., 2010). Genetic-environment interactions may have a role in this regard (Eisenberg et al., 2010).

The associations of both obesity and air pollution with several age-related diseases remain poorly understood with regard to causality and underlying mechanisms. Exposure to both, excess body fat and particulate matter, is accompanied by systemic low-grade inflammation as well as alterations in insulin/insulin-like growth factor signaling and cell cycle control. Understanding the causality of exposure disease associations and differences in susceptibilities to environment and lifestyle is an important aspect for effective prevention (Probst-Hensch, 2010).

A case-control study evaluated the effects of urban pollution on the lipid balance of members of a municipal police force in comparison with controls. Mean and frequency distributions of HDL-cholesterol and triglycerides had significant difference between the exposed traffic police group and controls. This study suggested that some chemical agents, as carbon dioxide, of the urban pollution could cause dyslipidemia among exposed people (Tomao et al., 2002).

A study among asthmatic patients showed that with a 1-microg/m3 increase in coarse PM, triglycerides increased 4.8% (p = 0.02), and very low-density lipoprotein increased 1.15% (p = 0.01). This study suggested that small temporal increases in ambient coarse PM are sufficient to affect lipid profile in adults with asthma (Yeatts et al., 2007).

Hypercholesterolemia may potentiate diesel exhaust-related endothelial gene regulation. These regulated transcripts may implicate pathways involved in the acceleration of atherosclerosis by air pollution (Maresh et al., 2011). The systemic pro-inflammatory and pro-thrombotic response to the inhalation of fine and ultrafine particulate matters may be associated with platelet activation (Poursafa & Kelishadi, 2010 platelets).

A study conducted in Greece, explored the relations between ambient environmental factors and arterial stiffness, peripheral and central hemodynamics in a cohort of 1222 participants.It found that the exposure to lower environmental temperatures is related to impaired hemodynamics not only to the periphery but also to the aorta. In men, PM10 levels were associated with intensified amplitude of the reflection wave resulting in significant alterations in central-pulse pressure (Adamopoulos et al., 2010).

A study examined the associations of PM2.5 with heart rate variability, a marker of autonomic function, and whether metabolic syndrome modified these associations. It found significant correlations; which were stronger among individuals with metabolic syndrome than among those without it. This study proposed that autonomic dysfunction may be a mechanism through which PM exposure affects cardiovascular risk, especially among persons with metabolic syndrome (Park et al., 2010).

Exposure to high and low air temperatures are associated with cardiovascular mortality, the underlying mechanisms are still under investigation. In a cohort in the US, 478 men with a mean age of 74.2 years were followed up from 1995 to 2008. Associations of three temperature variables, i.e. ambient, apparent, and dew point temperature with serum lipid profile were studied with linear mixed models by including possible confounders such as air pollution and a random intercept for each individual. HDL decreased -1.76%, and -5.58% for each 5°C increase in mean ambient temperature. For the same increase in mean ambient temperature, LDL increased by 1.74% and 1.87%. Similar results were also found for apparent and dew point temperatures. No changes were found in total cholesterol or triglycerides in relation to temperature increase. This study suggested that changes in HDL and LDL levels, which are associated with an increase in ambient temperature, may be among the underlying mechanisms of temperature-related cardiovascular mortality (Halonen et al., 2011).

A study in Taiwan found that increased 1-year average ozone, PM and nitrogen dioxide were associated with elevated blood pressure, total cholesterol, fasting glucose, and HbA1c. PM2.5 was more significantly associated with end-point variables than other gaseous pollutants (Chuang et al., 2011). A study on the association of blood markers of cardiovascular risk and air pollution in a national sample of the U.S. population found that PM_{10}, but not gaseous air pollutants, is associated with blood markers of cardiovascular risk (Schwartz, 2001). In a study in Italy, the carboxyhaemoglobin concentration had an inverse correlation with HDL-C (Biava et al., 1992). In addition to the outdoor environment, the health hazards of indoor pollution should be considered (Kaplan, 2010).

In recent years, global climate change has affected many biological and environmental factors. Of its most important effects are the increasing levels of atmospheric carbon dioxide, ultraviolet radiation, and ocean temperatures. In turn, they have resulted in decreased marine phytoplankton growth and reduced synthesis of omega-3 polyunsaturated fatty acids. It is suggested that the detrimental effects of climate change on the oceans may reduce the availability of dietary omega-3, which may have detrimental effects on serum lipid profile (Kang, 2011).

4. Conclusion

Climate change may alter concentrations of air pollutants or alterations in mechanisms of pollutant transport and thus influence individual and public health. The potential impacts of climate change and air pollution on lipid disorders is considered as an important area of investigation. This is of special concern for low- and middle-income countries, where the burden of air pollution and climate-related health disorders, and the burden of non-communicable diseases are emerging. Effects of environmental factors on dyslipidemia should be considered in primordial and primary prevention of chronic diseases from early life.

5. References

Adamopoulos D, Vyssoulis G, Karpanou E, Kyvelou SM, Argacha JF, Cokkinos D, Stefanadis C, van de Borne P.Environmental determinants of blood pressure, arterial stiffness, and central hemodynamics. J Hypertens 2010;28(5):903-9.

Bell ML, Goldberg R, Hogrefe C, et al. Climate change, ambient ozone, and health in 50 US cities. Climatic Change 2007; 82:61-76.

Biava PM, Audisio R, Centonze A, Barbieri A, Bisanti L, Duca G. [An epidemiological study of the health conditions of Milan traffic police with respect to pollution from vehicular traffic]. Lav 1992;83(3):249-58.

Brook RD, Franklin B, Cascio W. Expert Panel on Population and Prevention Science of the American Heart Association. Air pollution and cardiovascular disease: a statement for healthcare professionals from the Expert Panel on Population and Prevention Science of the American Heart Association. Circulation 2004; 109: 2655-71.

Chen B, Kan H. Air pollution and population health: a global challenge.Environ Health Prev Med 2008;13:94-101.

Chuang KJ, Yan YH, Cheng TJ. Effect of air pollution on blood pressure, blood lipids, and blood sugar: a population-based approach. J Occup Environ Med 2010;52(3):258-62.

Eisenberg DT, Kuzawa CW, Hayes MG. Worldwide allele frequencies of the human apolipoprotein E gene: climate, local adaptations, and evolutionary history. Am J Phys Anthropol 2010;143(1):100-11.

Evensen KA, Steinshamn S, Tjønna AE, Stølen T, Høydal MA, Wisløff U, et al. Effects of preterm birth and fetal growth retardation on cardiovascular risk factors in young adulthood. Early Hum Dev 2008: 85:239-45.

Halonen JI, Zanobetti A, Sparrow D, Vokonas PS, Schwartz J. Outdoor temperature is associated with serum HDL and LDL. Environ Res 2011 ;111(2):281-7.

Han X, Naeher LP. A review of traffic-related air pollution exposure assessment studies in the developing world. Environ Int 2006; 32:106-20.

Jacob D, Winner D. Effect of climate change on air quality. Atmospheric Environ 2009; 43:51-63.

Kang JX.Omega-3: a link between global climate change and human health. Biotechnol Adv. 2011;29(4):388-90.

Kaplan C. Indoor air pollution from unprocessed solid fuels in developing countries. Reviews on Environmental Health 2010 ; 25(3) : 221-42.

Kargarfard M, Poursafa P, Rezanejad S, Mousavinasab F. Effects of exercise in polluted air on the aerobic power, serum lactate level and cell blood count of active individuals. Int J Prev Med 2011; 2(3): 145-50.

Kelishadi R, Mirghaffari N, Poursafa P, Gidding SS. Lifestyle and environmental factors associated with inflammation, oxidative stress and insulin resistance in children. Atherosclerosis 2009; 203: 311-9.

Kelishadi R, Poursafa P. Air pollution and non-respiratory health hazards for children. Arch Med Sci.2010; 6: 483-95.

Mansourian M, Javanmard SH, Poursafa P, Kelishadi R. Air pollution and hospitalization for respiratory diseases among children in Isfahan, Iran. Ghana Med J. 2010; 44(4):138-43.

Maresh JG, Campen MJ, Reed MD, Darrow AL, Shohet RV. Hypercholesterolemia potentiates aortic endothelial response to inhaled diesel exhaust. Inhal Toxicol2011;23(1):1-10.

Park SK, Auchincloss AH, O'Neill MS, Prineas R, Correa JC, Keeler J, Barr RG, Kaufman JD, Diez Roux AV. Particulate air pollution, metabolic syndrome, and heart rate variability: the multi-ethnic study of atherosclerosis (MESA). Environ Health Perspect. 2010 Oct;118(10):1406-11.

Poursafa P, Kelishadi R. Air pollution, platelet activation and atherosclerosis. Inflamm Allergy Drug Targets 2010;9 (5):387-92.

Poursafa P, Kelishadi R, Lahijanzadeh A, Modaresi M, Javanmard SH, Assari R, et al. The relationship of air pollution and surrogate markers of endothelial dysfunction in a population-based sample of children. BMC Public Health 2011;11:115.

Poursafa P, Kelishadi R, Moattar F, Rafiei L, Amin MM, Lahijanzadeh A, et al. Genetic variation in the association of air pollutants with a biomarker of vascular injury in children and adolescents in Isfahan, Iran. J Res Med Sci 2011;16(6)

Probst-Hensch NM. Chronic age-related diseases share risk factors: do they share pathophysiological mechanisms and why does that matter? Swiss Med Wkly 2010 1;140: w13072.

Samet J, Krewski D. Health effects associated with exposure to ambient air pollution. J Toxicol Environ Health A 2007; 70:227-42.

Schwartz J. Air pollution and blood markers of cardiovascular risk. Environ Health Perspect. 2001;109 Suppl 3:405-9

Sinclair KD, Lea RG, Rees WD, Young LE.The developmental origins of health and disease: current theories and epigenetic mechanisms. Soc Reprod Fertil 2007;Suppl. 64:425-43.

Sheffield PE, Landrigan PJ. Global climate change and children's health: threats and strategies for prevention. Environ Health Perspect 2011;119(3):291-8.

Subramaniam V. Seasonal variation in the incidence of preeclampsia and eclampsia in tropical climatic conditions. BMC Womens Health. 2007;7:18

Tomao E, Tiziana PB, Rosati V, Marcellini L, Tomei F. The effects of air pollution on the lipid balance of traffic police personnel. Ann Saudi Med 2002;22(5-6):287-90.

Yeatts K, Svendsen E, Creason J, Alexis N, Herbst M, Scott J, Kupper L, Williams R, Neas L, Cascio W, Devlin RB, Peden DB. Coarse particulate matter (PM2.5-10) affects heart rate variability, blood lipids, and circulating eosinophils in adults with asthma. Environ Health Perspect. 2007;115(5):709-14.

Wegesser TC, Pinkerton KE, Last JA. California Wildfires of 2008: coarse and fine particulate matter toxicity. Environ Health Perspect 2009; 117:893-7

7

Functions of OSBP/ORP Family Proteins and Their Relation to Dyslipidemia

Hiroshi Koriyama, Hironori Nakagami,
Tomohiro Katsuya and Ryuichi Morishita
Osaka University
Japan

1. Introduction

The pathway of intracellular cholesterol synthesis, uptake and efflux is much affected by both the positive and the negative feedbacks from direct interaction between cholesterol and its oxygenated derivatives (oxysterols) as well as the regulatory factors such as the sterol-regulatory-element-binding protein (SREBP)– cleavage-activating protein–Insig complex (Radhakrishnan, Ikeda et al. 2007), 3-hydroxy-3-methylglutaryl-CoA (HMG-CoA) reductase (Sever, Song et al. 2003) and liver X receptors (LXRs) (Chen, Chen et al. 2007). Since these regulatory factors are located in the compartments with comparatively low cholesterol density, they can react promptly on acute changes in local cholesterol or oxysterol density. While much is known about the interaction between these regulatory factors and cholesterol, only little has been studied about the mechanism to deliver the cholesterol or oxysterol to its appropriate compartments.

Therefore, there arises a possibility that oxysterol-binding protein/oxysterol-binding protein-related protein (OSBP/ORP) family may regulate such processes by binding oxyterol and/or cholesterol and by functioning as a cholesterol sensor or cholesterol transporter. According to the study about the family members, it is now becoming clear that they affect the regulation such as the cholesterol or triglyceride level.

For comprehensive information on OSBP/ORP family, please refer to several good reviews already published (Fairn and McMaster 2008; Ngo, Colbourne et al. 2010; Raychaudhuri and Prinz 2010; Vihervaara, Jansen et al. 2011). This review focuses more on the family's association with dyslipidemia from a perspective of the individual features of the structure, the expression, the cellular localization, the molecular functions, and the epidemiologial study-based information of each member.

2. Overview of functions of OSBP/ORP family proteins and their relation to dyslipidemia

It has become widely known that each member of OSBP/ORP family respectively affects diverse processes considered to have an association with dyslipidemia, such as intracellular trafficking of cholesterol or neutral lipid. The first presented is a brief overview of the members as a whole before the individual explanation of each member.

OSBP negatively regulates ATP-binding cassette transporter A1 (ABCA1) protein stability (Bowden and Ridgway 2008). OSBP induces upregulation of SREBP-1c and enhances hepatic lipogenesis (Yan, Lehto et al. 2007).

ORP1L forms a RILP-Rab7-ORP1L complex (Johansson, Rocha et al. 2007) and is involved in both protein and lipid transport functions of the late endocytic compartments (Vihervaara, Uronen et al. 2011).

ORP1S and ORP2 enhance plasma membrane (PM)-to-lipid droplet (LD) sterol transport (Jansen, Ohsaki et al. 2011). ORP2 presents on LD and has a functional role in the regulation of neutral lipid metabolism, possibly as a factor that integrates the cellular metabolism of triglycerides (TG) with that of cholesterol (Hynynen, Suchanek et al. 2009).

ORP3 may play an important role in efficient directed membrane trafficking (Lehto, Mayranpaa et al. 2008). But the direct evidence that ORP3 functions to regulate dyslipidemia is yet to be reported.

ORP4 in an interaction with intermediate filaments inhibits an intracellular cholesterol-transport pathway mediated by vimentin (Wang, JeBailey et al. 2002).

ORP5 may cooperate with Niemann-Pick C1 (NPC1) to mediate the exit of cholesterol from endosomes/lysosomes (Du, Kumar et al. 2011).

ORP6 is identified as one of the candidate genes that are possibly involved in the regulation of high-density lipoprotein (HDL) cholesterol levels (North, Martin et al. 2003).

SNPs near ORP7 gene show a genome-wide significant association with low-density lipoprotein (LDL) cholesterol (Teslovich, Musunuru et al. 2010).

ORP8 negatively regulates ABCA1 expression and macrophage cholesterol efflux (Yan, Mayranpaa et al. 2008). ORP8 has the capacity to modulate lipid homeostasis and SREBP activity, probably through an indirect mechanism required Nup62 (Zhou, Li et al. 2011). The OSBPL8-ZDHHC17 region (chr12) is detected for HDL cholesterol identified by one new SNP with genome-wide significance (Ma, Yang et al. 2010).

ORP9 and ORP11 are dimerized and may act as an intracellular lipid sensor or transporter (Zhou, Li et al. 2010).

ORP10 suppresses hepatic lipogenesis and very-low-density lipoprotein production (Perttila, Merikanto et al. 2009). ORP10 is genetically associated with both TG (Perttila, Merikanto et al. 2009) and LDL cholesterol level (Koriyama, Nakagami et al. 2010).

SNPs in the ORP11 gene is associated with LDL cholesterol levels, hyperglycemia / diabetes as well as with metabolic syndrome per se (Bouchard, Faucher et al. 2009).

2.1 Phylogenetic distribution and molecular structure of OSBP/ORP family

As a result of differential promoter usage and splicing, there are 16 major OSBP/ORP family members. The human ORP family is divided into six subfamilies based on the gene structure and amino acid sequence homology (Fig. 1). Some of the proteins, for example ORP1 and ORP4, have both short (S) and long (L) variants.

A feature in common for all ORPs is a conserved C-terminal OSBP-related domain (ORD), which contains the highly conserved "OSBP-fingerprint (OF)" sequence EQVSHHPP (Fig. 1). Most of the human ORPs belong to the long subtype have a pleckstrin homology domain (PH domain), which bind phosphoinositides (PIPs). This interaction controls the subcellular localization of the proteins. 12 out of the 16 major mammalian OSBP/ORP family members contain a FFAT motif, which is a short sequence that binds VAMP associated proteins (VAPs), integral membrane proteins of the ER. Instead of an ER targeting FFAT motif, ORP5 and ORP8 contain a putative C-terminal transmembrane segment, which anchors these proteins in the ER. The human ORP1L have at their N-terminus ankyrin repeats, which interacts with the active GTP-bound form of Rab7 on late endosomes, and thus mediates targeting of the protein to late endosomes.

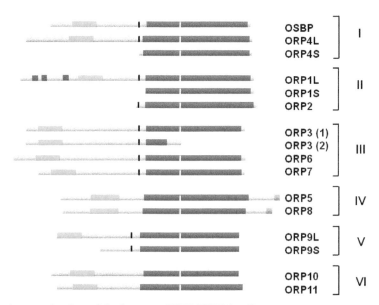

Fig. 1. Domain organization of the humam OSBP/ORP family.

Human OSBP/ORP family members are arranged into subfamilies I-VI. The color codes are: red, OSBP-related domain (ORD); yellow, OSBP-fingerprint (OF) motif; green, pleckstrin homology (PH) domain; Blue, ankirin repeats; black, VAP targeting motif (FFAT motif); Orange, transmembrane domain. L and S in the protein names indicate long and short variants, respectively.

2.2 OSBP

Structure, Tissue distribution and Intracellular localization: OSBP belongs to the subfamily I of OSBP/ORP homologues. OSBP has an ORD, a PH domain and an FFAT motif. OSBP shares the highest degree of similarity with ORP4 and dimerizes with ORP4. In the transfected cells, some of the OSBP was distributed diffusely in the cytoplasm, and some was bound to small vesicles near the nucleus. Upon addition of 25-hydroxycholesterol, most of the OSBP became concentrated in the Golgi apparatus (Ridgway, Dawson et al. 1992).

Molecular functions related to dyslipidemia: OSBP is the founding member of the OSBP/ORP family. Human OSBP was cloned in 1990 (Levanon, Hsieh et al. 1990) and was studied intensively (Ridgway, Dawson et al. 1992; Lagace, Byers et al. 1997; Ridgway, Badiani et al. 1998; Ridgway, Lagace et al. 1998; Storey, Byers et al. 1998; Lagace, Byers et al. 1999; Mohammadi, Perry et al. 2001; Levine and Munro 2002).

Yan et al. reported that adenovirus-mediated hepatic overexpression of OSBP induced a marked increase of VLDL TG. Also, the liver tissue TG were elevated in the AdOSBP-injected mice, and their TG secretion rate was increased by 70%. The messenger RNAs for enzymes of fatty acid synthesis and their transcriptional regulator, SREBP-1c, as well as the

Insig-1 mRNA, were upregulated two-fold in the OSBP expressing livers. Silencing of OSBP in hepatocytes suppressed the induction of SREBP1-c by insulin and resulted in a reduction of TG synthesis. These results demonstrate that OSBP regulates hepatic TG metabolism and suggest the involvement of OSBP in the insulin signaling pathways that control hepatic lipogenesis (Yan, Lehto et al. 2007).

Bowden et al. revealed that suppression of OSBP in Chinese hamster ovary cells by RNA interference resulted in increased ABCA1 protein expression and cholesterol efflux activity following induction with oxysterols or the synthetic LXR agonist TO901317. OSBP knockdown in J774 macrophages also increased ABCA1 expression in the presence and absence of LXR agonists. Their results demonstrate that OSBP opposes the activity of LXR by negatively regulating ABCA1 activity in the cytoplasm by sterol-binding domain-dependent protein destabilization (Bowden and Ridgway 2008).

Cephalostatin 1, OSW-1, ritterazine B and schweinfurthin A are natural products that potently, and in some cases selectively, inhibit the growth of cultured human cancer cell lines. Recently, Burgett et al. have discovered that these molecules target OSBP and its closest paralog, ORP4L, and have named these natural products ORPphilins (Burgett, Poulsen et al. 2011). By uncovering the cellular targets of the ORPphilins, they have revealed that OSBP and ORP4L are involved in cancer cell survival.

They also show that ORPphilins perturb the cellular localization of OSBP and affect sphingomyelin biosynthesis. The ORPphilins are powerful probes of OSBP and ORP4L that will be useful in uncovering their cellular functions and their roles in human diseases.

Epidemiological study: Epidemiological study of OSBP is not reported yet.

2.3 OSBPL1B (ORP1L)
Structure, Tissue distribution and Intracellular localization: ORP1L belongs to the subfamily II of OSBP/ORP homologues. ORP1L has an ORD, an FFAT motif, a PH domain and three ankyrin repeats.

While macrophages, brain, and lung are the areas where ORP1L is expressed most predominantly, it is also found in colon, kidney, and liver (Johansson, Bocher et al. 2003). ORP1L localizes to late endosomes.

Molecular functions related to dyslipidemia: Johansson et al. reported that ORP1L binds to Rab7, modifies its functional cycle, and can interfere with LE/lysosome organization and endocytic membrane trafficking (Johansson, Lehto et al. 2005).

They show that the GTPase Rab7, when bound to GTP, simultaneously binds to ORP1L and RILP to form a RILP-Rab7-ORP1L complex, which is required for the perinuclear localization of late endosomes/lysosomes (Johansson, Rocha et al. 2007). The later study of Rocha et al., went deeper in examining these processes more in detail. They found that the cholesterol levels in late endosomes are sensed by ORP1L and are lower in peripheral vesicles. Under low cholesterol conditions, ORP1L conformation induces the formation of endoplasmic reticulum (ER)- late endosome membrane contact sites. At these sites, the ER protein VAP (VAMP [vesicle-associated membrane protein]-associated ER protein) can interact in trans with the Rab7-RILP complex to remove p150 (Glued) and associated motors. late endosomes then move to the microtubule plus end. Under high cholesterol conditions, as in Niemann-Pick type C disease, this process is prevented, and late endosomes accumulate at the microtubule minus end as the result of dynein motor activity. These data explain how the ER and cholesterol control the association of late endosomes with motor proteins and their positioning in cells (Rocha, Kuijl et al. 2009).

Recently, Vihervaara et al. have shown that ORP1L silencing in macrophage foam cells inhibits the efflux of lipoprotein-derived endocytosed cholesterol to apolipoprotein A-I, providing evidence for the involvement of ORP1L in both protein and lipid transport functions of the late endocytic compartments (Vihervaara, Uronen et al. 2011).

The multivesicular body(MVB) sorting pathway is known to be involved in many processes, including growth factor receptor down-regulation, exosome secretion, antigen presentation, the budding of enveloped viruses, and cytokinesis. Recently, Kobuna et al. have shown that knockdown of ORP1L induces the formation of enlarged MVBs in HeLa cells. They suggest that the proper cholesterol level of late endosomes/lysosomes generated by ORPs is required for normal MVB formation and MVB–mediated membrane protein degradation (Kobuna, Inoue et al. 2010).

Epidemiological study: Epidemiological study of ORP1L is not reported yet.

2.4 OSBPL1A (ORP1S) and OSBPL2 (ORP2)

Structure, Tissue distribution and Intracellular localization: ORP1S and ORP2 belong to the subfamily II of OSBP/ORP homologues. ORP1S and ORP2 have an ORD and an FFAT motif but lack PH domain.

ORP1S is expressed predominantly in skeletal muscle and heart (Johansson, Bocher et al. 2003). ORP2 is expressed ubiquitously in mammalian tissues. Highest mRNA levels of ORP2 are present in specific parts of the central nervous system (cerebellum, pituitary gland, pons, and putamen) as well as in leukocytes, placenta, and pancreas (Laitinen, Lehto et al. 2002).

ORP1S has been reported to be largely cytosolic (Johansson, Bocher et al. 2003) and ORP2 localizes, in addition to a cytosolic fraction, on the surface of lipid droplets (LDs) and also the plasma membrane (PM) (Hynynen, Suchanek et al. 2009).

Molecular functions related to dyslipidemia: In the earlier study of Hynynen et al., overexpression of ORP2 induces enhancement of [14C]cholesterol efflux to all extracellular acceptors, which results in a reduction of cellular free cholesterol. They also show that ORP2 binds PtdIns(3,4,5)P(3) and enhances endocytosis.

In their recent study, Hynynen et al. discover that ORP2 localizes not only cytosolic fraction but also on cytoplasmic LDs and reveal its function in neutral lipid metabolism. They show that the ORP2 LD association depends on sterol binding: Treatment with 5 mM 22(R)OHC inhibits the LD association, while a mutant defective in sterol binding is constitutively LD bound. Silencing of ORP2 using RNA interference slows down cellular TG hydrolysis. Furthermore, ORP2 silencing increases the amount of [14C]cholesteryl esters but only under conditions in which lipogenesis and LD formation are enhanced by treatment with oleic acid (Hynynen, Suchanek et al. 2009). These results identify ORP2 as a sterol receptor present on LD and provide an evidence for its role in the regulation of neutral lipid metabolism, possibly as a factor that integrates the cellular metabolism of TG with that of cholesterol.

By overexpressing all mammalian ORPs, Jansen et al. found that especially ORP1S and ORP2 enhanced PM-to-LD sterol transport. This reflected the stimulation of transport from the PM to the ER, rather than from the ER to LDs. Double knockdown of ORP1S and ORP2 inhibited sterol transport from the PM to the ER and LDs, suggesting a physiological role for these ORPs in the process (Jansen, Ohsaki et al. 2011). These findings suggest that ORP1S and ORP2 are essential in controlling cellular neutral lipid and cholesterol and has a strong association with the pathophysiology of dyslipidemia.

Epidemiological study: Epidemiological studies of ORP1S or ORP2 are not reported yet.

2.5 OSBPL3 (ORP3)

Structure, Tissue distribution and Intracellular localization: ORP3 belongs to the subfamily III of OSBP/ORP homologues. ORP3 has an ORD, a PH domain and an FFAT motif. A total of eight isoforms of ORP3 were demonstrated with alternative splicing (Collier, Gregorio-King et al. 2003). In human tissues there was specific isoform distribution, with most tissues expressing varied levels of isoforms with the complete ORD; while only whole brain, kidney, spleen, thymus, and thyroid expressed high levels of the isoforms associated with the truncated ORD. The expression in cerebellum, heart, and liver of most isoforms was negligible. Lehto et al described that ORP3 was expressed at high levels in kidney tubule epithelia and in the human embryonic kidney cell line HEK293 (Lehto, Mayranpaa et al. 2008).

They also described that the endogenous ORP3 protein in HEK293 cells localized at the ER and the PM, especially thin filopodial cell-surface projections.

Molecular functions related to dyslipidemia: The direct evidence that ORP3 functions to regulate Dyslipidemia is yet to be reported.

ORP3 interacts with R-Ras, a small GTPase regulating cell adhesion, spreading and migration (Lehto, Mayranpaa et al. 2008). Gene silencing of ORP3 and overexpression of ORP3 in HEK293 cells or primary macrophages demonstrate the function of ORP3 as part of the machinery that controls the actin cytoskeleton, cell polarity and cell adhesion. These functional evidences, together with the abundant expression of ORP3 in polarized cell types, suggest that ORP3 may play an important role in efficient directed membrane trafficking.

Epidemiological study: Epidemiological study of ORP3 is not reported yet.

2.6 OSBPL4 (ORP4, OSBP2, HLM)

Structure, Tissue distribution and Intracellular localization: ORP4 belongs to the subfamily I of OSBP/ORP homologues. ORP4 has an ORD, a PH domain and an FFAT motif. ORP4 shares the highest degree of similarity with OSBP and dimerizes with OSBP.

Two ORP4 cDNAs were identified: a full-length ORP4 containing a PH domain and an ORD (designated ORP4-L), and a splice variant in which the PH domain and part of the ORD were deleted (designated ORP4-S). ORP4 mRNA and protein expression overlapped partially with OSBP and were restricted to brain, heart, muscle and kidney(Wang, JeBailey et al. 2002).

Immunofluorescence localization in stably transfected Chinese hamster ovary cells showed that ORP4-S co-localized with vimentin and caused the intermediate filament network to bundle or aggregate. ORP4-L displayed a diffuse staining pattern that did not overlap with vimentin except when the microtubule network was disrupted with nocodazole.

Molecular functions related to dyslipidemia: Cells overexpressing ORP4S had a 40% reduction in the esterification of low-density-lipoprotein-derived cholesterol, demonstrating that ORP4 in an interaction with intermediate filaments inhibits an intracellular cholesterol-transport pathway mediated by vimentin (Wang, JeBailey et al. 2002).

ORP4L bound [3H]25-hydroxycholesterol with high affinity and specificity. However, sterol-binding or a mutation that ablated sterol-binding did not influence the interaction of GST-ORP4 with vimentin (Wyles, Perry et al. 2007). Thus the precise mechanism about what ORP4L senses to regulate intracellular cholesterol-transport pathway still remains unidentified.

Epidemiological study: Epidemiological study of ORP4 is not reported yet.

2.7 OSBPL5 (ORP5)

Structure, Tissue distribution and Intracellular localization: ORP5 belongs to the subfamily IV of OSBP/ORP homologues. ORP5 has an ORD, a PH domain and a transmembrane domain. ORP5 localizes to the ER.

Molecular functions related to dyslipidemia: Knocking down ORP5 causes cholesterol accumulation in late endosomes and lysosomes, which is reminiscent of the cholesterol trafficking defect in Niemann Pick C (NPC) fibroblasts (Du, Kumar et al. 2011). Cholesterol appears to accumulate in the limiting membranes of endosomal compartments in ORP5-depleted cells, whereas depletion of NPC1 or both ORP5 and NPC1 results in luminal accumulation of cholesterol. Moreover, trans-Golgi resident proteins mislocalize to endosomal compartments upon ORP5 depletion, which depends on a functional NPC1.

Niemann-Pick type C (NPC) disease is most often caused by mutations in the NPC1 gene, whose protein product is believed to facilitate the egress of cholesterol and other lipids from late endosomes and lysosomes to other cellular compartments (Boadu and Francis 2006).

The results of the research by Du et al. establish the first link between NPC1 and a cytoplasmic sterol carrier, and suggest that ORP5 may cooperate with NPC1 to mediate the exit of cholesterol from endosomes/lysosomes.

Epidemiological study: Epidemiological study of ORP5 is not reported yet.

2.8 OSBPL6 (ORP6)

Structure, Tissue distribution and Intracellular localization: ORP6 belongs to the subfamily III of OSBP/ORP homologues. ORP6 has an ORD, a PH domain and an FFAT motif. ORP6 shows the highest expression in brain and skeletal muscle (Lehto, Tienari et al. 2004). Endogenous ORP6 associated predominantly with the nuclear envelope. When expressed from the cDNA in cultured cells, ORP6 was distributed between the cytosol and ER membranes, with a minor portion found at the PM.

Molecular functions related to dyslipidemia: The direct evidence that ORP6 functions to regulate Dyslipidemia is yet to be reported.

Epidemiological study: Using the Framingham Heart Study data set, a quantitative trait locus in the chromosome 2q was found to be significantly involved in variations of HDL cholesterol levels. ORP6 is identified as one of the candidate genes that are possibly involved in the regulation of HDL cholesterol levels in this region (North, Martin et al. 2003).

2.9 OSBPL7 (ORP7)

Structure, Tissue distribution and Intracellular localization: ORP7 belongs to the subfamily III of OSBP/ORP homologues. ORP7 has an ORD, a PH domain and a an FFAT motif. ORP7 shows the highest expression in the gastrointestinal tract (Lehto, Tienari et al. 2004). When expressed from the cDNA in cultured cells, ORP7 was distributed between the cytosol and ER membranes, with a minor portion found at the PM. The N-terminal portion of the proteins, containing a PH domain, has markedly strong PM targeting specificity, while the C-terminal half remains largely cytosolic. The dual targeting of the proteins indicates a putative role in communication between the ER and the PM.

Molecular functions related to dyslipidemia: Recently, Zhong et al. identified by yeast two-hybrid screening an interaction partner of ORP7, GATE-16, which (i) regulates the function and stability of Golgi SNARE of 28kDa (GS28), and (ii) plays a role in autophagosome biogenesis (Zhong, Zhou et al. 2011).

GATE-16 is a ubiquitin-like low molecular weight peripheral membrane protein which was initially reported to localize at the Golgi complex and to regulate docking/fusing reactions in intra-Golgi traffic and Golgi assembly from mitotic fragments via interactions with NSF and the Golgi v-SNARE GS28 (Sagiv, Legesse-Miller et al. 2000). GS28 was identified as a SNARE protein, the majority of which is associated with the cis-Golgi, and is implicated in both ER-Golgi and intra-Golgi transport (Subramaniam, Peter et al. 1996). In the presence of NSF, SNAP and ATP, GATE-16 interacts with GS28, apparently maintaining GS28 in a transport competent form and protecting it from proteolysis.

Zhong et al. revealed that ORP7 knockdown in 293A cells resulted in a 40% increase of GS28 protein while ORP7 overexpression had the opposite effect. Similar to ORP7 overexpression, treatment of cells with 25-hydroxycholesterol (25-OH) resulted in GS28 destabilization, which was potentiated by excess ORP7 and inhibited by ORP7 silencing. Their results suggest that ORP7 negatively regulates GS28 protein stability via sequestration of GATE-16, and may mediate the effect of 25-OH on GS28 and Golgi function.

Epidemiological study: It is reported that SNPs near ORP7 gene show genome-wide significant association with LDL cholesterol (Teslovich, Musunuru et al. 2010).

2.10 OSBPL8 (ORP8)

Structure, Tissue distribution and Intracellular localization: ORP8 belongs to the subfamily IV of OSBP/ORP homologues. ORP8 has an ORD, a PH domain and a transmembrane domain. ORP8 is expressed at the highest levels in macrophages, liver, spleen, kidney, and brain (Yan, Mayranpaa et al. 2008). ORP8 is localized in the ER via its C-terminal transmembrane domain.

Molecular functions related to dyslipidemia: It is reported that silencing of ORP8 by RNA interference in THP-1 macrophages increased the expression of ABCA1 and concomitantly cholesterol efflux to lipid-free apolipoprotein A-I. Experiments employing an ABCA1 promoter-luciferase reporter confirmed that ORP8 silencing enhances ABCA1 transcription. These data identify ORP8 as a negative regulator of ABCA1 expression and macrophage cholesterol efflux. But the precise mechanism to regulate the expression of ABCA1 has not been revealed.

Recently, Zhou et al. investigated the action of ORP8 in hepatic cells in vivo and in vitro. They found that adenoviral overexpression of ORP8 in mouse liver induced a decrease of cholesterol, phospholipids, and triglycerides in serum (-34%, -26%, -37%, respectively) and liver tissue (-40%, -12%, -24%), coinciding with reduction of nuclear (n)SREBP-1 and -2 and mRNA levels of their target genes. Consistently, excess ORP8 reduced nSREBPs in HuH7 cells, and ORP8 overexpression or silencing by RNA interference moderately suppressed or induced the expression of SREBP-1 and SREBP-2 target genes, respectively. In accordance, cholesterol biosynthesis was reduced by ORP8 overexpression and enhanced by ORP8 silencing in [(3)H]acetate pulse-labeling experiments.

They also performed yeast two-hybrid, bimolecular fluorescence complementation (BiFC), and co-immunoprecipitation analyses, and revealed the nuclear pore component Nup62 as an interaction partner of ORP8. They showed that the impact of overexpressed ORP8 on nSREBPs and their target mRNAs was inhibited in cells depleted of Nup62.

These results reveal that ORP8 has the capacity to modulate lipid homeostasis and SREBP activity, probably through an indirect mechanism required Nup62.

Epidemiological study: Ma et al. performed a genome-wide association analysis of total cholesterol and HDL cholesterol levels using the Framingham heart study data. In that study, single-locus effects and pairwise epistasis effects of 432,096 SNP markers were tested for their significance on log-transformed total cholesterol and HDL cholesterol levels. As a result, the OSBPL8-ZDHHC17 region (chr12) was detected for HDL cholesterol identified by one new SNP with genome-wide significance (Ma, Yang et al. 2010).

2.11 OSBPL9 (ORP9)

Structure, Tissue distribution and Intracellular localization: ORP9 belongs to the subfamily V of OSBP/ORP homologues. ORP9 has an ORD, a PH domain and an FFAT motif. VAP binding FFAT motif and PH domains target ORP9 to the ER and a Golgi-COPII compartment, respectively (Wyles and Ridgway 2004).

Molecular functions related to dyslipidemia: Ngo et al. demonstrate that ORP9L partitioning between the trans-Golgi/trans-Golgi network (TGN), and the ER is mediated by a phosphatidylinositol 4-phosphate (PI-4P)-specific PH domain and VAP, respectively (Ngo and Ridgway 2009). In vitro, ORP9L mediates PI-4P-dependent cholesterol transport between liposomes, suggesting that its primary function in vivo is sterol transfer between the Golgi and ER. Depletion of ORP9L by RNAi caused Golgi fragmentation, inhibition of vesicular somatitus virus glycoprotein transport from the ER and accumulation of cholesterol in endosomes/lysosomes. These findings indicate that ORP9 maintains the integrity of the early secretory pathway by mediating transport of sterols between the ER and trans-Golgi/TGN.

It is also reported that ORP9, in interaction with ORP11, may act as an intracellular lipid sensor or transporter (Zhou, Li et al. 2010). (see also ORP11.)

Epidemiological study: Epidemiological study of ORP9 is not reported yet.

2.12 OSBPL10 (ORP10)

Structure, Tissue distribution and Intracellular localization: ORP10 belongs to the subfamily VI of OSBP/ORP homologues. ORP10 has an ORD and a PH domain but does not have an FFAT motif or a transmembrane domain.

ORP10 was shown to associate dynamically with microtubules, being consistent with its involvement in intracellular transport or organelle positioning (Perttila, Merikanto et al. 2009).

Immunofluorescence localization in transiently transfected bovine aorta endothelial cells showed that EGFP-ORP10 co-localized with alpha-tubulin (Fig. 2 c, g) and not with actin (Fig. 2 a, e) or vimentin (Fig. 2 b, f). The microtubules co-localize with EGFP-ORP10 show the aberrant bundled structures. These structures were disrupted by treatment with nocodazol (Fig. 2 d, h).

Molecular functions related to dyslipidemia: Silencing of ORP10 increased the incorporation of [(3)H]acetate into cholesterol and both [(3)H]acetate and [(3)H]oleate into triglycerides and enhanced the accumulation of secreted apolipoprotein B100 in growth medium, suggesting that ORP10 suppresses hepatic lipogenesis and very-low-density lipoprotein production.

Epidemiological study: We examined the association between polymorphisms in the ORP10 gene and risk factors for the metabolic syndrome in the Tanno and Sobetsu Study in Japan (Koriyama, Nakagami et al. 2010).

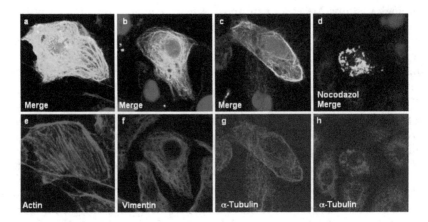

Fig. 2. Intracellular localization of ORP10.

As a result, we found that the LDL cholesterol of individuals with the rs2290532 (D254N) polymorphism was significantly greater in subjects with the CC+CT genotype than in subjects with the TT genotype (124.3+/-1.3 vs. 111.6+/-4.1 mg per 100 ml, P=0.009) (Fig. 3). Comparison of the genotype frequency in both groups indicated that the genotype associated with low risk (TT) reduced the risk of hyper-LDL cholesterolemia significantly (P=0.003), with an odds ratio of 0.35 (95% confidence interval=0.17-0.76). These findings suggest that the rs2290532 (D254N) polymorphism in OSBPL10 may predispose individuals with this SNP to hyper-LDL cholesterolemia.

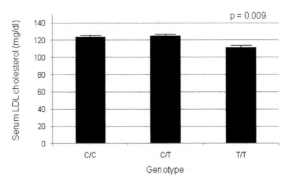

Fig. 3. Relation of rs2290532 of ORP10 with serum LDL cholesterol.

Perttila et al. also reported that the analysis of variants in ORP10 gene revealed suggestive linkage of ORP10 single-nucleotide polymorphisms (SNPs) with extreme end high TG (>90th percentile) trait. They carried out an association analysis in a metabolic syndrome subcohort (Genmets) of Health2000 examination survey (N = 2,138), revealing an association of multiple ORP10 SNPs with high serum TG levels (>95th percentile).

The result proves that ORP10 is genetically associated with both TG and LDL cholesterol levels. Though it is estimated that microtubule dependent intracellular transport of vesicles plays an important role in that process, the mechanism to control TG and LDL cholesterol levels is yet to be explained. A further analysis is highly expected.

2.13 OSBPL11 (ORP11)

Structure, Tissue distribution and Intracellular localization: ORP11 belongs to the subfamily VI of OSBP/ORP homologues. ORP11 has an ORD and a PH domain but does not have an FFAT motif or a transmembrane domain. ORP11 is present at the highest levels in human ovary, testis, kidney, liver, stomach, brain, and adipose tissue. Immunohistochemistry demonstrates abundant ORP11 in the epithelial cells of kidney tubules, testicular tubules, caecum, and skin. ORP11 dimerizes with ORP9 and localizes at the Golgi-late endosome interface (Zhou, Li et al. 2010).

Molecular functions related to dyslipidemia: Cells overexpressing ORP11 displayed lamellar lipid bodies associated with vacuolar structures or the Golgi complex, indicating a disturbance of lipid trafficking. Similar multilamellar membranes arise in endo-lysosomal compartments in phospholipidosis occurring, for instance, upon incubation of macrophage with oxidized low-density lipoprotein, or associated with inheritable lysosomal storage disorders, situations in which normal lipid transport is disturbed. These findings indicate that ORP11, in interaction with ORP9, may act as an intracellular lipid sensor or transporter.

Epidemiological study: it is reported that ORP11 is significantly overexpressed in the visceral adipose tissue of obese men with metabolic syndrome (Bouchard, Faucher et al. 2009). Furthermore, they found SNPs in the ORP11 gene to be associated with several cardiovascular risk factors in obese individuals. IVS12+95 T>C, a newly discovered SNP of the study, was associated with LDL cholesterol levels (OR = 1.63; P < 0.001), hyperglycemia/diabetes (OR = 1.48; P < 0.004) as well as with metabolic syndrome per se (OR = 1.56; P < 0.01). These results suggest that ORP11 is involved in cholesterol and glucose metabolism in obese individuals.

3. Conclusion

Since OSBP/ORP family involves functional redundancy as well as overlap tissue expression and intracellular localization, the function of each family member has been mostly left unrevealed. Various studies including the genome-wide association study, however, have succeeded to prove the direct association between the individual members and dyslipidemia. Analyses on the individual members have also made it clear that the members affect the regulation of cholesterol and triglyceride level in interaction with diverse molecules.

Nevertheless, the precise molecular mechanism of the process still remains unascertained. The recent findings such as the identification of the small molecule which associates with OSBP are expected to act as a convenient tool to clarify the more detailed functions of OSBP/ORP family in future.

4. Acknowledgment

Work in the authors' group is supported by a Grant-in-Aid for Scientific Research from Japan Society for the Promotion of Science and research grants from Takeda Science Foundation.

5. References

Boadu, E. and G. A. Francis (2006). "The role of vesicular transport in ABCA1-dependent lipid efflux and its connection with NPC pathways." J Mol Med (Berl) 84(4): 266-275.

Bouchard, L., G. Faucher, et al. (2009). "Association of OSBPL11 gene polymorphisms with cardiovascular disease risk factors in obesity." Obesity (Silver Spring) 17(7): 1466-1472.

Bowden, K. and N. D. Ridgway (2008). "OSBP negatively regulates ABCA1 protein stability." J Biol Chem 283(26): 18210-18217.

Burgett, A. W., T. B. Poulsen, et al. (2011). "Natural products reveal cancer cell dependence on oxysterol-binding proteins." Nat Chem Biol.

Chen, W., G. Chen, et al. (2007). "Enzymatic reduction of oxysterols impairs LXR signaling in cultured cells and the livers of mice." Cell Metab 5(1): 73-79.

Collier, F. M., C. C. Gregorio-King, et al. (2003). "ORP3 splice variants and their expression in human tissues and hematopoietic cells." DNA Cell Biol 22(1): 1-9.

Du, X., J. Kumar, et al. (2011). "A role for oxysterol-binding protein-related protein 5 in endosomal cholesterol trafficking." J Cell Biol 192(1): 121-135.

Fairn, G. D. and C. R. McMaster (2008). "Emerging roles of the oxysterol-binding protein family in metabolism, transport, and signaling." Cell Mol Life Sci 65(2): 228-236.

Hynynen, R., M. Suchanek, et al. (2009). "OSBP-related protein 2 is a sterol receptor on lipid droplets that regulates the metabolism of neutral lipids." J Lipid Res 50(7): 1305-1315.

Jansen, M., Y. Ohsaki, et al. (2011). "Role of ORPs in sterol transport from plasma membrane to ER and lipid droplets in mammalian cells." Traffic 12(2): 218-231.

Johansson, M., V. Bocher, et al. (2003). "The two variants of oxysterol binding protein-related protein-1 display different tissue expression patterns, have different intracellular localization, and are functionally distinct." Mol Biol Cell 14(3): 903-915.

Johansson, M., M. Lehto, et al. (2005). "The oxysterol-binding protein homologue ORP1L interacts with Rab7 and alters functional properties of late endocytic compartments." Mol Biol Cell 16(12): 5480-5492.

Johansson, M., N. Rocha, et al. (2007). "Activation of endosomal dynein motors by stepwise assembly of Rab7-RILP-p150Glued, ORP1L, and the receptor betalll spectrin." J Cell Biol 176(4): 459-471.

Kobuna, H., T. Inoue, et al. (2010). "Multivesicular body formation requires OSBP-related proteins and cholesterol." PLoS Genet 6(8).

Koriyama, H., H. Nakagami, et al. (2010). "Variation in OSBPL10 is associated with dyslipidemia." Hypertens Res 33(5): 511-514.

Lagace, T. A., D. M. Byers, et al. (1997). "Altered regulation of cholesterol and cholesteryl ester synthesis in Chinese-hamster ovary cells overexpressing the oxysterol-binding protein is dependent on the pleckstrin homology domain." Biochem J 326 (Pt 1): 205-213.

Lagace, T. A., D. M. Byers, et al. (1999). "Chinese hamster ovary cells overexpressing the oxysterol binding protein (OSBP) display enhanced synthesis of sphingomyelin in response to 25-hydroxycholesterol." J Lipid Res 40(1): 109-116.

Laitinen, S., M. Lehto, et al. (2002). "ORP2, a homolog of oxysterol binding protein, regulates cellular cholesterol metabolism." J Lipid Res 43(2): 245-255.

Lehto, M., M. I. Mayranpaa, et al. (2008). "The R-Ras interaction partner ORP3 regulates cell adhesion." J Cell Sci 121(Pt 5): 695-705.

Lehto, M., J. Tienari, et al. (2004). "Subfamily III of mammalian oxysterol-binding protein (OSBP) homologues: the expression and intracellular localization of ORP3, ORP6, and ORP7." Cell Tissue Res 315(1): 39-57.

Levanon, D., C. L. Hsieh, et al. (1990). "cDNA cloning of human oxysterol-binding protein and localization of the gene to human chromosome 11 and mouse chromosome 19." Genomics 7(1): 65-74.

Levine, T. P. and S. Munro (2002). "Targeting of Golgi-specific pleckstrin homology domains involves both PtdIns 4-kinase-dependent and -independent components." Curr Biol 12(9): 695-704.

Ma, L., J. Yang, et al. (2010). "Genome-wide association analysis of total cholesterol and high-density lipoprotein cholesterol levels using the Framingham heart study data." BMC Med Genet 11: 55.

Mohammadi, A., R. J. Perry, et al. (2001). "Golgi localization and phosphorylation of oxysterol binding protein in Niemann-Pick C and U18666A-treated cells." J Lipid Res 42(7): 1062-1071.

Ngo, M. and N. D. Ridgway (2009). "Oxysterol binding protein-related Protein 9 (ORP9) is a cholesterol transfer protein that regulates Golgi structure and function." Mol Biol Cell 20(5): 1388-1399.

Ngo, M. H., T. R. Colbourne, et al. (2010). "Functional implications of sterol transport by the oxysterol-binding protein gene family." Biochem J 429(1): 13-24.

North, K. E., L. J. Martin, et al. (2003). "HDL cholesterol in females in the Framingham Heart Study is linked to a region of chromosome 2q." BMC Genet 4 Suppl 1: S98.

Perttila, J., K. Merikanto, et al. (2009). "OSBPL10, a novel candidate gene for high triglyceride trait in dyslipidemic Finnish subjects, regulates cellular lipid metabolism." J Mol Med (Berl) 87(8): 825-835.

Radhakrishnan, A., Y. Ikeda, et al. (2007). "Sterol-regulated transport of SREBPs from endoplasmic reticulum to Golgi: oxysterols block transport by binding to Insig." Proc Natl Acad Sci U S A 104(16): 6511-6518.

Raychaudhuri, S. and W. A. Prinz (2010). "The diverse functions of oxysterol-binding proteins." Annu Rev Cell Dev Biol 26: 157-177.

Ridgway, N. D., K. Badiani, et al. (1998). "Inhibition of phosphorylation of the oxysterol binding protein by brefeldin A." Biochim Biophys Acta 1390(1): 37-51.

Ridgway, N. D., P. A. Dawson, et al. (1992). "Translocation of oxysterol binding protein to Golgi apparatus triggered by ligand binding." J Cell Biol 116(2): 307-319.

Ridgway, N. D., T. A. Lagace, et al. (1998). "Differential effects of sphingomyelin hydrolysis and cholesterol transport on oxysterol-binding protein phosphorylation and Golgi localization." J Biol Chem 273(47): 31621-31628.

Rocha, N., C. Kuijl, et al. (2009). "Cholesterol sensor ORP1L contacts the ER protein VAP to control Rab7-RILP-p150 Glued and late endosome positioning." J Cell Biol 185(7): 1209-1225.

Sagiv, Y., A. Legesse-Miller, et al. (2000). "GATE-16, a membrane transport modulator, interacts with NSF and the Golgi v-SNARE GOS-28." EMBO J 19(7): 1494-1504.

Sever, N., B. L. Song, et al. (2003). "Insig-dependent ubiquitination and degradation of mammalian 3-hydroxy-3-methylglutaryl-CoA reductase stimulated by sterols and geranylgeraniol." J Biol Chem 278(52): 52479-52490.

Storey, M. K., D. M. Byers, et al. (1998). "Cholesterol regulates oxysterol binding protein (OSBP) phosphorylation and Golgi localization in Chinese hamster ovary cells: correlation with stimulation of sphingomyelin synthesis by 25-hydroxycholesterol." Biochem J 336 (Pt 1): 247-256.

Subramaniam, V. N., F. Peter, et al. (1996). "GS28, a 28-kilodalton Golgi SNARE that participates in ER-Golgi transport." Science 272(5265): 1161-1163.

Teslovich, T. M., K. Musunuru, et al. (2010). "Biological, clinical and population relevance of 95 loci for blood lipids." Nature 466(7307): 707-713.

Vihervaara, T., M. Jansen, et al. (2011). "Cytoplasmic oxysterol-binding proteins: sterol sensors or transporters?" Chem Phys Lipids 164(6): 443-450.

Vihervaara, T., R. L. Uronen, et al. (2011). "Sterol binding by OSBP-related protein 1L regulates late endosome motility and function." Cell Mol Life Sci 68(3): 537-551.

Wang, C., L. JeBailey, et al. (2002). "Oxysterol-binding-protein (OSBP)-related protein 4 binds 25-hydroxycholesterol and interacts with vimentin intermediate filaments." Biochem J 361(Pt 3): 461-472.

Wyles, J. P., R. J. Perry, et al. (2007). "Characterization of the sterol-binding domain of oxysterol-binding protein (OSBP)-related protein 4 reveals a novel role in vimentin organization." Exp Cell Res 313(7): 1426-1437.

Wyles, J. P. and N. D. Ridgway (2004). "VAMP-associated protein-A regulates partitioning of oxysterol-binding-protein-related protein-9 between the endoplasmic reticulum and Golgi apparatus." Exp Cell Res 297(2): 533-547.

Yan, D., M. Lehto, et al. (2007). "Oxysterol binding protein induces upregulation of SREBP-1c and enhances hepatic lipogenesis." Arterioscler Thromb Vasc Biol 27(5): 1108-1114.

Yan, D., M. I. Mayranpaa, et al. (2008). "OSBP-related protein 8 (ORP8) suppresses ABCA1 expression and cholesterol efflux from macrophages." J Biol Chem 283(1): 332-340.

Zhong, W., Y. Zhou, et al. (2011). "OSBP-related protein 7 interacts with GATE-16 and negatively regulates GS28 protein stability." Exp Cell Res.

Zhou, T., S. Li, et al. (2011). "OSBP-related protein 8 (ORP8) regulates plasma and liver tissue lipid levels and interacts with the nucleoporin Nup62." PLoS One 6(6): e21078.

Zhou, Y., S. Li, et al. (2010). "OSBP-related protein 11 (ORP11) dimerizes with ORP9 and localizes at the Golgi-late endosome interface." Exp Cell Res 316(19): 3304-3316.

Adipose Tissue and Skeletal Muscle Plasticity in Obesity and Metabolic Disease

Jozef Ukropec[1] and Barbara Ukropcova[1,2]
[1]Institute of Experimental Endocrinology Slovak Academy of Sciences,
[2]Institute of Pathological Physiology, Faculty of Medicine Comenius University,
Slovakia

1. Introduction

Obesity and lack of physical activity are two major factors contributing considerably to the pathogenesis of many chronic diseases so prevalent in contemporary human population. Adipose tissue and skeletal muscle are therefore the primary organs one would immediately suggest to target in an attempt to battle metabolic disease progression. Fine tuning of the physiological processes within the two organs have a large potential to modulate (i) energy balance, (ii) lipid storage-utilization efficiency as well as (iii) central and peripheral actions in the brain, gastrointestinal system or liver which are integrated by the endocrine activity of the two energy balance maintaining tissues.

2. Adipose tissue in metabolic health and disease

Despite the fact that the primary role of adipose tissue is an effective lipid storage and timely regulation of its release and that these processes could, in a simplified adipocentric view, be the primary determinants of the dyslipidemia and metabolic disease progression, adipose tissue has a broad range of other regulatory functions exerted *via* its autocrine, paracrine and endocrine actions. Adipose tissue secretory products, "adipokines", could modulate food intake, energy expenditure, or tissue oxidative capacity (Trayhurn et al. 1998; Ukropec et al. 2001; Ahima & Lazar 2008; Henry & Clarke 2008; Friedman 2011). In addition, adipose tissue dynamically changes its structure (*tissue remodeling, lipid composition*), function (*lipid storage & lipolysis*) as well as endocrine action in response to different physiological (*fasting / refeeding, exercise, microgravity*) and pathophysiological (*obesity, prediabetes, diabetes, cachexia, lipodystrophy, growth hormone deficiency*) conditions (Ukropec et al. 2008; Itoh et al. 2011; Pietilainen et al. 2011). It is important to understand that adipose tissue is a mixture of very different cell-types. Apart from approximately 50% of mature lipid-laden adipocytes it contains various stromal cells including preadipocytes, endothelial cells, fibroblasts, pluripotent stem cells and immune cells which substantially influence its function (Bjorntorp 1974; Sethi & Vidal-Puig 2007; Divoux & Clement 2011). Extreme enlargement of the fat cell size, such as we have recently observed in individuals with growth hormone deficiency, is perhaps the best early marker of the obesity related - metabolic disease development (Ukropec et al. 2008a) (Fig. 1.). Adipose tissue with enlarged adipocytes, expressing markers of the local tissue microhypoxia but not responding to it properly and attracting large amount of activated immunocompetent cells, has recently been termed "pathogenic adipose tissue" (Bays et al. 2008; Ukropec et al. 2008b).

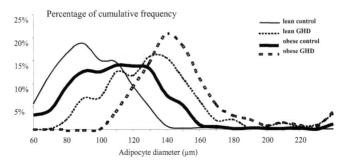

Fig. 1. Fat cell size in obesity and in growth hormone deficiency (GHD), percentage of cumulative frequency (Y axis), (Ukropec et al. 2008a).

The tissue damage due to overwhelming adipocytes with lipids, largely exceeding their lipid storage capacity, changes the adipokine secretory profile and leads to uncontrolled release of a large amount of lipids into circulation while the capacity of the adipose tissue adaptive remodeling is compromised. This is followed by the accumulation of lipids in tissues not designed for the lipid storage such as liver, skeletal muscle, pancreatic beta cells or lung which largely interferes with their physiological functions and accelerates the development of metabolic disease (Bays et al. 2008; Foster et al. 2010; Unger et al. 2010). Limited expandability of the adipose tissue seems to determine individual propensity to the development of metabolic disease (Arner, P. et al. 2011). Adaptive expansion of the adipose tissue is enabled by combination of adipocyte hypertrophy and hyperplasia. Expansion of adipose tissue requires quite extensive tissue remodeling, in order to maintain adequate energy and oxygen supply, active neuronal network as well as integrity and functional properties of cellular membranes (Itoh et al. 2011; Pietilainen et al. 2011). Broader knowledge of the fat cell life-cycle dynamics is critical for our understanding the pathophysiological mechanisms limiting adipose tissue hyperplastic expansion. In 2008, Arner's group analyzed the adipocyte turnover by detecting the genomic DNA incorporation of atmospheric ^{14}C derived from above-ground nuclear bomb tests in period between 1955 and 1963. This work revealed that approximately 10% of fat cells are renewed per year at all adult ages and levels of BMI and that neither adipocyte death nor generation rate is altered in early onset obesity. It seemed that the steady production of adipocytes in adults results in a stable size of the constantly turning over adipocyte population (Spalding et al. 2008). More recent work by these authors examining morphology of the subcutaneous adipose tissue from 764 individuals with broad range of BMI (18-60 kg.m²) defines hyperplasia and hypertrophy as a difference between measured adipocyte volume and volume predicted by the curve-like fit, for adipocyte volume and body fat mass (Fig. 2.). In this analysis occurrence of hyperplasia or hypertrophy correlated with fasting plasma insulin and insulin sensitivity. In addition, total adipocyte number was greatest in individuals with pronounced hyperplasia, and smallest in those with pronounced hypertrophy. The absolute number of new adipocytes generated each year was 70% lower in patients with hypertrophy than with hyperplasia. Whereas the relative death rate (~ 10% per year) or mean age of adipocytes (~ 10 years) was not correlated with adipocyte morphology (Arner, E. et al. 2010).

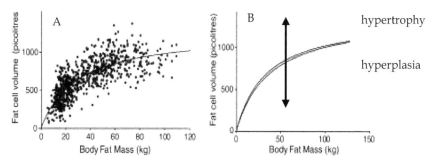

Fig. 2. (A) Graph depicts large variability in adipose tissue morphology in individuals with identical body fat mass (764 subjects). (B) Level of hyperplasia is represented by adequately lowered morphology value while hypertrophy is associated with parallel increase in morphology value defined as a difference between measured and expected adipocyte volume given by the curve-like fit , for given body fat mass (Arner, E. et al. 2010).

Insulin sensitivity could therefore govern adipose tissue morphology towards beneficial hyperplastic state at the population level. Conversely, defects in insulin action are interconnected with the hypertrophic adipocytes, and higher risk of lipid flooding the nonadipose tissues. Absolute numbers of adipocytes as well as their capacity to expand and store lipids are quite difficult to modulate. Morbid obesity and lipodystrophy represent the two medical conditions associated with excessive hypertriglyceridemia, hepatic steatosis, and disordered muscle glucose metabolism, due to defected ability of adipose tissue to store lipids or the selective loss of adipose tissue respectively. Activation of adipogenic programme by PPARγ agonists or chronic leptin treatment improves insulin-stimulated hepatic and peripheral glucose metabolism in obese and lipodystrophic patients respectively (Petersen et al. 2002; Rieusset et al. 2002; Van Gaal et al. 2003). Adipogenesis is necessary to increase the adipose tissue cellularity (hyperplastic adaptive change) and lipid storage capacity; it is largely dependent on the signal transducers and activators of transcription (STAT) pathway. In brief, transcription factors C/EBPα, C/EBPβ, and PPARγ control adipogenesis by regulating STAT5B and STAT5A. Regulation of PPARγ-STAT5 by C/EBPβ signaling seems to be the crucial adipogenesis - initiating cascade of the various adipogenic genes (Jung et al. 2011). Activation of adipogenic program should be paralleled with the extracellular matrix remodeling. As mentioned above, adipocytes are embedded in a unique extracellular matrix which main function is to provide mechanical support, in addition to participating in a variety of signaling events. Extracellular matrix requires remodeling to accommodate growing adipocytes in the expanding adipose tissue. We have recently participated in the research by Christian Wolfrum's laboratory investigating regulatory processes related to adipose tissue hyperplasia. In this work, the transcription factor retinoid-related orphan receptor γ (RORγ) was identified as an important regulator of adipocyte development through regulation of its newly identified target gene matrix metallopeptidase-3. RORγ might serve as a novel predictor for the risk of metabolic complications in obesity as well as a pharmaceutical target for the treatment of obesity-associated diseases (Meissburger et al. 2011).

Khan et al., recently proposed that "adipose tissue fibrosis" is a hallmark of metabolically challenged adipocytes. Authors observed that the absence of collagen VI, the highly enriched extracellular matrix component of adipose tissue, results in the uninhibited expansion of individual adipocytes, which is paradoxically associated with substantial improvements in whole-body energy homeostasis, both with high-fat diet exposure and in the ob/ob background. Weakening the extracellular scaffold of adipocytes seems to enable their stress-free expansion during states of positive energy balance, which is consequently associated with an improved inflammatory profile (Khan et al. 2009). Further support to the notion that metabolic deregulation is rather due to lipid-leakage than the adipocyte hypertrophy *per se* comes from the experiment where mice lacking leptin were made to overexpress adiponectin. This led to the modest increase in circulating levels of full-length adiponectin and to subsequent normalization of glucose and insulin levels, dramatic improvement of glucose tolerance and positive effect on serum triglyceride levels. Adiponectin in fact completely rescued the diabetic phenotype in ob/ob mice. These mice displayed increased expression of PPARγ target genes and a reduction in macrophage infiltration in adipose tissue and systemic inflammation. Adiponectin expressing ob/ob mice, however, were morbidly obese, with significantly higher levels of adiposity and adipocyte hypertrophy than their ob/ob littermates. Adiponectin seems to act as a peripheral "starvation" signal promoting the storage of triglycerides preferentially in adipose tissue. As a consequence, reduced triglyceride levels in the liver and muscle convey improved systemic insulin sensitivity despite adipocyte hypertrophy (Kim et al. 2007).

2.1 Specificities of subcutaneous and visceral adipose tissue

In contrast to visceral adipose tissue, which is often blamed from inducing detrimental metabolic effects, subcutaneous adipose tissue has the potential to benefit lipid and glucose metabolism. It has been repeatedly shown that differences in regional body fat distribution determine the propensity for the development of obesity related metabolic complications (Tchernof 2007). Accumulation of fat in the visceral region (mesentery, omentum, retroperitoneum), that in fact corresponds to central obesity (determined by increased waist circumference) is associated with cardiovascular disease and type 2 diabetes, independently on overall obesity (Wajchenberg 2000; Hamdy et al. 2006; Pischon et al. 2008). The amount of visceral fat increases with age in both genders but man in general have greater visceral adiposity than women (Wajchenberg 2000). Consistent with this notion, removal of visceral adipose tissue (omentectomy) decreases glucose and insulin levels in humans (Thorne et al. 2002). By contrast peripheral obesity – increased subcutaneous adipose tissue mass, mainly in the region of buttock and thighs seem to be associated with improved insulin sensitivity and lower risk for type 2 diabetes mellitus (Snijder et al. 2003; Koska et al. 2008). One possible explanation for the detrimental effect of visceral fat accumulation comes from its unfortunate anatomical location (Arner, P. 1998; Bergman et al. 2006), but second theory based on adipose tissue transplantation experiments blames rather the tissue internal properties such as unfavorable secretory profile (Matsuzawa et al. 1999).

Adipose tissue transplantation experiments have been primarily used as a tool to study physiology for human reconstructive surgery, but they provide important information on differences between visceral and subcutaneous adipose tissue which opens the vision of the adipose tissue or adipose tissue derived stem cells transplantation for the treatment of obesity and metabolic disorders.

2.2 Brown adipose tissue in human physiology

Humans and other mammals have two types of adipose tissue that contribute to control of the whole body energy metabolism. The above discussed white adipose tissue, "the bad guy" associated with obesity, is necessary for energy storage. Brown adipose, "the good guy", contains a lots of mitochondria and is ready to burn energy to generate heat in response to cold or dietary intake, keeping the body warm and slim (Cannon & Nedergaard 2004). Until recently, physiologically relevant amount of brown fat was only found in newborns. However, accumulating evidence indicates that adult humans – or at least significant portion of us retain physiologically relevant amount of brown fat (van Marken Lichtenbelt et al. 2009; Vijgen et al. 2011; Virtanen & Nuutila 2011). This provides an exciting possibility to precisely regulate the adaptive thermogenic process in humans, which could dissipate energy and lower the obesity related metabolic burden. Brown adipose tissue activity in humans was determined with the aid of ^{18}F-fluorodeoxyglucose positron-emission tomography and computing tomography mainly in the supraclavicular region of cold-exposed individuals. Importantly, specimens of the adipose tissue from the supraclavicular region of adult humans with active brown adipose tissue were positive for UCP1 protein (Fig. 3.) (van Marken Lichtenbelt et al. 2009; Zingaretti et al. 2009). Vision of translating this knowledge into the clinical practice is quite reachable (Nedergaard & Cannon 2010; Tseng et al. 2010). Clinical importance could be significant, despite the fact that the volume of active brown adipose tissue tends to be lower in the overweight or obese than in the lean individuals (van Marken Lichtenbelt et al. 2009), and that it decreases with age (Cypess et al. 2009). Interestingly, applying the personalized cooling protocol for maximal nonshivering conditions to morbidly obese individuals could still increase brown adipose tissue activity (Vijgen et al. 2011).

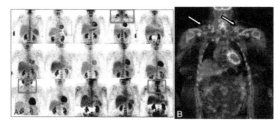

Fig. 3. Metabolically activated brown adipose tissue in supraclavicular region (arrows, B) in morbidly obese individuals after personalized cooling protocol (Vijgen et al. 2011).

2.3 Metabolic activation of the white adipose tissue

It has recently been shown that brown adipocytes and muscle cells share the common origin and in this respect they are quite distinct from white adipocytes (Tseng et al. 2008; Seale & Lazar 2009). The question remains, what is the origin of "brown fat-like white (brite) " adipocytes containing UCP1 which could be induced in white fat depots under certain pohysiological (cold exposure) (Fig. 4.) or pharmacological (activation of SNS, agonists of PPARγ) conditions (Granneman et al. 2005; Li et al. 2005; Ukropec et al. 2006). Nedegaard`s laboratory had recently reported that chronic treatment with the PPARγ agonist rosiglitazone promotes not only the expression of PGC1α and mitochondriogenesis but also a catecholamine – inducible UCP1 gene expression in a significant subset of the white adipocytes, giving them the genuine, thermogenic capacity.

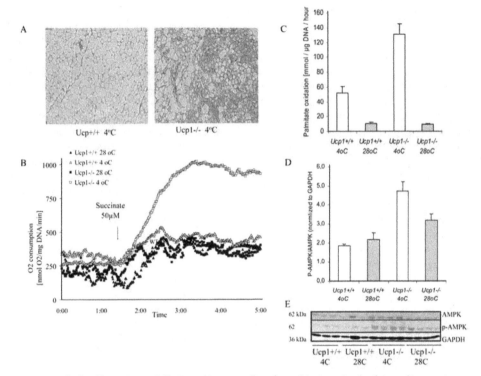

Fig. 4. Metabolically activated "brite adipocytes" as found in inguinal white adipose tissue of mice lacking the UCP1-thermogenesis after gradual exposure to cold.
(A) histomorphology, (B) O_2 consumption by oxymetry, (C) adipose tissue *ex vivo* palmitate oxidation, (D&E) evidence for AMPK activation (Ukropec et al. 2006).

In collaboration with laboratory of dr. Kvatnansky we have recently observed that catecholamines, important regulators of lipolysis in adipose tissue, could be produced within adipocytes. Adipocytes isolated from mesenteric adipose tissue expressed genes encoding the catecholamine biosynthetic enzymes and produced catecholamines *de novo*. Administration of tyrosine hydroxylase inhibitor, alpha-methyl-p-tyrosine, significantly reduced concentration of catecholamines in isolated adipocytes *in vitro* (Fig. 5.). We therefore hypothesized that the sympathetic innervation of adipose tissue is not the only source of catecholamines and that adipocyte-derived catecholamines could dynamically modulate metabolic or thermogenic properties of the white adipose tissue perhaps by enhancing "brite adipocyte" function (Vargovic et al. 2011).

3. Adipocentric view on the pathophysiology of metabolic disease

The prevalence of obesity and its consequent pathologies in modern society is of serious health concern. Although the expansion of adipose tissue mass during pathological obesity is in itself not a grave problem, rather it is the ensuing pathologies resultant of this state, including development of hypertension, type 2 diabetes and cardiac myopathies, that impacts peoples lives and health services worldwide.

Clearly not all obese individuals develop metabolic and cardiovascular complications; here we discuss several regulatory mechanisms representing a base for the strategies to prevent metabolic disease development.

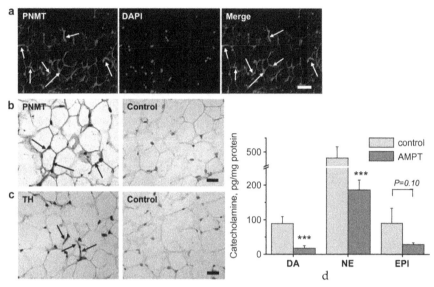

Fig. 5. Adipocytes have internal catecholamine production capacity. Adipose tissue contains mRNA and proteins specific for tyrosine hydroxylase (TH) and phenylethanolamine N-methyltransferase PNMT as shown on histological sections probed with specific PNMT (a,b) and TH (c) antibodies, scale bar: 20 μm. (d) Adipocytes freshly isolated from mesenteric adipose tissue produce dopamine (DA), norepinephrine (NE) and epinephrine (EPI) into the media. Production of catecholamines is largely inhibited by addition of alpha-methyl-p-tyrosine (AMPT) – competitive inhibitor of TH activity (Vargovic et al. 2011).

3.1 Hypoxia

Hypothesis that adipose tissue populated by large adipocytes contains the local microhypoxia suffering areas, which has a profound effect on the tissue metabolic and inflammatory phenotype, has been largely accepted. Hypoxia is one of the major triggers strongly inhibiting adipocyte differentiation. Tissue hypoxia in obesity is associated with the defects in the nutrient and oxygen supply into the tissue, related to a defective blood flow regulation which might be perpetuated by the increased fat cell size (Yun et al. 2002). This is happening in spite of the almost unlimited capacity of adipose tissue to expand in a non-transformed form, which is a very unique property of adipose tissue that cannot be seen in any other organ. To accomplish this adipose tissue requires potent mechanisms to remodel, acutely and chronically, as it can rapidly reach the diffusional limit of oxygen; molecular response to hypoxia is therefore an early determinant that limits healthy adipose tissue expansion. Proper expansion requires a highly coordinated response among many different cell types, including endothelial precursor cells, immune cells, and preadipocytes (Sun et al. 2011). It has also been demonstrated that mitochondrial oxidative apparatus is essential for the white fat adipocyte differentiation (De Pauw et al. 2009). Beside their key role in ATP production, mitochondria constitute the primary source of reactive oxygen species (ROS), which have a great potential to influence the tissue plasticity.

ROS are not only considered a negative factors contributing to degenerative processes and ageing, but also a physiological signal molecules participating in the oxygen sensing mechanisms (Chandel & Budinger 2007). Mitochondrial ROS production influences the size of the white adipocytes, and ROS are in fact antiadipogenic signaling molecules triggering the hypoxia-dependent inhibition of adipocyte differentiation (Carriere et al. 2004). In addition, decreased oxygen availability stimulates the programming of cellular metabolism towards increased glycolysis and fatty acid and triacylglyceride synthesis (Halperin et al. 1969; Kinnula et al. 1978). Hypoxia-inducible factor (HIF), dimers composed of HIF1α, HIF2α or HIF3α (collectively HIFα) and HIF1β/ARNT subunits, play a key role in the coordination of these metabolic adaptations (Trayhurn et al. 2008; Krishnan et al. 2009). HIFα subunits are constitutively expressed but degraded under normoxia due to prolyl hydroxylase activity, which marks them for recognition by the von Hippel-Lindau (VHL) tumor suppressor protein pVHL, that acts as part of an E3 ubiquitin ligase complex to target HIFα subunit for proteasomal degradation. Loss of pVHL function or hypoxia leads to accumulation of HIFα, dimerization with HIFα/ARNT and the activation of numerous hypoxia-inducible genes (Krek 2000; Semenza 2001). Previous work by Krek`s laboratory provided the seminal observation that hypoxia activated pVHL and HIF1α oxygen sensing system affects normal physiological function of heart and pancreatic beta cells by triggering the changes in the glucose and fatty acid metabolism (Zehetner et al. 2008; Krishnan et al. 2009). Interestingly, hypoxia present in atherosclerotic lesions contributes to the pro-inflammatory lipid-loaded foam cells formation, as it decreases expression of enzymes involved in β-oxidation and increases expression of enzymes related to fatty acid synthesis and lipid droplet formation. The aforementioned processes possibly stimulate progression of the atherosclerotic plaque formation (Bostrom et al. 2007). Finally, tissue hypoxia largely modulates adipocytokine production and possibly contributes to the adipose tissue inflammation in obesity (Hosogai et al. 2007; Wang et al. 2007; Ukropec et al. 2008).

3.2 Inflammation – Macrophage, adipocyte and preadipocyte plasticity

Chronic low level of inflammation present in the "pathogenic" adipose tissue has been found to have adverse effects on the adipose tissue physiological functions contributing thus to the metabolic disease. It has been shown that increase in both body fat mass and adipocyte cell size are directly related to the number of macrophages found in the adipose tissue (Wellen & Hotamisligil 2005; Weisberg et al. 2006; Goossens 2008). A net pro-inflammatory response of the adipose tissue may result from adipose tissue secretion of pro-inflammatory factors; adipose tissue secretion of factors that stimulate other tissues to produce inflammatory factors; and decreased production of anti-inflammatory factors. Although the contribution of specific cell types to inflammation is uncertain, evidence is mounting that implicates adipose tissue macrophages as the significant contributor to inflammation in insulin resistant adipose tissue (Kanda et al. 2006; Neels & Olefsky 2006). There are controversial reports related to the importance of the CC chemokine ligand 2 (CCL2, monocyte chemoattractant protein-1) for the macrophage-recruitment and activation in obesity (Kamei et al. 2006; Inouye et al. 2007). Interestingly CCL2 has also been proposed to affect metabolism independently of its macrophage-recruiting capabilities (Inouye et al. 2007). There is also preliminary data indicating that the tissue infiltration by macrophages depends upon the expression of osteopontin, an extracellular matrix protein and pro-inflammatory cytokine which promotes the monocyte chemotaxis and cell motility. Mice exposed to a high-fat diet exhibited increased plasma osteopontin level, and elevated expression of osteopontin in macrophages recruited into adipose tissue. In addition, obese mice lacking osteopontin displayed improved insulin sensitivity in the absence of an effect on the diet-induced obesity, body composition or energy expenditure. These mice further demonstrated decreased macrophage infiltration into adipose tissue, which may reflect both impaired macrophage motility and attenuated monocyte recruitment by stromal vascular cells. Finally, obese osteopontin-deficient mice exhibited decreased markers of inflammation, both in adipose tissue and systemically (Nomiyama et al. 2007).

Adipose tissue resident macrophages show significant heterogeneity in their properties and activation state, reflecting the local metabolic and immune microenvironment (Gordon & Taylor 2005). Different stimuli activate macrophages to express distinct patterns of chemokines, surface markers and enzymes that ultimately generate the diversity of macrophage function seen in inflammatory and non-inflammatory settings. It has recently been proposed that adipose tissue macrophages, which accumulate with obesity and are implicated in insulin resistance switch their phenotype from one of an alternatively activated (M2) to pro-inflammatory (M1) cells (Lumeng et al. 2007). Characteristic features of the IFN-γ induced pro-inflammatory (M1) macrophages include enhanced MHC class II expression, but distinctive up-regulation of i-NOS. Alternative activation of macrophages (M2) is strongly associated with extracellular parasitic infections, allergy, humoral immunity, and fibrosis. It is characterized by up-regulation of the endocytic lecithin-like receptors and arginase rather than i-NOS (Gordon 2007). Therefore, the alternatively activated (M2) macrophages seem to have high capacity for the tissue remodeling and repair.

It had been recently proposed that PPARγ is required for maturation of alternatively activated macrophages (M2), which could also participate to its insulin sensitizing effect (Odegaard et al. 2007). Disruption of PPARγ in myeloid cells impaired alternative macrophage activation and predisposed to the development of diet-induced obesity, insulin resistance, and glucose intolerance. This might be related to the concomitant down-regulation of oxidative phosphorylation gene expression in skeletal muscle and liver (Odegaard et al. 2007). Phenotype of macrophages in the pathogenic-hypoxic adipose tissue might also be regulated by HIF-1 since the functional loss of HIF-1α resulted in a dramatic reduction of the intracellular ATP stores in macrophages to approximately 15-20%, most likely due to the inhibition of the HIF-1α regulated glycolytic energy generation (Cramer & Johnson 2003; Cramer et al. 2003). It could be hypothesized that resident alternatively activated macrophages have a beneficial role in regulating nutrient homeostasis and suggest that macrophage polarization towards the alternative state might be a useful strategy for treating type 2 diabetes, by modulating adipose tissue phenotype.

Fatty acid binding proteins (FABPs), which are common to adipocytes and macrophages, could also play an important role in metabolic and inflammatory disease, and might therefore represent desirable therapeutic targets for metabolic syndrome (Erbay et al. 2007). Macrophage-derived foam cells express the adipocyte fatty acid-binding protein (FABP) aP2 that plays an important role in regulating the development of insulin resistance in obesity. It has been shown that macrophages deficient in aP2 display alterations in the inflammatory cytokine production. Through its distinct actions in adipocytes and macrophages, aP2 links together the features of the metabolic syndrome including insulin resistance, obesity, inflammation, and atherosclerosis (Linton & Fazio 2003).

3.3 Phospholipid membrane composition

In the last decades, free radical processes delineated an interdisciplinary field linking chemistry to biology and medicine. Free radical mechanisms became of importance as molecular basis of physiological and pathological conditions. Lipids, in particular unsaturated fatty acids, are susceptible to free radical attack. The reactivity of the double bond toward free radicals is well known; in particular the reversible addition of radical species to this functionality determines the cis-trans double bond isomerization. Since the prevalent geometry displayed by unsaturated fatty acids in eukaryotes is cis, the occurrence of the cis-trans isomerization by free radicals corresponds to the loss of an important structural information linked to biological activity (Ferreri & Chatgilialoglu 2009). Formation of trans isomers of unsaturated fatty acid in biological membranes can have important meaning and consequences connected to radical stress associated with nutritional overload and mitochondrial defects. It might, together with changes in membrane lipid composition (Pietilainen et al. 2011), substantially modulate lipid membrane biophysical characteristics such as thickness, fluidity, protein lateral diffusion capacity, permeability to small molecules in expanding adipocytes and contribute thus to the development of metabolic disease in obesity.

3.4 Pollutants and metabolic health

Physical inactivity and unhealthy diet are well recognized environmental influences largely increasing the risk for metabolic disease development. Recent advances in detecting the presence of various persistent organic pollutants in the surrounding world as well as within our bodies, prompted us to evaluate its possible role in pathogenesis of different endocrine and metabolic pathological states (Langer et al. 2003; Langer et al. 2007; Langer 2010; Langer et al. 2010; Ukropec et al. 2010; Langer et al. 2011).

A heavily polluted area of Eastern Slovakia was targeted by the PCBrisk cross-sectional survey to search for possible links between environmental pollution and both prediabetes and diabetes. Associations of serum levels of five persistent organic pollutants (POPs), namely polychlorinated biphenyls (PCBs), 2,2'-bis(4-chlorophenyl)-1,1-dichloroethylene (p,p'-DDE), 2,2'-bis(4-chlorophenyl)-1,1,1-trichloro-ethane (p,p'-DDT), hexachlorobenzene (HCB) and beta-hexachlorocyclohexane (β-HCH), with prediabetes and diabetes were investigated in 2,047 adults. Prevalence of prediabetes and diabetes increased in a dose-dependent manner, with individuals in upper quintiles of individual POPs showing striking increases in prevalence of prediabetes (Fig. 6.) Interestingly, unlike PCBs, DDT and DDE, increased levels of HCB and β-HCH seemed not to be associated with increased prevalence of diabetes (Ukropec et al. 2010). Cumulative effect of all five persistent organic pollutants (sum of orders) more than tripled the prevalence of prediabetes while that of diabetes was increased more than six times as compared to the referent quintile composed of individuals with lowest levels of pollutants in serum. We as well as the others have clearly shown that increasing serum concentrations of individual persistent organic pollutants considerably increased prevalence of prediabetes and diabetes in a dose-dependent manner. Interaction of industrial and agricultural pollutants in increasing prevalence of prediabetes or diabetes is likely (Hong et al. 2010; Ukropec et al. 2010; Howard & Lee 2011; Lee, D. H. et al. 2011; Lee, D. H. et al. 2011; Lee, H. K. 2011).

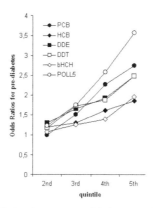

Fig. 6. The prevalence of prediabetes increases with increased circulating levels of PCBs (sum 15 congeners of polychlorinated biphenyls); DDE (2,2'-bis(4-chlorophenyl)-1,1-dichloroethylene); DDT (2,2'-bis(4-chlorophenyl)-1,1,1-trichloro-ethane); HCB (hexachlorobenzene) and b-HCH (beta-hexachlorocyclohexane); POLL5 represents the sum of orders for all 5 pollutants. Odds ratios were adjusted for age, gender and BMI.

4. Skeletal muscle in metabolic health and disease

Skeletal muscle represents a large mass of tissue, and its primary function is to use energy, though quite inefficiently, to enable us the 3D life, voluntary positioning and moving our bodies in a surrounding space. This makes an active muscle to be the most effective energy burner. In addition to obvious metabolic consequences, regular exercise activates central reward mechanisms and makes us happy (Figure 7.) (Sher 1998; Boecker et al. 2008).

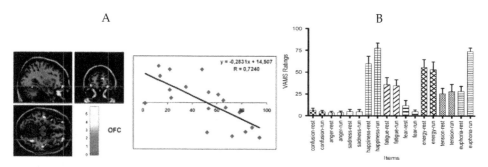

Fig. 7. Correlation of opidergic ligand 6-O-(2-[18F]fluoroethyl)-6-O-desmethyldiprenorphine binding in right orbitofrontal cortex (OFC) with the visual analog mood scale (for euphoria) in runners (**A**) and effect of exercise on the individual's mood expressed in the visual analog mood scale (**B**) (Boecker et al. 2008).

More importantly, inadequate physical activity, associated with defects in mitochondrial function and changes in ultrastructure as well as muscle endocrine properties, largely contributes to the imbalance between energy intake and energy expenditure and is tightly associated with many chronic metabolic and cardiovascular diseases (Bluher & Zimmer 2010; Pedersen 2011). Physical activity is a key factor to bring individuals living in a modern society with plenty of palatable food choices to energy balance. The mechanisms that tie muscle activity to health are unclear. Generation of "exercise pill" targeting organ systems involved in facultative thermogenesis had been envisaged (Himms-Hagen 2004). And results of studies aimed at identifying the endocrine properties of exercising muscle are encouraging our thinking in this respect. In our recent study we observed on the sample of 71 individuals with a broad range of BMI that overweight and obesity is associated with decreased physical activity. This might be not so surprising. But low physical activity level was also associated with decreased insulin sensitivity, increased fat cell size and expanded visceral adiposity all independent on BMI (Fig. 8.). In addition, the basic metabolic rate was positively and respiratory quotient negatively associated with the duration of the daily physical activity representing thus a direct link between physical activity and major determinants of energy homeostasis (Ukropcova et al., unpublished observations).

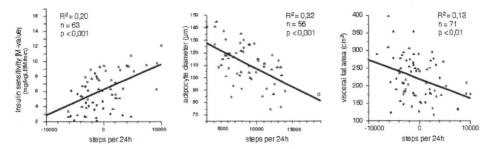

Fig. 8. Free-living ambulatory activity (number of steps in 24h) correlates with insulin sensitivity, modulates adipocyte diameter as well as visceral adiposity (Ukropcova et al., unpublished observations).

This complements the previous observations by others indicating that inactivity initiates unique cellular processes that are qualitatively different from the exercise responses. Inactivity physiology studies are beginning to raise a new concern with potentially major clinical and public health significance. Sedentary lifestyle threatens our society. The average nonexercising person may become even more metabolically unfit in the coming years if they sit too much and thereby lower the normally high volume of intermittent nonexercise physical activity in everyday life (Fig. 8) (Hamilton et al. 2007; Levine et al. 2008). Dynamic interrelations of skeletal muscle and adipose tissue during exercise are necessary to support muscle performance. This requires precise spacio-temporal management of the adipose tissue metabolic flux. The transcriptional coactivator PGC1α has recently been shown to regulate several exercise-associated aspects of muscle function. There is mounting evidence suggesting that this transcription factor controls muscle plasticity, suppresses a broad inflammatory response and integrates many beneficial effects of exercise on metabolic health (Handschin & Spiegelman 2008).

4.1 Exercise and skeletal muscle endocrinology

The recent identification of skeletal muscle as an endocrine organ that produces and releases biologically active substances, "myokines", expands our knowledge on how the endocrine, immune and nervous systems contribute to the maintenance of homeostasis, especially when energy demands are increased (Pedersen & Febbraio 2008). To date, only a few muscle cell-secreted proteins with auto-, para-, or endocrine functions have been identified. It could be hypothesized that skeletal muscle releases a large number of biologically active substances which participate to cell-to-cell and organ-to-organ cross-talk. It also has to be noted that specific biological functions of known myokines are very incompletely understood.

Certain myokines, such as calprotectin (Mortensen et al. 2008), IL15 (Nielsen & Pedersen 2007) and IL6 (Jonsdottir et al. 2000), are acutely induced by muscle contraction but might not necessarily be increased in response to muscle training (Pedersen & Febbraio 2008; Haugen et al. 2010). Exercise training involves multiple adaptations including increased pre-exercise skeletal muscle glycogen content (Kirwan et al. 1990), enhanced activity of key enzymes involved in β-oxidation (Schantz 1986), increased sensitivity of adipose tissue to epinephrine-induced lipolysis (Crampes et al. 1986), and increased muscle capacity to oxidize fat (Holloszy & Booth 1976; Phillips et al. 1996). It could therefore be hypothesized that secretory activity of muscle subjected to inadequate physical activity would be qualitatively and quantitatively distinct from that of the trained athlete, and that it could simply be regulated by e.g. the glycogen level (Keller et al. 2001; Steensberg et al. 2001), reactive oxygen species production (Kosmidou et al. 2002; Steensberg et al. 2007) or by modulating biological availability of various forms of lipids (Peter et al. 2009), such as found in obesity.

Previous reports indicate that calprotectin, IL6 and IL15 might contribute to homeostatic control of glucose and lipid metabolism (Van Hall et al. 2003; Febbraio et al. 2004). In addition, fibroblast growth factor-21 (FGF-21), the potent metabolic regulator, shown to improve glucose metabolism and insulin sensitivity in animal models, had recently been found to be expressed and secreted *in vitro* from murine muscle cells and *in vivo* from human muscle in response to insulin stimulation (hyperinsulinemic-euglycemic clamp) (Hojman et al. 2009). Follistatin-like 1 (Fstl-1) is another myokine whose functional significance in physiological and pathological processes is incompletely understood. Preliminary evidence indicates that Fstl-1 promotes endothelial cell function and stimulates revascularization in response to ischemic insult through its ability to activate Akt-eNOS signaling in muscle (Ouchi et al. 2008). Interleukin-8 is a CXC family chemokine increased in human muscle in response to concentric exercise (Akerstrom et al. 2005), which has also been shown to have angiogenic actions associated with activation of CXCR2 receptors in the human microvascular endothelial cells (Bek et al. 2002; Frydelund-Larsen et al. 2007). Recent report by Drevon's laboratory describes interleukin-7 as a novel myokine affecting myogenesis *in vitro* in human primary muscle cells. Interleukin-7 is up-regulated by exercise training in male individuals undergoing a strength training program (Haugen et al. 2010).

4.2 Mitochondrial biogenesis in skeletal muscle – Energetic remodeling of muscle phenotype in obesity, insulin resistance and exercise

Mitochondria are energy power plants of the cells, believed to have evolved over billions of years from invading prokaryotic oxygen utilizing "quite energizing" eubacterium to early eucaryotic cells, giving the life on earth new energy spark (Lanza & Nair 2010). Their structure and function is orchestrated by a strict coordination of nuclear and mitochondrial genome. Of ~1.000 mitochondrial proteins, only 13 are encoded by the mitochondrial genome, remaining proteins are translated from nuclear genome and transported across the inner mitochondrial membrane (Lanza & Nair 2010). Mitochondria cover majority of energetic needs of cells by coupling substrate oxidation with ATP formation, the process known as oxidative phosphorylation. This process also generates reactive oxygen species (ROS). It has been estimated that 0.2 – 2% of oxygen taken up by the cell is converted into ROS (Harper et al. 2004). Mechanisms for detoxifying the ROS are quite well developed in a eukaryotic cell which is another reason for their long lasting partnership with "dangerous" mitochondria. Sustained excessive production may accumulate amount of ROS exceeding the antioxidant capacity of the specific cell, eventually leading to cell damage and death (Harman 1956). During recent years, mitochondria , though not only those found in skeletal muscle, were put on the spot as organelles involved in aging and associated chronic civilization diseases such as Alzheimer's disease (Reddy 2009), some forms of cancer, obesity and type 2 diabetes (Johannsen & Ravussin 2009).

4.2.1 Mitochondria in obesity, insulin resistance and type 2 diabetes
Recent evidence indicates that insulin resistance in skeletal muscle might develop due to the reduced capacity of mitochondria to oxidize lipids (Bjorntorp et al. 1967; Kelley et al. 2002; Petersen et al. 2004; Ukropcova et al. 2007) and reduced capacity for insulin-stimulated ATP-synthesis (Petersen et al. 2005). Obese individuals and subjects with type 2 diabetes are characterized also by reduced adiponectin signaling (Kern et al. 2003; Civitarese et al. 2004; Rasmussen et al. 2006), lower rates of fasting lipid utilization and impaired switch to carbohydrate oxidation in response to insulin (Kelley et al. 1999; Kelley & Mandarino 2000; Ukropcova et al. 2005; Ukropcova et al. 2007). Recent studies using microarray expression analysis reported a decrease in the expression of genes involved in mitochondrial biogenesis in skeletal muscle of individuals with insulin resistance (Patti et al. 2003) and T2D (Mootha et al. 2003). Further studies in insulin resistant subjects and individuals with type 2 diabetes have shown reduced mitochondrial content, lower electron transport chain activity in total mitochondria and in intramyofibrilar and subsarcolemal mitochondrial fractions (Kelley et al. 2002; Ritov et al. 2005). Taken together, these data support the hypothesis that insulin resistance in human skeletal muscle arises from lowering mitochondrial number and functional capacity. Another hypothesis challenges this paradigm; it is supported by observations that increased fatty acid availability is associated with increased mitochondrial fat oxidation. However, mitochondrial overload with energy rich substrates highlights the pathophysiological role of ROS and that of products of incomplete mitochondrial oxidation rather than simple lowering of mitochondrial functional capacity (Koves et al. 2008; Holloszy 2009). The importance of mitochondria for energy homeostasis makes this organelle an exciting target for investigation and better understanding to regulation of mitochondrial biogenesis and function would help us to understand its putative role in the pathogenesis of obesity and insulin resistance.

4.2.2 Exercise and ageing keep constant battle for healthy mitochondria
Exercise is one of the two physiological stimuli known to increase production of new mitochondria and to improve mitochondrial efficiency. In our work, we have shown that caloric restriction, the only officially acknowledged physiological stimulus demonstrated to

prolong lifespan, is also inducing mitochondrial biogenesis in human skeletal muscle (Civitarese et al. 2007). Many scientists are on a quest, pursuing the vision of exercise mimicking pill, capable of induction of mitochondrial biogenesis *in vivo*. „Exercise in a pill" (another option would be a pill mimicking caloric restriction) is by many considered a putatively great tool to combat obesity and civilization diseases. However, healthy lifestyle intervention, with sufficient physical activity and matching caloric intake still proves to be the most natural and effective way how to stay fit, healthy and with increased chances to live up to be a hundred.

4.2.3 Adipose tissue and skeletal muscle interplay

Our organism can be viewed as a very complex society of tissues that need to communicate with one another in order to maintain metabolic health. Tissue cross-talk plays the central role in the regulation of food intake, energy expenditure, oxidative capacity, adaptation to changes in physical activity, nutritional status etc. As mentioned above, adipose tissue (as well as many other tissues in our body) is (are) a (the) source of many biologically active substances with autocrine, paracrine and endocrine activities, exerting effects over many different neighboring as well as distant tissues and organs.

Adiponectin is the most studied adipocytokine which is in relatively high quantities secreted from adipose tissue into the bloodstream. Adiponectin has very positive effects on our metabolic health as it activates glucose and fatty acid metabolism and improves insulin sensitivity. Adiponectin levels are inversely correlated with body fat mass and positively with insulin sensitivity (Hara et al. 2005) and it also displays anti-atherogenic and anti-inflammatory effects (Antoniades et al. 2009). This hormone was first characterized in mice as a transcript overexpressed in preadipocytes (precursors of fat cells) differentiating into adipocytes. The human homologue was identified as the most abundant transcript in adipose tissue. Contrary to expectations and despite being produced in adipose tissue, adiponectin was found to be decreased in obesity. The gene was localized to chromosome 3p27, a region highlighted as affecting genetic susceptibility to T2D and obesity. Supplementation by differing forms of adiponectin was able to improve insulin control, blood glucose and triglyceride levels in mouse models. The question remains what are the mechanisms underlying positive effects of adiponectin on metabolism?

The molecular mechanisms leading to mitochondrial dysfunction in obesity and T2D remain largely unknown. Bergeron et al (Bergeron et al. 2001) demonstrated that activation of cAMP-activated protein kinase (AMPK) increases both mitochondrial biogenesis and oxidative capacity in skeletal muscle of rodents. In animal models of T2D, the activation of AMPK by adiponectin increases muscle and hepatic fat oxidation and improves insulin sensitivity (Yamauchi et al. 2001). Studies in obese and diabetic rhesus monkey demonstrate that plasma adiponectin level declines in the early phases of obesity and in parallel to the progressive development of insulin resistance (Hotta et al. 2001). Furthermore, circulating plasma adiponectin levels and the expression of both adiponectin receptors are reduced in subjects with a family history of diabetes (Civitarese et al. 2004), while prospective studies in Pima Indians show that high concentrations of adiponectin is protective against the development of T2D (Lindsay et al. 2002). Collectively, these data define a pathway in skeletal muscle by which adiponectin contributes to energy homeostasis by modulating mitochondrial number and function (Civitarese et al. 2006). Early defects in the secretion of adiponectin or in adiponectin signaling might contribute to the lower mitochondrial content and/or function in the prediabetic state. Interestingly and in accordance with our results, it has been recently demonstrated that an adiponectin-like molecule, a recombinant globular domain of adiponectin (rgAd110-244), has a significant therapeutic potential to treat insulin resistance in mice fed a high fat diet for 3 months (Sulpice et al. 2009). This makes adiponectin derivatives a promising new treatment for T2D.

It appears that adiponectin is also produced by skeletal muscle and that globular adiponectin is capable of inducing the differentiation and fusion of muscle cells in vitro (Fiaschi et al. 2009). Mimicking of pro-inflammatory settings or exposure to oxidative stress strongly increases the production of adiponectin from differentiating primary muscle cells. These data suggest a novel function of adiponectin, coordinating the myogenic differentiation program.

4.2.4 Mitochondrial biogenesis in muscle cells – Lipids and exercise

Fatty acids are known to be the ligands of various transcription factors involved in the regulation of metabolism and mitochondrial biogenesis (Gilde & Van Bilsen 2003). It has been shown previously that fatty acids as well as a diet with an increased fat content is capable of inducing mitochondrial biogenesis both in vitro and in vivo (Watt et al. 2006; Hancock et al. 2008). In our work, we have tested the effect of chronic, 4-day long exposure to palmitate on metabolic phenotypes of human primary skeletal muscle cells. We observed an increase in number of active mitochondria as measured by incorporation of mitotracker (fluorescencent dye selectively activated within respiring mitochondria) as well as increased expression of genes involved in mitochondrial biogenesis, increase in the capacity for fatty acid oxidation (Ukropcova et al. 2005, Ukropcova et al, unpublished observation). At this moment we can only speculate on the mechanisms behind this oxidation boosting effect of palmitate. However, it has been shown that fatty acids are capable of activating AMP activated protein kinase (AMPK) in skeletal muscle (Watt et al. 2006). AMPK signaling is activated in energy deficit states and it primarily saves the cell by inducing *de novo* mitochondrial biogenesis. It cooperates with transcription factor PGC1α, overexpression of which has been demonstrated to enhance both lipid oxidation and synthesis (Espinoza et al. 2010). Another possibility is that palmitate is a ligand for the transcription factors involved in the regulation of cell´s oxidative capacity, such as PPARδ (Gilde & Van Bilsen 2003). Animal (Hancock et al. 2008) as well as clinical studies (Bajaj et al. 2007) also support the role of fatty acids for PGC1α regulation at the level of gene expression. We and others have indicated that saturated fatty acids (e.g. palmitate) contribute to the regulation of metabolism by self-promoting their utilization *via* increased oxidative capacity of the skeletal muscle cell.

In addition, dynamic interrelations of skeletal muscle and adipose tissue during exercise are necessary to support muscle performance and adipose tissue energy fluxes management. The transcriptional coactivator PGC1α has also been shown to regulate several exercise-associated aspects of muscle function. It could be hypothesized that this protein controls muscle plasticity, suppresses a broad inflammatory response and mediates the beneficial effects of exercise on metabolic health (Handschin and Spiegelman 2008).

4.2.5 Caloric restriction induces mitochondrial biogenesis in skeletal muscle

Caloric restriction is a non-genetic manipulation that results in the lifespan extension of many different species, from yeasts to dogs, and even primates, and it is accompanied by delayed onset of chronic civilization diseases (Ball et al. 1947; Anderson et al. 2009). There are also hints that people who eat a calorie-restricted diet might live longer than those who overeat. People living in Okinawa, Japan, have a lower energy intake than the rest of the Japanese population and an extremely long life span (Willcox et al. 2007). In addition, calorie-restricted diets beneficially affect several biomarkers of aging, including decreased insulin sensitivity. Based on combined favorable changes in lipid and blood pressure, caloric restriction with or without exercise induces weight loss and favorably reduces risk for cardiovascular disease even in healthy non-obese individuals (Lefevre et al. 2009) and ameliorates the age-related loss of muscle mass, sarcopenia, in a variety a species (Marzetti et al. 2009). But how might caloric restriction slow aging? Some of the theories behind the lifespan extending effect of caloric restriction include (i) decreased oxidative damage, (ii) altered glucose utilization, (iii) increased insulin sensitivity, (iv) neuroendocrine changes and (v) enhanced stress responsiveness (Allard et al. 2009). Reduction of oxidative damage to proteins, lipids, and DNA is one of the leading theories, although the underlying mechanisms of this process are unclear. Cellular nutrient sensing systems seem to mediate many of the metabolic responses to caloric restriction, including the regulation of free radical production and oxidative stress. Mitochondria are the major consumers of cellular oxygen (~85%) and the predominant production site of free radicals, a by-product of oxidative phosphorylation. Studies in mammals have shown that caloric restriction reduces the generation of free radicals by mitochondria, in parallel to reductions in mitochondrial proton leak and whole-body energy expenditure. Paradoxically, caloric restriction induces mitochondrial proliferation in rodents (Lanza & Nair 2010), and either lowers (Handschin & Spiegelman 2008) or does not affect mitochondrial oxygen consumption (Lanza & Nair 2010). Low mitochondrial content seems to contribute to increased ROS production. When mitochondrial mass is reduced, mitochondria have increased "workload," leading to higher membrane potential and increased ROS production (Handschin & Spiegelman 2008; Lanza & Nair 2009; Lanza & Nair 2010). It has also been demonstrated that caloric restriction is strongly associated with an increased level and activation of sirtuins, namely the Sir2 histone deacetylase and its mammalian ortholog Sirt1. Sirtuins are members of the silent information regulator 2 (Sir2) family, a family of Class III histone/protein deacetylases. The enzymatic activity of most sirtuins has been shown to be dependent on nicotinamide dinucleotide, suggesting that the activity of these enzymes is dependent on the nutritive state of the organism (Allard et al. 2009). Specific Sirt1 activation mimics low energy levels and protects against diet-induced metabolic disorders by enhancing fat oxidation (Feige et al. 2008). PGC1α is a transcriptional coactivator playing a pivotal role in the regulation of mitochondrial biogenesis, which is known to be induced in response to exercise and caloric restriction (Fig. 8.). Research strongly supports the health benefits of exercise in humans of all ages. Increased exercise in the absence of other behavioral changes prevents the onset of many chronic diseases (Elbekai & El-Kadi 2005).

In our study we showed that short-term caloric deficit (caloric restriction with or without exercise) coordinately up-regulated the expression of genes involved in mitochondrial biogenesis in skeletal muscle resulting in increased mitochondrial content, improved whole body energy efficiency, and decreased DNA fragmentation in non-obese humans (Civitarese et al. 2007). Our results suggest that caloric restriction induces biogenesis of "efficient" mitochondria as an adaptive mechanism, which in turn lowers oxidative stress.

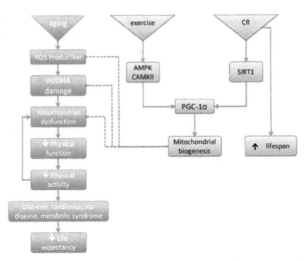

Fig. 9. The free radical theory of aging posits that a senescent phenotype is induced by accumulation of oxidative damage resulting from reactive oxygen species. Exercise and caloric restriction (CR) are two interventions that induce mitochondrial biogenesis through PGC-1α. Although exercise and CR increase average life expectancy by protecting against age-related comorbidities, only CR has been shown to increase maximal life span; an effect that seems to require the activation of sirtuins (Lanza & Nair 2010).

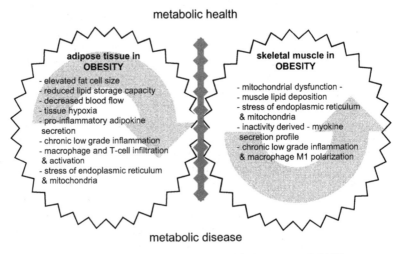

Fig. 10. Determinants of metabolic health and disease (Ukropec et al. 2008)

5. Conclusion

Ability of tissues to adapt morphologically and functionally to different physiological situations determines the overall metabolic health. Increased adipose tissue mass but mainly adipocyte lipid overload is responsible for the "pathogenic" adipose tissue phenotype. This phenotype, characteristic by extra-large unilocular adipocytes, further promotes tissue hypoxia and development of chronic persistent inflammation and metabolic stress. Pathogenic modification of the adipocyte modulates its metabolic, secretory and immunologic function leading to the development of metabolic disease (Fig. 10.). Inactive skeletal muscle, overloaded with fat could also contribute to metabolic imbalance by switching the fiber type towards less oxidative (less insulin sensitive) fibers, by lack of anti-inflammatory and insulin-sensitizing myokine production as well as by chronic inflammation associated with mitochondrial stress and stress of endoplasmic reticulum (Fig. 10.). Our environment greatly modifies our metabolic health by means of dietary influences and exercise activity which together with pathologies associated with hyperlipidemia, chronic systemic hypoxia and tissue inflammation determines adipose tissue and skeletal muscle metabolic and secretory phenotype and subsequently our metabolic health.

It is generally accepted that regular physical activity prevents metabolic and cardiovascular disease development, and supports healthy aging. Skeletal muscle has been shown to produce and secrete several bioactive factors (hormones) termed "myokines". Different spectra of myokines originating from either active "trained" or inactive "sedentary" skeletal muscles elicit distinct adaptive changes in immune system, metabolic balance and processes of cellular growth and differentiation in order to maintain the whole body homeostasis. This requires extensive communication of skeletal muscle with many different cells and organs but the nature of mechanisms that tie muscle activity to metabolic health is not completely understood. It seems to be essential (i) to identify myokines differentially expressed and secreted from muscle cells derived from healthy and obese individuals, and individuals with type 2 diabetes; to (ii) determine basic principles of the muscle cross-communication with adipocytes (differentiation) and endothelial cells (angiogenesis) in fostering tissue plasticity necessary for adaptation to obesity and type 2 diabetes; and (iii) to discover novel myokines and to investigate their physiological significance in cell culture models and *in vivo* in genetically modified animal models as well as in humans. Myokines may be involved in mediating the health beneficial effects of exercise and play important roles in the protection against chronic diseases associated with low-grade inflammation, insulin resistance, hyperlipidemia, such as cardiovascular disease, type-2-diabetes, and cancer. Extension of the knowledge on the mechanisms whereby regular exercise offers protection against chronic diseases in combination with clinical research serves as a foundation for the development of public health guidelines with regard to exercise. Moreover, identification of new myokines and understanding basic principles and mechanisms of their action will potentially provide pharmacological targets for the treatment of metabolic and cardiovascular disorders.

6. Acknowledgement

We would like to express our cordial gratitude to everybody who contributed to this work. There is too many people to thank. Above all we would like to acknowledge our parents and our wonderfull children Kiki and Jakub, our inspiration in everyday life. We would also like to thank the funding agencies: APVV grant agency (APVV 0122-06), European Foundation to Study Diabetes (EFSD New Horizons Collaborative Research Grant) and the 7th FP EC 2007-2.1.1-6. grant entitled „LipidomicNET" for their generous support.

7. References

Ahima, R.S. & Lazar, M.A. (2008). Adipokines and the peripheral and neural control of energy balance, *Mol Endocrinol*, vol.22, No.5, pp. 1023-1031, issn 0888-8809 (Print)

Akerstrom, T.; Steensberg, A.; Keller, P.; Keller, C.; Penkowa, M. & Pedersen, B.K. (2005). Exercise induces interleukin-8 expression in human skeletal muscle, *J Physiol*, vol.563, No.Pt 2, pp. 507-516, issn 0022-3751 (Print)

Allard, J.S.; Perez, E.; Zou, S. & De Cabo, R. (2009). Dietary activators of sirt1, *Mol Cell Endocrinol*, vol.299, No.1, pp. 58-63, issn 0303-7207 (Print)

Anderson, R.M.; Shanmuganayagam, D. & Weindruch, R. (2009). Caloric restriction and aging: Studies in mice and monkeys, *Toxicol Pathol*, vol.37, No.1, pp. 47-51, issn 1533-1601 (Electronic)

Antoniades, C.; Antonopoulos, A.S.; Tousoulis, D. & Stefanadis, C. (2009). Adiponectin: From obesity to cardiovascular disease, *Obes Rev*, vol.10, No.3, pp. 269-279, issn 1467-789X (Electronic)

Arner, E.; Westermark, P.O.; Spalding, K.L.; Britton, T.; Ryden, M.; Frisen, J.; Bernard, S. & Arner, P. (2010). Adipocyte turnover: Relevance to human adipose tissue morphology, *Diabetes*, vol.59, No.1, pp. 105-109, issn 1939-327X (Electronic)

Arner, P. (1998). Not all fat is alike, *Lancet*, vol.351, No.9112, pp. 1301-1302, issn 0140-6736 (Print)

Arner, P.; Arner, E.; Hammarstedt, A. & Smith, U. (2011). Genetic predisposition for type 2 diabetes, but not for overweight/obesity, is associated with a restricted adipogenesis, *PLoS One*, vol.6, No.4, p. e18284, issn 1932-6203 (Electronic)

Bajaj, M.; Medina-Navarro, R.; Suraamornkul, S.; Meyer, C.; Defronzo, R.A. & Mandarino, L.J. (2007). Paradoxical changes in muscle gene expression in insulin-resistant subjects after sustained reduction in plasma free fatty acid concentration, *Diabetes*, vol.56, No.3, pp. 743-752, issn 0012-1797 (Print)

Ball, Z.B.; Barnes, R.H. & Visscher, M.B. (1947). The effects of dietary caloric restriction on maturity and senescence, with particular reference to fertility and longevity, *Am J Physiol*, vol.150, No.3, pp. 511-519, issn 0002-9513 (Print)

Bays, H.E.; Gonzalez-Campoy, J.M.; Bray, G.A.; Kitabchi, A.E.; Bergman, D.A.; Schorr, A.B.; Rodbard, H.W. & Henry, R.R. (2008). Pathogenic potential of adipose tissue and metabolic consequences of adipocyte hypertrophy and increased visceral adiposity, *Expert Rev Cardiovasc Ther*, vol.6, No.3, pp. 343-368, issn 1744-8344 (Electronic)

Bek, E.L.; Mcmillen, M.A.; Scott, P.; Angus, L.D. & Shaftan, G.W. (2002). The effect of diabetes on endothelin, interleukin-8 and vascular endothelial growth factor-mediated angiogenesis in rats, *Clin Sci (Lond)*, vol.103 Suppl 48, pp. 424S-429S, issn 0143-5221 (Print)

Bergeron, R.; Ren, J.M.; Cadman, K.S.; Moore, I.K.; Perret, P.; Pypaert, M.; Young, L.H.; Semenkovich, C.F. & Shulman, G.I. (2001). Chronic activation of amp kinase results in nrf-1 activation and mitochondrial biogenesis, *Am J Physiol Endocrinol Metab*, vol.281, No.6, pp. E1340-1346, issn 0193-1849 (Print)

Bergman, R.N.; Kim, S.P.; Catalano, K.J.; Hsu, I.R.; Chiu, J.D.; Kabir, M.; Hucking, K. & Ader, M. (2006). Why visceral fat is bad: Mechanisms of the metabolic syndrome, *Obesity (Silver Spring)*, vol.14 Suppl 1, pp. 16S-19S, issn 1930-7381 (Print)

Bjorntorp, P.; Schersten, T. & Fagerberg, S.E. (1967). Respiration and phosphorylation of mitochondria isolated from the skeletal muscle of diabetic and normal subjects, *Diabetologia,* vol.3, No.3, pp. 346-352, issn 0012-186X (Print)

Bjorntorp, P. (1974). Size, number and function of adipose tissue cells in human obesity, *Horm Metab Res,* vol.Suppl 4, pp. 77-83, issn 0018-5043 (Print)

Bluher, M. & Zimmer, P. (2010). [metabolic and cardiovascular effects of physical activity, exercise and fitness in patients with type 2 diabetes], *Dtsch Med Wochenschr,* vol.135, No.18, pp. 930-934, issn 1439-4413 (Electronic)

Boecker, H.; Sprenger, T.; Spilker, M.E.; Henriksen, G.; Koppenhoefer, M.; Wagner, K.J.; Valet, M.; Berthele, A. & Tolle, T.R. (2008). The runner's high: Opioidergic mechanisms in the human brain, *Cereb Cortex,* vol.18, No.11, pp. 2523-2531, issn 1460-2199 (Electronic)

Bostrom, M.A.; Boyanovsky, B.B.; Jordan, C.T.; Wadsworth, M.P.; Taatjes, D.J.; De Beer, F.C. & Webb, N.R. (2007). Group v secretory phospholipase a2 promotes atherosclerosis: Evidence from genetically altered mice, *Arterioscler Thromb Vasc Biol,* vol.27, No.3, pp. 600-606, issn 1524-4636 (Electronic)

Cannon, B. & Nedergaard, J. (2004). Brown adipose tissue: Function and physiological significance, *Physiol Rev,* vol.84, No.1, pp. 277-359, issn 0031-9333 (Print)

Carriere, A.; Carmona, M.C.; Fernandez, Y.; Rigoulet, M.; Wenger, R.H.; Penicaud, L. & Casteilla, L. (2004). Mitochondrial reactive oxygen species control the transcription factor chop-10/gadd153 and adipocyte differentiation: A mechanism for hypoxia-dependent effect, *J Biol Chem,* vol.279, No.39, pp. 40462-40469, issn 0021-9258 (Print)

Civitarese, A.E.; Jenkinson, C.P.; Richardson, D.; Bajaj, M.; Cusi, K.; Kashyap, S.; Berria, R.; Belfort, R.; Defronzo, R.A.; Mandarino, L.J. & Ravussin, E. (2004). Adiponectin receptors gene expression and insulin sensitivity in non-diabetic mexican americans with or without a family history of type 2 diabetes, *Diabetologia,* vol.47, No.5, pp. 816-820, issn 0012-186X (Print)

Civitarese, A.E.; Ukropcova, B.; Carling, S.; Hulver, M.; Defronzo, R.A.; Mandarino, L.; Ravussin, E. & Smith, S.R. (2006). Role of adiponectin in human skeletal muscle bioenergetics, *Cell Metab,* vol.4, No.1, pp. 75-87, issn 1550-4131 (Print)

Civitarese, A.E.; Carling, S.; Heilbronn, L.K.; Hulver, M.H.; Ukropcova, B.; Deutsch, W.A.; Smith, S.R. & Ravussin, E. (2007). Calorie restriction increases muscle mitochondrial biogenesis in healthy humans, *PLoS Med,* vol.4, No.3, p. e76, issn 1549-1676

Cramer, T. & Johnson, R.S. (2003). A novel role for the hypoxia inducible transcription factor hif-1alpha: Critical regulation of inflammatory cell function, *Cell Cycle,* vol.2, No.3, pp. 192-193, issn 1538-4101 (Print)

Cramer, T.; Yamanishi, Y.; Clausen, B.E.; Forster, I.; Pawlinski, R.; Mackman, N.; Haase, V.H.; Jaenisch, R.; Corr, M.; Nizet, V.; Firestein, G.S.; Gerber, H.P.; Ferrara, N. & Johnson, R.S. (2003). Hif-1alpha is essential for myeloid cell-mediated inflammation, *Cell,* vol.112, No.5, pp. 645-657, issn 0092-8674 (Print)

Crampes, F.; Beauville, M.; Riviere, D. & Garrigues, M. (1986). Effect of physical training in humans on the response of isolated fat cells to epinephrine, *J Appl Physiol,* vol.61, No.1, pp. 25-29, issn 8750-7587 (Print)

Cypess, A.M.; Lehman, S.; Williams, G.; Tal, I.; Rodman, D.; Goldfine, A.B.; Kuo, F.C.; Palmer, E.L.; Tseng, Y.H.; Doria, A.; Kolodny, G.M. & Kahn, C.R. (2009). Identification and importance of brown adipose tissue in adult humans, *N Engl J Med*, vol.360, No.15, pp. 1509-1517, issn 1533-4406 (Electronic)

De Pauw, A.; Tejerina, S.; Raes, M.; Keijer, J. & Arnould, T. (2009). Mitochondrial (dys)function in adipocyte (de)differentiation and systemic metabolic alterations, *Am J Pathol*, vol.175, No.3, pp. 927-939, issn 1525-2191 (Electronic)

Divoux, A. & Clement, K. (2011). Architecture and the extracellular matrix: The still unappreciated components of the adipose tissue, *Obes Rev*, vol.12, No.5, pp. e494-503, issn 1467-789X (Electronic)

Elbekai, R.H. & El-Kadi, A.O. (2005). The role of oxidative stress in the modulation of aryl hydrocarbon receptor-regulated genes by as3+, cd2+, and cr6+, *Free Radic Biol Med*, vol.39, No.11, pp. 1499-1511, issn 0891-5849 (Print)

Erbay, E.; Cao, H. & Hotamisligil, G.S. (2007). Adipocyte/macrophage fatty acid binding proteins in metabolic syndrome, *Curr Atheroscler Rep*, vol.9, No.3, pp. 222-229, issn 1523-3804 (Print)

Espinoza, D.O.; Boros, L.G.; Crunkhorn, S.; Gami, H. & Patti, M.E. (2010). Dual modulation of both lipid oxidation and synthesis by peroxisome proliferator-activated receptor-gamma coactivator-1alpha and -1beta in cultured myotubes, *FASEB J*, vol.24, No.4, pp. 1003-1014, issn 1530-6860 (Electronic)

Febbraio, M.A.; Hiscock, N.; Sacchetti, M.; Fischer, C.P. & Pedersen, B.K. (2004). Interleukin-6 is a novel factor mediating glucose homeostasis during skeletal muscle contraction, *Diabetes*, vol.53, No.7, pp. 1643-1648, issn 0012-1797 (Print)

Feige, J.N.; Lagouge, M.; Canto, C.; Strehle, A.; Houten, S.M.; Milne, J.C.; Lambert, P.D.; Mataki, C.; Elliott, P.J. & Auwerx, J. (2008). Specific sirt1 activation mimics low energy levels and protects against diet-induced metabolic disorders by enhancing fat oxidation, *Cell Metab*, vol.8, No.5, pp. 347-358, issn 1932-7420 (Electronic)

Ferreri, C. & Chatgilialoglu, C. (2009). Membrane lipidomics and the geometry of unsaturated fatty acids from biomimetic models to biological consequences, *Methods Mol Biol*, vol.579, pp. 391-411, issn 1940-6029 (Electronic)

Fiaschi, T.; Cirelli, D.; Comito, G.; Gelmini, S.; Ramponi, G.; Serio, M. & Chiarugi, P. (2009). Globular adiponectin induces differentiation and fusion of skeletal muscle cells, *Cell Res*, vol.19, No.5, pp. 584-597, issn 1748-7838 (Electronic)

Foster, D.J.; Ravikumar, P.; Bellotto, D.J.; Unger, R.H. & Hsia, C.C. (2010). Fatty diabetic lung: Altered alveolar structure and surfactant protein expression, *Am J Physiol Lung Cell Mol Physiol*, vol.298, No.3, pp. L392-403, issn 1522-1504 (Electronic)

Friedman, J.M. (2011). Leptin and the regulation of body weigh, *Keio J Med*, vol.60, No.1, pp. 1-9, issn 1880-1293 (Electronic)

Frydelund-Larsen, L.; Penkowa, M.; Akerstrom, T.; Zankari, A.; Nielsen, S. & Pedersen, B.K. (2007). Exercise induces interleukin-8 receptor (cxcr2) expression in human skeletal muscle, *Exp Physiol*, vol.92, No.1, pp. 233-240, issn 0958-0670 (Print)

Gilde, A.J. & Van Bilsen, M. (2003). Peroxisome proliferator-activated receptors (ppars): Regulators of gene expression in heart and skeletal muscle, *Acta Physiol Scand*, vol.178, No.4, pp. 425-434, issn 0001-6772 (Print)

Goossens, G.H. (2008). The role of adipose tissue dysfunction in the pathogenesis of obesity-related insulin resistance, *Physiol Behav*, vol.94, No.2, pp. 206-218, issn 0031-9384

Gordon, S. & Taylor, P.R. (2005). Monocyte and macrophage heterogeneity, *Nat Rev Immunol*, vol.5, No.12, pp. 953-964, issn 1474-1733 (Print)

Gordon, S. (2007). The macrophage: Past, present and future, *Eur J Immunol*, vol.37 Suppl 1, pp. S9-17, issn 0014-2980 (Print)

Granneman, J.G.; Li, P.; Zhu, Z. & Lu, Y. (2005). Metabolic and cellular plasticity in white adipose tissue i: Effects of beta3-adrenergic receptor activation, *Am J Physiol Endocrinol Metab*, vol.289, No.4, pp. E608-616, issn 0193-1849 (Print)

Halperin, M.L.; Connors, H.P.; Relman, A.S. & Karnovsky, M.L. (1969). Factors that control the effect of ph on glycolysis in leukocytes, *J Biol Chem*, vol.244, No.2, pp. 384-390, issn 0021-9258 (Print)

Hamdy, O.; Porramatikul, S. & Al-Ozairi, E. (2006). Metabolic obesity: The paradox between visceral and subcutaneous fat, *Curr Diabetes Rev*, vol.2, No.4, pp. 367-373, issn 1573-3998 (Print)

Hamilton, M.T.; Hamilton, D.G. & Zderic, T.W. (2007). Role of low energy expenditure and sitting in obesity, metabolic syndrome, type 2 diabetes, and cardiovascular disease, *Diabetes*, vol.56, No.11, pp. 2655-2667, issn 1939-327X (Electronic)

Hancock, C.R.; Han, D.H.; Chen, M.; Terada, S.; Yasuda, T.; Wright, D.C. & Holloszy, J.O. (2008). High-fat diets cause insulin resistance despite an increase in muscle mitochondria, *Proc Natl Acad Sci U S A*, vol.105, No.22, pp. 7815-7820, issn 1091-6490 (Electronic)

Handschin, C. & Spiegelman, B.M. (2008). The role of exercise and pgc1alpha in inflammation and chronic disease, *Nature*, vol.454, No.7203, pp. 463-469, issn 1476-4687 (Electronic)

Hara, K.; Yamauchi, T. & Kadowaki, T. (2005). Adiponectin: An adipokine linking adipocytes and type 2 diabetes in humans, *Curr Diab Rep*, vol.5, No.2, pp. 136-140, issn 1534-4827 (Print)

Harman, D. (1956). Aging: A theory based on free radical and radiation chemistry, *J Gerontol*, vol.11, No.3, pp. 298-300, issn 0022-1422 (Print)

Harper, M.E.; Bevilacqua, L.; Hagopian, K.; Weindruch, R. & Ramsey, J.J. (2004). Ageing, oxidative stress, and mitochondrial uncoupling, *Acta Physiol Scand*, vol.182, No.4, pp. 321-331, issn 0001-6772 (Print)

Haugen, F.; Norheim, F.; Lian, H.; Wensaas, A.J.; Dueland, S.; Berg, O.; Funderud, A.; Skalhegg, B.S.; Raastad, T. & Drevon, C.A. (2010). Il-7 is expressed and secreted by human skeletal muscle cells, *Am J Physiol Cell Physiol*, vol.298, No.4, pp. C807-816, issn 1522-1563 (Electronic)

Henry, B.A. & Clarke, I.J. (2008). Adipose tissue hormones and the regulation of food intake, *J Neuroendocrinol*, vol.20, No.6, pp. 842-849, issn 1365-2826 (Electronic)

Himms-Hagen, J. (2004). Exercise in a pill: Feasibility of energy expenditure targets, *Curr Drug Targets CNS Neurol Disord*, vol.3, No.5, pp. 389-409, issn 1568-007X (Print)

Hojman, P.; Pedersen, M.; Nielsen, A.R.; Krogh-Madsen, R.; Yfanti, C.; Akerstrom, T.; Nielsen, S. & Pedersen, B.K. (2009). Fibroblast growth factor-21 is induced in human skeletal muscles by hyperinsulinemia, *Diabetes*, vol.58, No.12, pp. 2797-2801, issn 1939-327X (Electronic)

Holloszy, J.O. & Booth, F.W. (1976). Biochemical adaptations to endurance exercise in muscle, *Annu Rev Physiol*, vol.38, pp. 273-291, issn 0066-4278 (Print)

Holloszy, J.O. (2009). Skeletal muscle "Mitochondrial deficiency" Does not mediate insulin resistance, *Am J Clin Nutr,* vol.89, No.1, pp. 463S-466S, issn 1938-3207 (Electronic)

Hong, S.; Lee, H.J.; Kim, S.J. & Hahm, K.B. (2010). Connection between inflammation and carcinogenesis in gastrointestinal tract: Focus on tgf-beta signaling, *World J Gastroenterol,* vol.16, No.17, pp. 2080-2093, issn 1007-9327 (Print)

Hosogai, N.; Fukuhara, A.; Oshima, K.; Miyata, Y.; Tanaka, S.; Segawa, K.; Furukawa, S.; Tochino, Y.; Komuro, R.; Matsuda, M. & Shimomura, I. (2007). Adipose tissue hypoxia in obesity and its impact on adipocytokine dysregulation, *Diabetes,* vol.56, No.4, pp. 901-911, issn 0012-1797 (Print)

Hotta, K.; Funahashi, T.; Bodkin, N.L.; Ortmeyer, H.K.; Arita, Y.; Hansen, B.C. & Matsuzawa, Y. (2001). Circulating concentrations of the adipocyte protein adiponectin are decreased in parallel with reduced insulin sensitivity during the progression to type 2 diabetes in rhesus monkeys, *Diabetes,* vol.50, No.5, pp. 1126-1133, issn 0012-1797 (Print)

Howard, S.G. & Lee, D.H. (2011). What is the role of human contamination by environmental chemicals in the development of type 1 diabetes?, *J Epidemiol Community Health,* issn 1470-2738 (Electronic)

Chandel, N.S. & Budinger, G.R. (2007). The cellular basis for diverse responses to oxygen, *Free Radic Biol Med,* vol.42, No.2, pp. 165-174, issn 0891-5849 (Print)

Inouye, K.E.; Shi, H.; Howard, J.K.; Daly, C.H.; Lord, G.M.; Rollins, B.J. & Flier, J.S. (2007). Absence of cc chemokine ligand 2 does not limit obesity-associated infiltration of macrophages into adipose tissue, *Diabetes,* vol.56, No.9, pp. 2242-2250, issn 1939-327X (Electronic)

Itoh, M.; Suganami, T.; Hachiya, R. & Ogawa, Y. (2011). Adipose tissue remodeling as homeostatic inflammation, *Int J Inflam,* vol.2011, p. 720926, issn 2042-0099 (Electronic)

Johannsen, D.L. & Ravussin, E. (2009). The role of mitochondria in health and disease, *Curr Opin Pharmacol,* vol.9, No.6, pp. 780-786, issn 1471-4973 (Electronic)

Jonsdottir, I.H.; Schjerling, P.; Ostrowski, K.; Asp, S.; Richter, E.A. & Pedersen, B.K. (2000). Muscle contractions induce interleukin-6 mrna production in rat skeletal muscles, *J Physiol,* vol.528 Pt 1, pp. 157-163, issn 0022-3751 (Print)

Jung, H.S.; Lee, Y.J.; Kim, Y.H.; Paik, S.; Kim, J.W. & Lee, J.W. (2011). Peroxisome proliferator-activated receptor gamma/signal transducers and activators of transcription 5a pathway plays a key factor in adipogenesis of human bone marrow-derived stromal cells and 3t3-l1 preadipocytes, *Stem Cells Dev,* issn 1557-8534 (Electronic)

Kamei, N.; Tobe, K.; Suzuki, R.; Ohsugi, M.; Watanabe, T.; Kubota, N.; Ohtsuka-Kowatari, N.; Kumagai, K.; Sakamoto, K.; Kobayashi, M.; Yamauchi, T.; Ueki, K.; Oishi, Y.; Nishimura, S.; Manabe, I.; Hashimoto, H.; Ohnishi, Y.; Ogata, H.; Tokuyama, K.; Tsunoda, M.; Ide, T.; Murakami, K.; Nagai, R. & Kadowaki, T. (2006). Overexpression of monocyte chemoattractant protein-1 in adipose tissues causes macrophage recruitment and insulin resistance, *J Biol Chem,* vol.281, No.36, pp. 26602-26614, issn 0021-9258 (Print)

Kanda, H.; Tateya, S.; Tamori, Y.; Kotani, K.; Hiasa, K.; Kitazawa, R.; Kitazawa, S.; Miyachi, H.; Maeda, S.; Egashira, K. & Kasuga, M. (2006). Mcp-1 contributes to macrophage infiltration into adipose tissue, insulin resistance, and hepatic steatosis in obesity, *J Clin Invest,* vol.116, No.6, pp. 1494-1505, issn 0021-9738 (Print)

Keller, C.; Steensberg, A.; Pilegaard, H.; Osada, T.; Saltin, B.; Pedersen, B.K. & Neufer, P.D. (2001). Transcriptional activation of the il-6 gene in human contracting skeletal muscle: Influence of muscle glycogen content, *FASEB J*, vol.15, No.14, pp. 2748-2750, issn 1530-6860 (Electronic)

Kelley, D.E.; Goodpaster, B.; Wing, R.R. & Simoneau, J.A. (1999). Skeletal muscle fatty acid metabolism in association with insulin resistance, obesity, and weight loss, *Am J Physiol*, vol.277, No.6 Pt 1, pp. E1130-1141, issn 0002-9513 (Print)

Kelley, D.E. & Mandarino, L.J. (2000). Fuel selection in human skeletal muscle in insulin resistance: A reexamination, *Diabetes*, vol.49, No.5, pp. 677-683, issn 0012-1797

Kelley, D.E.; He, J.; Menshikova, E.V. & Ritov, V.B. (2002). Dysfunction of mitochondria in human skeletal muscle in type 2 diabetes, *Diabetes*, vol.51, No.10, pp. 2944-2950, issn 0012-1797 (Print)

Kern, P.A.; Di Gregorio, G.B.; Lu, T.; Rassouli, N. & Ranganathan, G. (2003). Adiponectin expression from human adipose tissue: Relation to obesity, insulin resistance, and tumor necrosis factor-alpha expression, *Diabetes*, vol.52, No.7, pp. 1779-1785, issn 0012-1797 (Print)

Khan, T.; Muise, E.S.; Iyengar, P.; Wang, Z.V.; Chandalia, M.; Abate, N.; Zhang, B.B.; Bonaldo, P.; Chua, S. & Scherer, P.E. (2009). Metabolic dysregulation and adipose tissue fibrosis: Role of collagen vi, *Mol Cell Biol*, vol.29, No.6, pp. 1575-1591, issn 1098-5549 (Electronic)

Kim, J.Y.; Van De Wall, E.; Laplante, M.; Azzara, A.; Trujillo, M.E.; Hofmann, S.M.; Schraw, T.; Durand, J.L.; Li, H.; Li, G.; Jelicks, L.A.; Mehler, M.F.; Hui, D.Y.; Deshaies, Y.; Shulman, G.I.; Schwartz, G.J. & Scherer, P.E. (2007). Obesity-associated improvements in metabolic profile through expansion of adipose tissue, *J Clin Invest*, vol.117, No.9, pp. 2621-2637, issn 0021-9738 (Print)

Kinnula, V.L.; Savolainen, M.J. & Hassinen, I. (1978). Hepatic triacylglycerol and fatty-acid biosynthesis during hypoxia in vivo, *Acta Physiol Scand*, vol.104, No.2, pp. 148-155, issn 0001-6772 (Print)

Kirwan, J.P.; Costill, D.L.; Flynn, M.G.; Neufer, P.D.; Fink, W.J. & Morse, W.M. (1990). Effects of increased training volume on the oxidative capacity, glycogen content and tension development of rat skeletal muscle, *Int J Sports Med*, vol.11, No.6, pp. 479-483, issn 0172-4622 (Print)

Koska, J.; Stefan, N.; Votruba, S.B.; Smith, S.R.; Krakoff, J. & Bunt, J.C. (2008). Distribution of subcutaneous fat predicts insulin action in obesity in sex-specific manner, *Obesity (Silver Spring)*, vol.16, No.9, pp. 2003-2009, issn 1930-7381 (Print)

Kosmidou, I.; Vassilakopoulos, T.; Xagorari, A.; Zakynthinos, S.; Papapetropoulos, A. & Roussos, C. (2002). Production of interleukin-6 by skeletal myotubes: Role of reactive oxygen species, *Am J Respir Cell Mol Biol*, vol.26, No.5, pp. 587-593, issn 1044-1549 (Print)

Koves, T.R.; Ussher, J.R.; Noland, R.C.; Slentz, D.; Mosedale, M.; Ilkayeva, O.; Bain, J.; Stevens, R.; Dyck, J.R.; Newgard, C.B.; Lopaschuk, G.D. & Muoio, D.M. (2008). Mitochondrial overload and incomplete fatty acid oxidation contribute to skeletal muscle insulin resistance, *Cell Metab*, vol.7, No.1, pp. 45-56, issn 1550-4131 (Print)

Krek, W. (2000). Vhl takes hif's breath away, *Nat Cell Biol*, vol.2, No.7, pp. E121-123, issn 1465-7392 (Print)

Krishnan, J.; Suter, M.; Windak, R.; Krebs, T.; Felley, A.; Montessuit, C.; Tokarska-Schlattner, M.; Aasum, E.; Bogdanova, A.; Perriard, E.; Perriard, J.C.; Larsen, T.; Pedrazzini, T. & Krek, W. (2009). Activation of a hif1alpha-ppargamma axis underlies the integration of glycolytic and lipid anabolic pathways in pathologic cardiac hypertrophy, *Cell Metab*, vol.9, No.6, pp. 512-524, issn 1932-7420 (Electronic)

Langer, P.; Kocan, A.; Tajtakova, M.; Petrik, J.; Chovancova, J.; Drobna, B.; Jursa, S.; Pavuk, M.; Koska, J.; Trnovec, T.; Sebokova, E. & Klimes, I. (2003). Possible effects of polychlorinated biphenyls and organochlorinated pesticides on the thyroid after long-term exposure to heavy environmental pollution, *J Occup Environ Med*, vol.45, No.5, pp. 526-532, issn 1076-2752 (Print)

Langer, P.; Kocan, A.; Tajtakova, M.; Petrik, J.; Chovancova, J.; Drobna, B.; Jursa, S.; Radikova, Z.; Koska, J.; Ksinantova, L.; Huckova, M.; Imrich, R.; Wimmerova, S.; Gasperikova, D.; Shishiba, Y.; Trnovec, T.; Sebokova, E. & Klimes, I. (2007). Fish from industrially polluted freshwater as the main source of organochlorinated pollutants and increased frequency of thyroid disorders and dysglycemia, *Chemosphere*, vol.67, No.9, pp. S379-385, issn 0045-6535 (Print)

Langer, P. (2010). The impacts of organochlorines and other persistent pollutants on thyroid and metabolic health, *Front Neuroendocrinol*, vol.31, No.4, pp. 497-518, issn 1095-6808 (Electronic)

Langer, P.; Kocan, A.; Drobna, B.; Susienkova, K.; Radikova, Z.; Huckova, M.; Imrich, R.; Ksinantova, L. & Klimes, I. (2010). Polychlorinated biphenyls and testosterone: Age and congener related correlation approach in heavily exposed males, *Endocr Regul*, vol.44, No.3, pp. 109-114, issn 1210-0668 (Print)

Langer, P.; Kocan, A.; Drobna, B.; Huckova, M.; Radikova, Z.; Susienkova, K.; Imrich, R. & Ukropec, J. (2011). Alpha-fetoprotein, carcinoembryonic antigen and beta2-microglobulin in adult population highly exposed to organochlorinated pollutants (pcb, dde and hcb), *Endocr Regul*, vol.45, No.3, pp. 149-155, issn 1210-0668 (Print)

Lanza, I.R. & Nair, K.S. (2009). Muscle mitochondrial changes with aging and exercise, *Am J Clin Nutr*, vol.89, No.1, pp. 467S-471S, issn 1938-3207 (Electronic)

Lanza, I.R. & Nair, K.S. (2010). Mitochondrial function as a determinant of life span, *Pflugers Arch*, vol.459, No.2, pp. 277-289, issn 1432-2013 (Electronic)

Lee, D.H.; Lind, L.; Jacobs, D.R., Jr.; Salihovic, S.; Van Bavel, B. & Lind, P.M. (2011). Associations of persistent organic pollutants with abdominal obesity in the elderly: The prospective investigation of the vasculature in uppsala seniors (pivus) study, *Environ Int*, issn 1873-6750 (Electronic)

Lee, D.H.; Lind, P.M.; Jacobs, D.R., Jr.; Salihovic, S.; Van Bavel, B. & Lind, L. (2011). Polychlorinated biphenyls and organochlorine pesticides in plasma predict development of type 2 diabetes in the elderly: The prospective investigation of the vasculature in uppsala seniors (pivus) study, *Diabetes Care*, vol.34, No.8, pp. 1778-1784, issn 1935-5548 (Electronic)

Lee, H.K. (2011). Mitochondrial dysfunction and insulin resistance: The contribution of dioxin-like substances, *Diabetes Metab J*, vol.35, No.3, pp. 207-215, issn 2233-6087

Lefevre, M.; Redman, L.M.; Heilbronn, L.K.; Smith, J.V.; Martin, C.K.; Rood, J.C.; Greenway, F.L.; Williamson, D.A.; Smith, S.R. & Ravussin, E. (2009). Caloric restriction alone and with exercise improves cvd risk in healthy non-obese individuals, *Atherosclerosis*, vol.203, No.1, pp. 206-213, issn 1879-1484 (Electronic)

Levine, J.A.; Mccrady, S.K.; Lanningham-Foster, L.M.; Kane, P.H.; Foster, R.C. & Manohar, C.U. (2008). The role of free-living daily walking in human weight gain and obesity, *Diabetes*, vol.57, No.3, pp. 548-554, issn 1939-327X (Electronic)

Li, P.; Zhu, Z.; Lu, Y. & Granneman, J.G. (2005). Metabolic and cellular plasticity in white adipose tissue ii: Role of peroxisome proliferator-activated receptor-alpha, *Am J Physiol Endocrinol Metab*, vol.289, No.4, pp. E617-626, issn 0193-1849 (Print)

Lindsay, R.S.; Funahashi, T.; Hanson, R.L.; Matsuzawa, Y.; Tanaka, S.; Tataranni, P.A.; Knowler, W.C. & Krakoff, J. (2002). Adiponectin and development of type 2 diabetes in the pima indian population, *Lancet*, vol.360, No.9326, pp. 57-58, issn 0140-6736 (Print)

Linton, M.F. & Fazio, S. (2003). Macrophages, inflammation, and atherosclerosis, *Int J Obes Relat Metab Disord*, vol.27 Suppl 3, pp. S35-40, issn 0307-0565 (Print)

Lumeng, C.N.; Bodzin, J.L. & Saltiel, A.R. (2007). Obesity induces a phenotypic switch in adipose tissue macrophage polarization, *J Clin Invest*, vol.117, No.1, pp. 175-184, issn 0021-9738 (Print)

Marzetti, E.; Lees, H.A.; Wohlgemuth, S.E. & Leeuwenburgh, C. (2009). Sarcopenia of aging: Underlying cellular mechanisms and protection by calorie restriction, *Biofactors*, vol.35, No.1, pp. 28-35, issn 0951-6433 (Print)

Matsuzawa, Y.; Funahashi, T. & Nakamura, T. (1999). Molecular mechanism of metabolic syndrome x: Contribution of adipocytokines adipocyte-derived bioactive substances, *Ann N Y Acad Sci*, vol.892, pp. 146-154, issn 0077-8923 (Print)

Meissburger, B.; Ukropec, J.; Roeder, E.; Beaton, N.; Geiger, M.; Teupser, D.; Civan, B.; Langhans, W.; Nawroth, P.P.; Gasperikova, D.; Rudofsky, G. & Wolfrum, C. (2011). Adipogenesis and insulin sensitivity in obesity are regulated by retinoid-related orphan receptor gamma, *EMBO Mol Med*, issn 1757-4684 (Electronic)

Mootha, V.K.; Lindgren, C.M.; Eriksson, K.F.; Subramanian, A.; Sihag, S.; Lehar, J.; Puigserver, P.; Carlsson, E.; Ridderstrale, M.; Laurila, E.; Houstis, N.; Daly, M.J.; Patterson, N.; Mesirov, J.P.; Golub, T.R.; Tamayo, P.; Spiegelman, B.; Lander, E.S.; Hirschhorn, J.N.; Altshuler, D. & Groop, L.C. (2003). Pgc-1alpha-responsive genes involved in oxidative phosphorylation are coordinately downregulated in human diabetes, *Nat Genet*, vol.34, No.3, pp. 267-273, issn 1061-4036 (Print)

Mortensen, O.H.; Andersen, K.; Fischer, C.; Nielsen, A.R.; Nielsen, S.; Akerstrom, T.; Aastrom, M.B.; Borup, R. & Pedersen, B.K. (2008). Calprotectin is released from human skeletal muscle tissue during exercise, *J Physiol*, vol.586, No.14, pp. 3551-3562, issn 1469-7793 (Electronic)

Nedergaard, J. & Cannon, B. (2010). The changed metabolic world with human brown adipose tissue: Therapeutic visions, *Cell Metab*, vol.11, No.4, pp. 268-272, issn 1932-7420

Neels, J.G. & Olefsky, J.M. (2006). Inflamed fat: What starts the fire?, *J Clin Invest*, vol.116, No.1, pp. 33-35, issn 0021-9738 (Print)

Nielsen, A.R. & Pedersen, B.K. (2007). The biological roles of exercise-induced cytokines: Il-6, il-8, and il-15, *Appl Physiol Nutr Metab*, vol.32, No.5, pp. 833-839, issn 1715-5312

Nomiyama, T.; Perez-Tilve, D.; Ogawa, D.; Gizard, F.; Zhao, Y.; Heywood, E.B.; Jones, K.L.; Kawamori, R.; Cassis, L.A.; Tschop, M.H. & Bruemmer, D. (2007). Osteopontin mediates obesity-induced adipose tissue macrophage infiltration and insulin resistance in mice, *J Clin Invest*, vol.117, No.10, pp. 2877-2888, issn 0021-9738 (Print)

Odegaard, J.I.; Ricardo-Gonzalez, R.R.; Goforth, M.H.; Morel, C.R.; Subramanian, V.; Mukundan, L.; Red Eagle, A.; Vats, D.; Brombacher, F.; Ferrante, A.W. & Chawla, A. (2007). Macrophage-specific ppargamma controls alternative activation and improves insulin resistance, *Nature*, vol.447, No.7148, pp. 1116-1120, issn 1476-4687

Ouchi, N.; Oshima, Y.; Ohashi, K.; Higuchi, A.; Ikegami, C.; Izumiya, Y. & Walsh, K. (2008). Follistatin-like 1, a secreted muscle protein, promotes endothelial cell function and revascularization in ischemic tissue through a nitric-oxide synthase-dependent mechanism, *J Biol Chem*, vol.283, No.47, pp. 32802-32811, issn 0021-9258 (Print)

Patti, M.E.; Butte, A.J.; Crunkhorn, S.; Cusi, K.; Berria, R.; Kashyap, S.; Miyazaki, Y.; Kohane, I.; Costello, M.; Saccone, R.; Landaker, E.J.; Goldfine, A.B.; Mun, E.; Defronzo, R.; Finlayson, J.; Kahn, C.R. & Mandarino, L.J. (2003). Coordinated reduction of genes of oxidative metabolism in humans with insulin resistance and diabetes: Potential role of pgc1 and nrf1, *Proc Natl Acad Sci U S A*, vol.100, No.14, pp. 8466-8471, issn 0027-8424 (Print)

Pedersen, B.K. & Febbraio, M.A. (2008). Muscle as an endocrine organ: Focus on muscle-derived interleukin-6, *Physiol Rev*, vol.88, No.4, pp. 1379-1406, issn 0031-9333 (Print)

Pedersen, B.K. (2011). Muscles and their myokines, *J Exp Biol*, vol.214, No.Pt 2, pp. 337-346, issn 1477-9145 (Electronic)

Peter, A.; Weigert, C.; Staiger, H.; Machicao, F.; Schick, F.; Machann, J.; Stefan, N.; Thamer, C.; Haring, H.U. & Schleicher, E. (2009). Individual stearoyl-coa desaturase 1 expression modulates endoplasmic reticulum stress and inflammation in human myotubes and is associated with skeletal muscle lipid storage and insulin sensitivity in vivo, *Diabetes*, vol.58, No.8, pp. 1757-1765, issn 1939-327X (Electronic)

Petersen, K.F.; Oral, E.A.; Dufour, S.; Befroy, D.; Ariyan, C.; Yu, C.; Cline, G.W.; Depaoli, A.M.; Taylor, S.I.; Gorden, P. & Shulman, G.I. (2002). Leptin reverses insulin resistance and hepatic steatosis in patients with severe lipodystrophy, *J Clin Invest*, vol.109, No.10, pp. 1345-1350, issn 0021-9738 (Print)

Petersen, K.F.; Dufour, S.; Befroy, D.; Garcia, R. & Shulman, G.I. (2004). Impaired mitochondrial activity in the insulin-resistant offspring of patients with type 2 diabetes, *N Engl J Med*, vol.350, No.7, pp. 664-671, issn 1533-4406 (Electronic)

Petersen, K.F.; Dufour, S. & Shulman, G.I. (2005). Decreased insulin-stimulated atp synthesis and phosphate transport in muscle of insulin-resistant offspring of type 2 diabetic parents, *PLoS Med*, vol.2, No.9, p. e233, issn 1549-1676 (Electronic)

Phillips, S.M.; Green, H.J.; Tarnopolsky, M.A.; Heigenhauser, G.F.; Hill, R.E. & Grant, S.M. (1996). Effects of training duration on substrate turnover and oxidation during exercise, *J Appl Physiol*, vol.81, No.5, pp. 2182-2191, issn 8750-7587 (Print)

Pietilainen, K.H.; Rog, T.; Seppanen-Laakso, T.; Virtue, S.; Gopalacharyulu, P.; Tang, J.; Rodriguez-Cuenca, S.; Maciejewski, A.; Naukkarinen, J.; Ruskeepaa, A.L.; Niemela, P.S.; Yetukuri, L.; Tan, C.Y.; Velagapudi, V.; Castillo, S.; Nygren, H.; Hyotylainen, T.; Rissanen, A.; Kaprio, J.; Yki-Jarvinen, H.; Vattulainen, I.; Vidal-Puig, A. & Oresic, M. (2011). Association of lipidome remodeling in the adipocyte membrane with acquired obesity in humans, *PLoS Biol*, vol.9, No.6, p. e1000623, issn 1545-7885

Pischon, T.; Boeing, H.; Hoffmann, K.; Bergmann, M.; Schulze, M.B.; Overvad, K.; Van Der Schouw, Y.T.; Spencer, E.; Moons, K.G.; Tjonneland, A.; Halkjaer, J.; Jensen, M.K.; Stegger, J.; Clavel-Chapelon, F.; Boutron-Ruault, M.C.; Chajes, V.; Linseisen, J.; Kaaks, R.; Trichopoulou, A.; Trichopoulos, D.; Bamia, C.; Sieri, S.; Palli, D.; Tumino, R.; Vineis, P.; Panico, S.; Peeters, P.H.; May, A.M.; Bueno-De-Mesquita, H.B.; Van Duijnhoven, F.J.; Hallmans, G.; Weinehall, L.; Manjer, J.; Hedblad, B.; Lund, E.; Agudo, A.; Arriola, L.; Barricarte, A.; Navarro, C.; Martinez, C.; Quiros, J.R.; Key, T.; Bingham, S.; Khaw, K.T.; Boffetta, P.; Jenab, M.; Ferrari, P. & Riboli, E. (2008). General and abdominal adiposity and risk of death in europe, N Engl J Med, vol.359, No.20, pp. 2105-2120, issn 1533-4406 (Electronic)

Rasmussen, M.S.; Lihn, A.S.; Pedersen, S.B.; Bruun, J.M.; Rasmussen, M. & Richelsen, B. (2006). Adiponectin receptors in human adipose tissue: Effects of obesity, weight loss, and fat depots, Obesity (Silver Spring), vol.14, No.1, pp. 28-35, issn 1930-7381

Reddy, P.H. (2009). Role of mitochondria in neurodegenerative diseases: Mitochondria as a therapeutic target in alzheimer's disease, CNS Spectr, vol.14, No.8 Suppl 7, pp. 8-13; discussion 16-18, issn 1092-8529 (Print)

Rieusset, J.; Touri, F.; Michalik, L.; Escher, P.; Desvergne, B.; Niesor, E. & Wahli, W. (2002). A new selective peroxisome proliferator-activated receptor gamma antagonist with antiobesity and antidiabetic activity, Mol Endocrinol, vol.16, No.11, pp. 2628-2644, issn 0888-8809 (Print)

Ritov, V.B.; Menshikova, E.V.; He, J.; Ferrell, R.E.; Goodpaster, B.H. & Kelley, D.E. (2005). Deficiency of subsarcolemmal mitochondria in obesity and type 2 diabetes, Diabetes, vol.54, No.1, pp. 8-14, issn 0012-1797 (Print)

Seale, P. & Lazar, M.A. (2009). Brown fat in humans: Turning up the heat on obesity, Diabetes, vol.58, No.7, pp. 1482-1484, issn 1939-327X (Electronic)

Semenza, G.L. (2001). Hif-1 and mechanisms of hypoxia sensing, Curr Opin Cell Biol, vol.13, No.2, pp. 167-171, issn 0955-0674 (Print)

Sethi, J.K. & Vidal-Puig, A.J. (2007). Thematic review series: Adipocyte biology. Adipose tissue function and plasticity orchestrate nutritional adaptation, J Lipid Res, vol.48, No.6, pp. 1253-1262, issn 0022-2275 (Print)

Sher, L. (1998). The endogenous euphoric reward system that reinforces physical training: A mechanism for mankind's survival, Med Hypotheses, vol.51, No.6, pp. 449-450, issn 0306-9877 (Print)

Schantz, P.G. (1986). Plasticity of human skeletal muscle with special reference to effects of physical training on enzyme levels of the nadh shuttles and phenotypic expression of slow and fast myofibrillar proteins, Acta Physiol Scand Suppl, vol.558, pp. 1-62, issn 0302-2994 (Print)

Snijder, M.B.; Dekker, J.M.; Visser, M.; Yudkin, J.S.; Stehouwer, C.D.; Bouter, L.M.; Heine, R.J.; Nijpels, G. & Seidell, J.C. (2003). Larger thigh and hip circumferences are associated with better glucose tolerance: The hoorn study, Obes Res, vol.11, No.1, pp. 104-111, issn 1071-7323 (Print)

Spalding, K.L.; Arner, E.; Westermark, P.O.; Bernard, S.; Buchholz, B.A.; Bergmann, O.; Blomqvist, L.; Hoffstedt, J.; Naslund, E.; Britton, T.; Concha, H.; Hassan, M.; Ryden, M.; Frisen, J. & Arner, P. (2008). Dynamics of fat cell turnover in humans, Nature, vol.453, No.7196, pp. 783-787, issn 1476-4687 (Electronic)

Steensberg, A.; Febbraio, M.A.; Osada, T.; Schjerling, P.; Van Hall, G.; Saltin, B. & Pedersen, B.K. (2001). Interleukin-6 production in contracting human skeletal muscle is influenced by pre-exercise muscle glycogen content, *J Physiol*, vol.537, No.Pt 2, pp. 633-639, issn 0022-3751 (Print)

Steensberg, A.; Keller, C.; Hillig, T.; Frosig, C.; Wojtaszewski, J.F.; Pedersen, B.K.; Pilegaard, H. & Sander, M. (2007). Nitric oxide production is a proximal signaling event controlling exercise-induced mrna expression in human skeletal muscle, *FASEB J*, vol.21, No.11, pp. 2683-2694, issn 1530-6860 (Electronic)

Sulpice, T.; Prunet-Marcassus, B.; Molveaux, C.; Cani, P.D.; Vitte, P.A.; Graber, P.; Dreano, M. & Burcelin, R. (2009). An adiponectin-like molecule with antidiabetic properties, *Endocrinology*, vol.150, No.10, pp. 4493-4501, issn 1945-7170 (Electronic)

Sun, K.; Kusminski, C.M. & Scherer, P.E. (2011). Adipose tissue remodeling and obesity, *J Clin Invest*, vol.121, No.6, pp. 2094-2101, issn 1558-8238 (Electronic)

Thorne, A.; Lonnqvist, F.; Apelman, J.; Hellers, G. & Arner, P. (2002). A pilot study of long-term effects of a novel obesity treatment: Omentectomy in connection with adjustable gastric banding, *Int J Obes Relat Metab Disord*, vol.26, No.2, pp. 193-199, issn 0307-0565 (Print)

Tchernof, A. (2007). Visceral adipocytes and the metabolic syndrome, *Nutr Rev*, vol.65, No.6 Pt 2, pp. S24-29, issn 0029-6643 (Print)

Trayhurn, P.; Hoggard, N.; Mercer, J.G. & Rayner, D.V. (1998). Hormonal and neuroendocrine regulation of energy balance--the role of leptin, *Arch Tierernahr*, vol.51, No.2-3, pp. 177-185, issn 0003-942X (Print)

Trayhurn, P.; Wang, B. & Wood, I.S. (2008). Hif-1alpha protein rather than mrna as a marker of hypoxia in adipose tissue in obesity: Focus on "Inflammation is associated with a decrease of lipogenic factors in omental fat in women," By poulain-godefroy et al, *Am J Physiol Regul Integr Comp Physiol*, vol.295, No.4, p. R1097; author reply R1098, issn 0363-6119 (Print)

Tseng, Y.H.; Kokkotou, E.; Schulz, T.J.; Huang, T.L.; Winnay, J.N.; Taniguchi, C.M.; Tran, T.T.; Suzuki, R.; Espinoza, D.O.; Yamamoto, Y.; Ahrens, M.J.; Dudley, A.T.; Norris, A.W.; Kulkarni, R.N. & Kahn, C.R. (2008). New role of bone morphogenetic protein 7 in brown adipogenesis and energy expenditure, *Nature*, vol.454, No.7207, pp. 1000-1004, issn 1476-4687 (Electronic)

Tseng, Y.H.; Cypess, A.M. & Kahn, C.R. (2010). Cellular bioenergetics as a target for obesity therapy, *Nat Rev Drug Discov*, vol.9, No.6, pp. 465-482, issn 1474-1784 (Electronic)

Ukropcova, B.; Mcneil, M.; Sereda, O.; De Jonge, L.; Xie, H.; Bray, G.A. & Smith, S.R. (2005). Dynamic changes in fat oxidation in human primary myocytes mirror metabolic characteristics of the donor, *J Clin Invest*, vol.115, No.7, pp. 1934-1941, issn 0021-9738

Ukropcova, B.; Sereda, O.; De Jonge, L.; Bogacka, I.; Nguyen, T.; Xie, H.; Bray, G.A. & Smith, S.R. (2007). Family history of diabetes links impaired substrate switching and reduced mitochondrial content in skeletal muscle, *Diabetes*, vol.56, No.3, pp. 720-727, issn 0012-1797 (Print)

Ukropec, J.; Sebokova, E. & Klimes, I. (2001). Nutrient sensing, leptin and insulin action, *Arch Physiol Biochem*, vol.109, No.1, pp. 38-51, issn 1381-3455 (Print)

Ukropec, J.; Anunciado, R.P.; Ravussin, Y.; Hulver, M.W. & Kozak, L.P. (2006). Ucp1-independent thermogenesis in white adipose tissue of cold-acclimated ucp1-/-mice, *J Biol Chem*, vol.281, No.42, pp. 31894-31908, issn 0021-9258 (Print)

Ukropec, J.; Penesova, A.; Skopkova, M.; Pura, M.; Vlcek, M.; Radikova, Z.; Imrich, R.; Ukropcova, B.; Tajtakova, M.; Koska, J.; Zorad, S.; Belan, V.; Vanuga, P.; Payer, J.; Eckel, J.; Klimes, I. & Gasperikova, D. (2008a). Adipokine protein expression pattern in growth hormone deficiency predisposes to the increased fat cell size and the whole body metabolic derangements, *J Clin Endocrinol Metab*, vol.93, No.6, pp. 2255-2262, issn 0021-972X (Print)

Ukropec, J.; Ukropcova, B.; Kurdiova, T.; Gasperikova, D. & Klimes, I. (2008b). Adipose tissue and skeletal muscle plasticity modulates metabolic health, *Arch Physiol Biochem*, vol.114, No.5, pp. 357-368, issn 1744-4160 (Electronic)

Ukropec, J.; Radikova, Z.; Huckova, M.; Koska, J.; Kocan, A.; Sebokova, E.; Drobna, B.; Trnovec, T.; Susienkova, K.; Labudova, V.; Gasperikova, D.; Langer, P. & Klimes, I. (2010). High prevalence of prediabetes and diabetes in a population exposed to high levels of an organochlorine cocktail, *Diabetologia*, vol.53, No.5, pp. 899-906, issn 1432-0428 (Electronic)

Unger, R.H.; Clark, G.O.; Scherer, P.E. & Orci, L. (2010). Lipid homeostasis, lipotoxicity and the metabolic syndrome, *Biochim Biophys Acta*, vol.1801, No.3, pp. 209-214, issn 0006-3002 (Print)

Van Gaal, L.F.; Mertens, I.L. & Abrams, P.J. (2003). Health risks of lipodystrophy and abdominal fat accumulation: Therapeutic possibilities with leptin and human growth hormone, *Growth Horm IGF Res*, vol.13 Suppl A, pp. S4-9, issn 1096-6374

Van Hall, G.; Jensen-Urstad, M.; Rosdahl, H.; Holmberg, H.C.; Saltin, B. & Calbet, J.A. (2003). Leg and arm lactate and substrate kinetics during exercise, *Am J Physiol Endocrinol Metab*, vol.284, No.1, pp. E193-205, issn 0193-1849 (Print)

Van Marken Lichtenbelt, W.D.; Vanhommerig, J.W.; Smulders, N.M.; Drossaerts, J.M.; Kemerink, G.J.; Bouvy, N.D.; Schrauwen, P. & Teule, G.J. (2009). Cold-activated brown adipose tissue in healthy men, *N Engl J Med*, vol.360, No.15, pp. 1500-1508, issn 1533-4406 (Electronic)

Vargovic, P.; Ukropec, J.; Laukova, M.; Cleary, S.; Manz, B.; Pacak, K. & Kvetnansky, R. (2011). Adipocytes as a new source of catecholamine production, *FEBS Lett*, vol.585, No.14, pp. 2279-2284, issn 1873-3468 (Electronic)

Vijgen, G.H.; Bouvy, N.D.; Teule, G.J.; Brans, B.; Schrauwen, P. & Van Marken Lichtenbelt, W.D. (2011). Brown adipose tissue in morbidly obese subjects, *PLoS One*, vol.6, No.2, p. e17247, issn 1932-6203 (Electronic)

Virtanen, K.A. & Nuutila, P. (2011). Brown adipose tissue in humans, *Curr Opin Lipidol*, vol.22, No.1, pp. 49-54, issn 1473-6535 (Electronic)

Wajchenberg, B.L. (2000). Subcutaneous and visceral adipose tissue: Their relation to the metabolic syndrome, *Endocr Rev*, vol.21, No.6, pp. 697-738, issn 0163-769X (Print)

Wang, B.; Wood, I.S. & Trayhurn, P. (2007). Dysregulation of the expression and secretion of inflammation-related adipokines by hypoxia in human adipocytes, *Pflugers Arch*, vol.455, No.3, pp. 479-492, issn 0031-6768 (Print)

Watt, M.J.; Steinberg, G.R.; Chen, Z.P.; Kemp, B.E. & Febbraio, M.A. (2006). Fatty acids stimulate amp-activated protein kinase and enhance fatty acid oxidation in l6 myotubes, *J Physiol*, vol.574, No.Pt 1, pp. 139-147, issn 0022-3751 (Print)

Weisberg, S.P.; Hunter, D.; Huber, R.; Lemieux, J.; Slaymaker, S.; Vaddi, K.; Charo, I.; Leibel, R.L. & Ferrante, A.W., Jr. (2006). Ccr2 modulates inflammatory and metabolic effects of high-fat feeding, *J Clin Invest,* vol.116, No.1, pp. 115-124, issn 0021-9738

Wellen, K.E. & Hotamisligil, G.S. (2005). Inflammation, stress, and diabetes, *J Clin Invest,* vol.115, No.5, pp. 1111-1119, issn 0021-9738 (Print)

Willcox, B.J.; Willcox, D.C.; Todoriki, H.; Fujiyoshi, A.; Yano, K.; He, Q.; Curb, J.D. & Suzuki, M. (2007). Caloric restriction, the traditional okinawan diet, and healthy aging: The diet of the world's longest-lived people and its potential impact on morbidity and life span, *Ann N Y Acad Sci,* vol.1114, pp. 434-455, issn 0077-8923 (Print)

Yamauchi, T.; Kamon, J.; Waki, H.; Terauchi, Y.; Kubota, N.; Hara, K.; Mori, Y.; Ide, T.; Murakami, K.; Tsuboyama-Kasaoka, N.; Ezaki, O.; Akanuma, Y.; Gavrilova, O.; Vinson, C.; Reitman, M.L.; Kagechika, H.; Shudo, K.; Yoda, M.; Nakano, Y.; Tobe, K.; Nagai, R.; Kimura, S.; Tomita, M.; Froguel, P. & Kadowaki, T. (2001). The fat-derived hormone adiponectin reverses insulin resistance associated with both lipoatrophy and obesity, *Nat Med,* vol.7, No.8, pp. 941-946, issn 1078-8956 (Print)

Yun, Z.; Maecker, H.L.; Johnson, R.S. & Giaccia, A.J. (2002). Inhibition of ppar gamma 2 gene expression by the hif-1-regulated gene dec1/stra13: A mechanism for regulation of adipogenesis by hypoxia, *Dev Cell,* vol.2, No.3, pp. 331-341, issn 1534-5807 (Print)

Zehetner, J.; Danzer, C.; Collins, S.; Eckhardt, K.; Gerber, P.A.; Ballschmieter, P.; Galvanovskis, J.; Shimomura, K.; Ashcroft, F.M.; Thorens, B.; Rorsman, P. & Krek, W. (2008). Pvhl is a regulator of glucose metabolism and insulin secretion in pancreatic beta cells, *Genes Dev,* vol.22, No.22, pp. 3135-3146, issn 0890-9369 (Print)

Zingaretti, M.C.; Crosta, F.; Vitali, A.; Guerrieri, M.; Frontini, A.; Cannon, B.; Nedergaard, J. & Cinti, S. (2009). The presence of ucp1 demonstrates that metabolically active adipose tissue in the neck of adult humans truly represents brown adipose tissue, *FASEB J,* vol.23, No.9, pp. 3113-3120, issn 1530-6860 (Electronic)

9

Disrupted VLDL Features and Lipoprotein Metabolism in Sepsis

Patricia Aspichueta, Nerea Bartolomé, Xabier Buqué,
María José Martínez, Begoña Ochoa and Yolanda Chico
Department of Physiology, Faculty of Medicine, University of the Basque Country
Spain

1. Introduction

Gram-negative sepsis is an increasingly clinical syndrome triggered by exposure to bacterial lipopolysaccharide (LPS) or endotoxin. It is associated with a plethora of physiological and biochemical changes, known as acute-phase response (APR), including disturbances in serum lipid and lipoprotein levels (Khovidhunkit et al., 2004). Within the blood, LPS is extracted by the acute phase reactant LPS-binding protein (LBP) and transferred to CD14 receptor on monocytes and macrophages. The CD14 associates with Toll like receptor 4, myeloid differentiation-2 and other proteins forming a receptor cluster that leads to LPS-induced activation (Triantafilou & Triantafilou, 2005), resulting in the release of soluble mediators, such as proinflammatory cytokines.

Kupffer cells (KC), the resident machrophages in the liver, secrete cytokines, particularly tumor necrosis factor α (TNF-α) and the interleukins (IL) IL-6 and IL-1β, that act as paracrine factors on neighboring hepatocytes and promote many of the metabolic changes that accompany the acute-phase response. One of the most striking changes associated to sepsis is the accumulation of triglycerides (TG) within very low density lipoprotein (VLDL) in the plasma, partly ascribed to an increased hepatic VLDL production and a decreased peripheral metabolism driven by pro-inflammatory cytokines. These metabolic alterations, clinically termed as the "lipemia of sepsis", have been postulated to be components of the innate defensive reaction against infection (Harris et al., 2000).

In this chapter we summarize the actual knowledge on sepsis induced alterations in VLDL metabolism, lipids and apoB availability and the involvement of inflammatory mediators.

2. Hiperlipemia of sepsis

Elevation of plasma lipid levels is an early hallmark of sepsis, clinically defined as lipemia of sepsis. The rise in circulating lipids is mainly caused by a rapid accumulation of triglycerides within very low density lipoproteins (Esteve et al., 2005; Khovidhunkit et al., 2004), although other lipids such as non-esterified fatty acids coming from peripheral tissue lipolysis (Khovidhunkit et al., 2004), or cholesterol, in the case of rodents, can also be elevated (Feingold et al., 1993). However, decreases in cholesterol associated to high density lipoproteins (HDL) have been reported as a characteristic associated to sepsis in primates and rodents (Khovidhunkit et al., 2004).

The accumulation of VLDL particles in plasma is attributable to complex disturbances in their metabolism, including increased hepatic production (Feingold et al., 1992; Khovidhunkit et al., 2004; Lanza-Jacoby et al., 1998) and depressed peripheral clearance in the bloodstream by lipoprotein lipase (LPL) depending upon the dose (Feingold et al., 1992; Khovidhunkit et al., 2004; Lanza-Jacoby et al., 1998). Initially, the sepsis-induced hypertriglyceridemia was thought to constitute a mechanism for supplying high-energy substrates to cells involved in host defence (Hardardottir et al., 1994). However, it is increasingly believed that TG-rich lipoproteins are also components of an innate, non-adaptive host immune reaction against infection in humans and animal models (Barcia & Harris, 2005; Harris et al., 2000; Harris et al., 2002).

Both in vitro (Levels et al., 2001; Van Lenten et al., 1986) and in vivo (Kitchens et al., 2003) studies have demonstrated that all lipoprotein classes are able to bind LPS, through their phospholipid (Kitchens et al., 2003) or apolipoprotein (Levels et al., 2001; Vreugdenhil et al., 2001) components, in such a way that lipoprotein-bound LPS is subsequently cleared from the circulation by hepatic parenchymal cells (Harris et al., 2002). Most of the LPS-binding ability corresponds to HDL particles (Levels et al., 2001); however, when levels of VLDL are increased and HDL diminished, as may occur in endotoxemia, the binding appears to shift towards VLDL (Kitchens & Thompson, 2003; Vreugdenhil et al., 2001) and partially depends on interacting with apolipoprotein B (apoB) (Vreugdenhil et al., 2001). Therefore, higher secretion levels of VLDL may be regarded as a protective mechanism against infection. We have shown in LPS-treated rats that plasma VLDL-apoB is rapidly elevated, and this can represent a defence mechanism to neutralize and remove LPS from the circulation (Fig. 1).

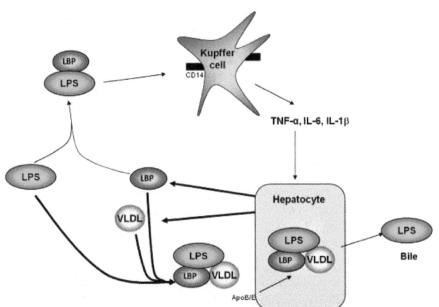

Fig. 1. Proposed role of VLDL in the host inflammatory response. Inflammatory mediators released from Kupffer cells act on hepatocytes inducing the production of VLDL and the synthesis of APR proteins, among them LBP. LBP mediates the binding of LPS to VLDL, the complex is taken up by the hepatocyte and LPS is eliminated through the bile.

Notwithstanding the beneficial role of VLDL, many of the sepsis-associated changes in lipoprotein characteristics and metabolism are similar to those promoting atherogenesis, and has been proposed that the APR associated changes in lipoproteins can be one possible link between infection/inflammation and atherosclerosis. During acute phase reaction, apart from changes in HDL-cholesterol, alterations in HDL associated proteins have been reported. These changes alter cholesterol reverse transport, leading to diminished HDL-cholesterol, and reduce their antioxidant properties (Esteve et al., 2005; Khovidhunkit et al., 2004). In fact, following acute infection low density lipoproteins (LDL) become more susceptible to oxidation (Memon et al., 2000).

One factor that may influence lipoprotein metabolism and is known to be altered during sepsis is food intake (Grunfeld et al., 1996). In order to avoid this variability, animals are food-deprived from the time of administration of endotoxin.

We have shown that endotoxin administration to fasted rats induced hipertriglyceridemia in a time-dependent pattern, related to different systemic fuels (Bartolome et al., 2010). Metabolic background is an important factor contributing to the sepsis-promoted VLDL abundance. We have demonstrated a biphasic response to endotoxin in systemic fuels of fasted rats, with two 12 h differentiated phases. We found that during the first phase serum fatty acids were markedly increased and glucose levels decreased, whereas in the second period hyperglycemia was recorded and fatty acid levels were bellow controls. Impaired glucose metabolism has been reported (McGuinness, 2005). During the second phase of the response we detected increased levels of insulin, that together with the high glucose levels indicate the reported sepsis induced insulin resistance (Andersen et al., 2004). It is well known that overproduction of VLDL is a characteristic of insulin-resistant states (Adeli et al., 2001).

	mean diamenter (nm)	Triglycerides		Cholesterol	
		8 h	18 h	8 h	18 h
VLDL	31,3-64	8,21**	3,16**	3,29***	2,24*
large	44,5-64	9,21***	2,74*	4,69***	2,37*
medium	36,8	6,62***	4,26**	2,89***	2,27*
small	31,3	5,83**	4,18**	1,76	2,00
LDL	16,7-28,6	3,66**	2,88**	0,97	1,36
large	28,6	4,37**	3,49*	1,37	1,78
medium	26,5	3,35**	2,87*	1,19	1,63
small	23	3,08**	2,61*	1,05	1,48
very small	16,7-20,7	3,82**	2,42**	0,83	1,21
HDL	7,6-15	4,64**	1,53*	0,98	0,72*
very large	13,5-15	7,28**	1,93**	1,11	0,72
large	12,1	5,78**	1,80**	1,03	0,69**
medium	10,9	4,15**	1,50**	0,79*	0,75**
small	9,8	4,84***	2,13**	0,83	0,76**
very small	7,6-8,8	4,12**	1,24	0,93	0,79*

Table 1. Fold-changes induced by LPS administration in triglyceride and cholesterol concentration in lipoprotein classes. Rats were injected with LPS and blood collected for lipoprotein triglyceride and total cholesterol measurements.

We analyzed the lipoprotein lipid profile in serum of rats after 8 or 18 h of LPS treatment (Table 1). We found that hypertriglyceridemia was associated with different VLDL, LDL and HDL subclasses depending on the metabolic background of the APR. Although TG increased in all lipoprotein classes, VLDL particles were the major contributors. We did find transient proatherogenic changes in VLDL particles. During the first phase of the APR hypertriglyceridemia was predominantly associated to large VLDL, which were increased 8 fold after 8 h (Bartolome et al., 2010). These large TG-rich VLDL particles, more than normal VLDL, are able to cross the endothelial barrier and interact with lipoprotein receptors in macrophages, initiating a sequence of events that result in the atherosclerotic lesion and, in addition they give rise to small-dense atherogenic LDL (Gianturco et al., 1998; Ginsberg, 2002; Taskinen, 2003). In addition, large TG-rich VLDL were also enriched in cholesterol, making them more proatherogenic.

In the second phase, the rise in serum VLDL-TG corresponded mainly to medium and small VLDL particles. Endotoxin did not affected serum total cholesterol, however changes occurs in lipoprotein subclasses. Total cholesterol increased in large and medium VLDL and HDL-cholesterol levels fell in all HDL subclasses.

3. Altered VLDL metabolism in sepsis

The assembly of VLDL particles is a complex and highly regulated process that occurs in the secretory pathway of hepatocytes. It represents an active export process of fuel carbons, mainly in the form of TG, and is an important route for cholesteryl ester and phospholipid secretion to the circulation. The biogenesis of VLDL has been mostly described as a two step process depending on the cellular availability of lipids, such as triglycerides, phospholipids, cholesterol, and cholesteryl esters, and it is absolutely dependent on the provision of functional apoB, which, in rodents, may be either the full length apoB-100 or the truncated form of apoB-48 (Davidson & Shelness, 2000). Firstly, during translocation to the lumen across the endoplasmic reticulum (ER) membrane, nascent apoB is lipidated by the essential chaperone microsomal triglyceride transfer protein (MTP) (Gordon & Jamil, 2000; Hussain et al., 2003; Liang & Ginsberg, 2001), originating a relatively small, dense, TG-poor lipoprotein particle. In the second stage, bulk of lipidation and final maturation of lipoprotein precursor occur in the ER and post-ER compartments to form mature VLDL (Gusarova et al., 2003; Kulinski et al., 2002). It is known that when MTP activity is low, or when lipid availability or synthesis is reduced, apoB is cotranslationally targeted for ER-associated degradation by both proteasome-dependent and non-dependent pathways (Fisher et al., 2001; Fisher & Ginsberg, 2002; Ginsberg & Fisher, 2009).

The apoB gene has been considered to be constitutively expressed (Pullinger et al., 1989) and VLDL assembly regulation as a post-transcriptional event. However, increasing evidence from in vivo and in vitro studies over the last years has shown changes in hepatic steady-state mRNA levels for apoB in several pathophysiological conditions, particularly under a variety of inflammatory conditions (Jura et al., 2004; Yokoyama et al., 1998).

VLDL secretion rate and composition can be modulated by a variety of factors, such as nutritional state (Gibbons & Burnham, 1991), endotoxin and proinflammatory cytokines (Aspichueta et al., 2006; Bartolome et al., 2007; Perez et al., 2006). Different mechanisms may be involved in the sepsis enhanced VLDL secretion (Fig. 2).

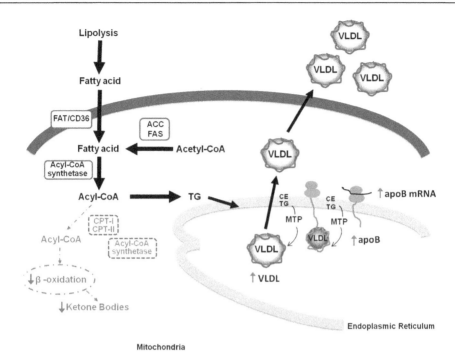

Fig. 2. Model of VLDL assembly and secretion during sepsis. FAT, fatty acid translocase; FAS, fatty acid synthase; ACC, Acetyl-CoA carboxylase; CPT, carnitine acyltransferase. Solid and blue arrows indicate increases, discontinuous and red arrows indicate decreases.

Our results suggest that specific mechanisms are involved in the temporal response to sepsis. In LPS treated rats we found that both fatty acids and hypertriglyceridemia, associated with VLDL-TG, peaked after 8 hours of endotoxin contact. During inflammation adipose tissue lipolysis is activated by pro-inflammatory mediators (Khovidhunkit et al., 2004; Zu et al., 2009) providing fatty acids for hepatic triglyceride synthesis, thus promoting VLDL secretion (Lanza-Jacoby et al., 1998). It has been reported that LPS enhance the expression of fatty acid translocase FAT/CD36, involved in fatty acid uptake (Memon et al., 1998a) and that endotoxin and cytokines suppressed mitochondrial acyl-CoA synthetase expression and activity (Memon et al., 1998b) but enhanced microsomal acyl-CoA synthetase. In addition, LPS administration to rats led to reduced carnitine acyltransferase I, lower ketogenic capacity (Takeyama et al., 1990) and decreased levels of serum ketone bodies (Bartolome et al., 2010). Evidences also established a relationship between increased de novo fatty acid synthesis and enhanced secretion of VLDL-TG in rodents treated with LPS or cytokines (Feingold et al., 1992; Lanza-Jacoby & Tabares, 1990). Taken all together, high amounts of fatty acids are directed away from mitochondrial oxidation and are available for their esterification into TG and secreted within VLDL. However, previous works done in our laboratory did not support the proposed hypothesis since levels of fatty acid synthase mRNA or rate of TG synthesis measured as the incorporation of [^{3}H]acetate or [^{3}H]oleate did not change after 18 h of LPS treatment (Aspichueta et al., 2006).

The high availability of lipids in the septic hepatocyte would protect apoB from degradation leading to an increased number of secreted VLDL particles (Phetteplace et al., 2000). In fact, we detected an elevation of 5 fold in the number of circulating VLDL particles, measured as apoB quantities, at 8 h from LPS administration, without any modification in apoB transcript level. The increment in VLDL-TG is of greater magnitude (8 fold), indicating that during the first phase of the septic response TG-rich VLDL particles accumulate in the circulation (Bartolome et al., 2010).

Different mechanisms seem to be involved in the second phase of septic response. The serum fatty levels drop below controls, which would suggest a lower availability of fatty acids of extrahepatic origin for hepatic VLDL-TG secretion.

Endotoxic rats showed a higher number (10 fold) of circulating VLDL particles in rats at 18 h, but the content of the lipid in each VLDL is reduced (Aspichueta et al., 2006; Bartolome et al., 2010). This was accompanied by high levels of *apob* gene transcript, which could provide for high apoB availability increasing the secretion of lipid poor VLDL particles. Using intact rats in the fasted state, injected with the LPL inhibitor Triton WR-1339, we have shown that the TG and cholesterol secreted into VLDL released by the liver to the blood in 2 h was not enhanced by LPS administration to the same extent as the VLDL-apoB production was (Aspichueta et al., 2005). In this way, hepatocytes isolated from 18 hour LPS-treated rats secreted TG-poor VLDL, and although secretion was highly stimulated, global triglyceride secretion in VLDL remained unchanged. This was related to unchanged rates of fatty acid esterification, measured as [^{3}H]oleate incorporation into TG (Aspichueta et al., 2005; Aspichueta et al., 2006).

In septic hypertriglyceridemic rats, 24 h after sepsis induction, the increase in plasma TG was associated to a decrease in VLDL-TG clearance rate, due to suppressed mRNA levels, protein mass and activity of LPL in peripheral tissues (Lanza-Jacoby et al., 1997; Lanza-Jacoby & Tabares, 1990). Thus, in the early phase of the septic reaction hypertriglyceridemia is mostly due to high VLDL secretion driven by availability of lipids in the hepatocyte; and during the second phase, hypertriglyceridemia would be the result of LPL inhibition, and the increase in apoB transcription would be responsible for the increased secretion of VLDL particles (Fig.3).

4. Zonation of VLDL secretion during sepsis

It has been suggested that parenchymal capacity for VLDL secretion is zonated. Zonation refers to a phenotypic heterogeneity that is well established in many essential liver functions (Jungermann & Katz, 1989). While some authors suggested that VLDL secretion might be higher in perivenous (PV) hepatocytes because of their higher capacity for fatty acid synthesis (Guzman & Castro, 1989), others proposed that it could be concentrated in the periportal (PP) area (Kang & Davis, 2000) since higher expression of the cholesterol synthesis rate-limiting enzyme 3-hydroxy-3-methylglutaryl-CoA reductase was found (Singer et al., 1984).

Zonation has also been evidenced in non parenchymal liver cells. Kupffer cells are more abundant and larger in the PP than in the PV zone (Bouwens et al., 1992), and expression of IL-6, a key cytokine acting on hepatocytes in response to endotoxin, occur preferentially in the PP region (Fang et al., 1998).

After 18 h of endotoxin treatment, highly pure rat PP and PV hepatocyte subpopulations, assessed by cytometry, were maintained in suspension for 2 h. Endotoxin treatment provoked zonation of VLDL secretion. The induction in VLDL-apoB secretion was markedly higher in PP hepatocytes (~90%) than in PV cells (~38%). In addition, the increase in the VLDL associated lipid, particularly in triglycerides, was lower than the enhance in apoB output, consequently producing changes in VLDL features which were triglyceride poor (Aspichueta et al., 2005). Endotoxin doubled apoB mRNA and increased by 50% MTP mRNA in PP hepatocytes when compared to their fasted controls, the increase in apoB genetic expression was of a lesser extend in PV cells. Regarding to de novo synthesis of lipids for VLDL assembly, the incorporation of [³H]acetate into TG and cholesterol did not change by endotoxin challenge.

We concluded that periportal and perivenous hepatocytes exhibited similar capabilities for VLDL assembly and secretion in normal conditions; and, only the endotoxic condition led PP hepatocytes to a marked increase in TG-poor VLDL secretion (Fig 4).

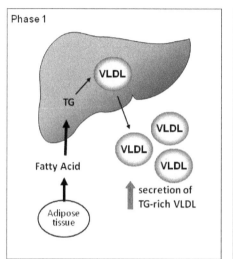
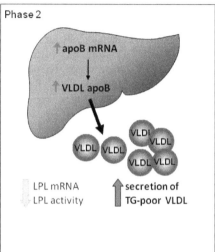

Fig. 3. Proposed model for the biphasic response to endotoxin in VLDL metabolism. In the first phase the stimulation of lipolysis provides fatty acids that are taken by the liver and esterified to be secreted into TG-rich VLDL. In the second phase apoB mRNA levels are increased providing the apolipoprotein for secretion of TG-poor VLDL.

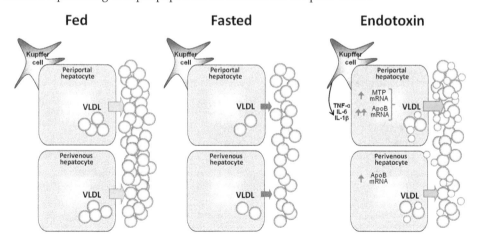

Fig. 4. Model of VLDL secretion by periportal and perivenous hepatocytes in fed state and 18 h after fasting or endotoxin treatment. Endotoxin effect when compared with the fasted state is marked with ⇨

5. Kupffer cell mediators and VLDL secretion

During the acute phase of the septic response, Kupffer cells, the resident macrophages in the liver, release a plethora of soluble bioactive molecules, among them soluble pro-inflammatory mediators as cytokines, particularly TNF-α, IL-6 and IL-1β. These cytokines would act locally on nearby hepatocytes as paracrine factors promoting VLDL secretion and many other metabolic changes that accompany the inflammatory reaction.

We confirmed a rapid release of TNF-α and IL-6 into the bloodstream in rats after 2 h of LPS injection (1 mg/Kg bw), whereas the IL-1β maximum level was observed at 6 h and the rise was less accentuated. Basal levels were recovered in all cases at 12 h from the LPS treatment (Bartolome et al., 2008).

Administration of cytokines to animals has been shown to mimic the sepsis induced alterations in lipid metabolism. TNF-α, IL-6 and IL-1β administered to rodents induce triglyceride synthesis and promote rises in VLDL-TG (Khovidhunkit et al., 2004). In the case of TNF-α and IL-6 administration, the hypertriglyceridemia has been reported to be secondary to higher lipolysis in peripheral tissues; consequently more fatty acids in blood are available and can be recruited by liver. In some studies, the three cytokines have been shown to stimulate hepatic de novo fatty acid synthesis (Feingold et al., 1989) and TG secretion (Feingold et al., 1991; Nonogaki et al., 1995), and decrease adipose tissue LPL activity (Feingold et al., 1994; Popa et al., 2007). Nevertheless, the reduction in LPL was delayed several hours with respect to hypertriglyceridemia (Esteve et al., 2005; Popa et al., 2007) and blockade of TNF-α or IL-6 function in septic mice inhibited hypertriglyceridemia without affecting LPL activity (Feingold et al., 1994).

In order to address the role of Kupffer cells in VLDL oversecretion during endotoxemia, we analyzed the response of rat primary hepatocytes to the direct effect of LPS-stimulated KC or unstimulated products. Hepatocytes were cultured for 8 h with the conditioned medium containing the mediators generated in 16 h by Kupffer cells after a previous 4 h culture with or without LPS. The exposure of hepatocytes to unstimulated KC conditioned medium resulted in doubled the secretion VLDL particles of normal composition. Cells cultured in LPS stimulated KC medium secreted further more VLDL particles that were enriched in PL (Bartolome et al., 2008). Regarding to apoB expression, KC products multiplied by two the abundance of apoB mRNA and no further increment was caused by specific LPS-triggered products. In any case was MTP mRNA modified. The high PL available would protect apoB from degradation, explaining the increase in apoB secretion in cells challenged by LPS-KC medium.

There are few studies investigating the direct effect of cytokines on VLDL secretion, and contradictory results have been reported using different cell types. In HepG2 cells IL-6 and IL-1β were found to reduce apoB secretion although apoB mRNA levels were increased (Yokoyama et al., 1998). However, in IL-6 treated murine hepatocytes, enhanced apoB synthesis, which corresponded with high apoB mRNA levels, was found to be the primary mechanism for increased lipoprotein secretion (Sparks et al., 2010). They also found that IL-6 did not alter the decay rate of apoB mRNA transcripts, concluding that it favours secretion of apoB-containing lipoproteins by increasing availability of apoB through changes in *apob* gene transcription (Sparks et al., 2010).

Our studies in rat hepatocyte cultures, have demonstrated that the inflammatory cytokines TNF-α, IL-6 and IL-1β, over a wide range of concentrations, enhanced VLDL-apoB secretion linked to upregulation of apoB mRNA expression (Bartolome et al., 2007; Bartolome et al.,

2008; Perez et al., 2006). IL-1β was the most potent and was the only one presenting a dose-response effect. The effect of the three cytokines was redundant, as the increase was not additive when they were combined. However, none of the treatments with cytokines modified the amount of TG and total lipids secreted as components of VLDL, suggesting that these particles are lipid poor.

We conclude that Kupffer cells play a role in the rise of VLDL secretion detected during the inflammatory processes and that the three cytokines TNF-α, IL-6 and IL-1β may be involved, nevertheless other Kupffer cells mediators are necessary to accomplish increased lipid association.

6. Higher apoB availability within the hepatocytes

As stated before, the assembly of VLDL is a complex process that depends on the availability of lipids and apoB (Davidson & Shelness, 2000).

Since we have found that under LPS treatment VLDL-apoB secretion was always increased, and given that not always enhanced apoB secretion is linked to high levels of apoB transcript, we hypothesized that during the acute phase response, transcriptional or post-transcriptional regulation affecting apoB mRNA levels might occur supplying more apoB for VLDL assembly.

During the first phase of the septic response we detected elevated circulating VLDL-apoB and -TG after 8 h of LPS treatment without altered apoB transcript levels. Taking into account that at this time point of the septic response, circulating fatty acid levels were elevated, we propose that fatty acid uptake by the liver is increased and large amounts of TG are synthesized. Since the N-terminus of apoB acquires neutral lipids in the endoplasmic reticulum membrane (Hussain et al., 2008), more nucleation sites are expected to be generated in apoB leading to increased apoB secretion. This could result in an increased hepatic secretion of triglycerides in VLDL particles, which would accumulate in the circulation, even in the absence of augmented levels of hepatic apoB mRNA (Bartolome et al., 2010).

In the second phase of the septic response, after 18 h of LPS challenge, enhanced VLDL-apoB secretion is accompanied by increased apoB mRNA levels (Bartolome et al., 2010). In addition, hepatocytes isolated 18 h after LPS administration presented higher levels of apoB transcript and secreted more VLDL particles, been this effect more marked in PP cells. At this time point of the septic response, lipid poor VLDL particles are secreted (Aspichueta et al., 2005) and lipid synthesis is not modified (Aspichueta et al., 2006). Therefore, the increase in *apob* gene transcript would provide the additional apoB necessary to enhance VLDL-apoB secretion. Similarly, the inflammatory cytokines TNF-α (Bartolome et al., 2007), IL1-β (Bartolome et al., 2010) and IL-6 (Perez et al., 2006) augmented the levels of apoB mRNA and secretion of VLDL particles without changing the amounts of lipid secreted in the VLDL.

Our hypothesis was that endotoxin-enhanced VLDL-apoB secretion was driven by higher transcription rates. However, we did not find a rise in transcription rate of *apob* gene when we measured the incorporation of $5'-[\alpha-^{32}P]$-UTP into newly synthesized RNA in liver nuclei from 16 h LPS-treated rats (Bartolome et al., 2010). We reported that global transcription rate in endotoxic liver was nearly two times higher than in control rats as expected in the acute phase response for up-regulating the positive proteins. However, the transcription rate of apoB gene was unaffected after 16 h of LPS challenge in the treated animals. It cannot be discarded that transcriptional activation may occur transiently during other stages of the APR.

Another aspect involved in regulating mRNA level is the modulation of mRNA stability through regulatory elements residing in the 3′- and 5′-untranslated region (UTR) and adequate RNA binding proteins. HuR is an important protein in stabilizing inflammatory AU-rich elements (ARE)-bearing RNAs. Human apoB mRNA has been reported to contain ARE sequences at 3′-UTRs and bioinformatic analysis of rat apoB transcript revealed the presence of AU-rich regions. Our results demonstrated the specific binding of stabilizing HuR protein to the rat apoB mRNA, although there were no superior binding in livers from LPS treated rats. Consequently, in our conditions it is not likely that apoB mRNA half-life was extended by HuR binding, but we can not discard a role for other stabilizing proteins or changes in the mRNA degradation pathway, but further analysis is need (Fig 5).

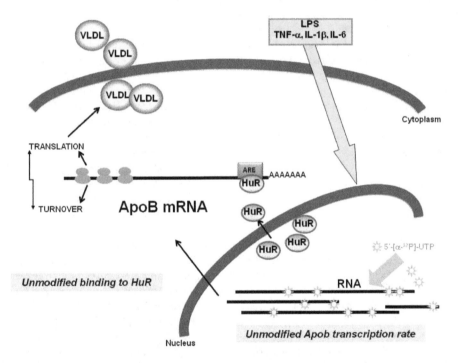

Fig. 5. Endotoxin induce increase in apoB mRNA without altering transcription rate or HuR protein binding.

7. Conclusion

During the septic response, altered VLDL metabolism is responsible for the lipemia of sepsis. Entotoxin promoted changes are biphasic. In the early stage hypertriglyceridemia is accompanied by increased circulating fatty acids levels and a rise in large TG-rich VLDL, whereas the later stage is characterized by high levels of hepatic apoB transcript and TG-poor VLDL accumulation. In the later stage, the endotoxin induced VLDL secretion is more accentuated in periportal cells. Kupffer cells released products directly promote VLDL assembly and secretion and increase apoB mRNA levels, among these products the cytokines TNF–α, IL-6 and IL-1β and other mediator/s could play a role in the enhancement of VLD secretion.

8. Acknowledgments

This work was supported by the Basque Government (IT336-10).

9. References

Adeli, K., Taghibiglou, C., Van Iderstine, SC., & Lewis, GF. (2001). Mechanisms of hepatic very low-density lipoprotein overproduction in insulin resistance. *Trends Cardiovasc. Med.*, Vol.11, No.5, pp. 170-176, ISSN 1050-1738

Andersen, SK., Gjedsted, J., Christiansen, C., & Tonnesen, E. (2004). The roles of insulin and hyperglycemia in sepsis pathogenesis. *J. Leukoc. Biol.*, Vol.75, No.3, pp. 413-421, ISSN 0741-5400

Aspichueta, P., Perez, S., Ochoa, B., & Fresnedo, O. (2005). Endotoxin promotes preferential periportal upregulation of VLDL secretion in the rat liver. *J. Lipid Res*, Vol.46, No.5, pp. 1017-1026, ISSN 0022-2275

Aspichueta, P., Perez-Agote, B., Perez, S., Ochoa, B., & Fresnedo, O. (2006). Impaired response of VLDL lipid and apoB secretion to endotoxin in the fasted rat liver. *J. Endotoxin. Res*, Vol.12, No.3, pp. 181-192, ISSN 0968-0519

Barcia, AM&Harris, HW. (2005). Triglyceride-rich lipoproteins as agents of innate immunity. *Clin. Infect. Dis.*, Vol.41 Suppl 7pp. S498-S503, ISSN 1058-4838

Bartolome, N., Arteta, B., Martinez, MJ., Chico, Y., & Ochoa, B. (2008). Kupffer cell products and interleukin 1beta directly promote VLDL secretion and apoB mRNA up-regulation in rodent hepatocytes. *Innate Immun.*, Vol.14, No.4, pp. 255-266, ISSN 1753-4259

Bartolome, N., Aspichueta, P., Martinez, MJ., Vazquez-Chantada, M., Martinez-Chantar, ML., Ochoa, B., & Chico, Y. (2010). Biphasic adaptative responses in VLDL metabolism and lipoprotein homeostasis during Gram-negative endotoxemia. *Innate. Immun.*, ISSN 1753-4259 Epub ahead of print

Bartolome, N., Rodriguez, L., Martinez, MJ., Ochoa, B., & Chico, Y. (2007). Upregulation of apolipoprotein B secretion, but not lipid, by tumor necrosis factor-alpha in rat hepatocyte cultures in the absence of extracellular fatty acids. *Ann. N. Y Acad. Sci.*, Vol.1096, pp. 55-69, ISSN 0077-8923

Bouwens, L., De, BP., Vanderkerken, K., Geerts, B., & Wisse, E. (1992). Liver cell heterogeneity: functions of non-parenchymal cells. *Enzyme*, Vol.46, No.1-3, pp. 155-168, ISSN 0013-9432

Davidson, NO&Shelness, GS. (2000). APOLIPOPROTEIN B: mRNA editing, lipoprotein assembly, and presecretory degradation. *Annu. Rev. Nutr.*, Vol.20pp. 169-193, ISSN 0199-9885

Esteve, E., Ricart, W., & Fernandez-Real, JM. (2005). Dyslipidemia and inflammation: an evolutionary conserved mechanism. *Clin. Nutr.*, Vol.24, No.1, pp. 16-31, ISSN 0261-5614

Fang, C., Lindros, KO., Badger, TM., Ronis, MJ., & Ingelman-Sundberg, M. (1998). Zonated expression of cytokines in rat liver: effect of chronic ethanol and the cytochrome P450 2E1 inhibitor, chlormethiazole. *Hepatology*, Vol.27, No.5, pp. 1304-1310, ISSN 0270-9139

Feingold, KR., Hardardottir, I., Memon, R., Krul, EJ., Moser, AH., Taylor, JM., & Grunfeld, C. (1993). Effect of endotoxin on cholesterol biosynthesis and distribution in serum lipoproteins in Syrian hamsters. *J. Lipid Res.*, Vol.34, No.12, pp. 2147-2158, ISSN 0022-2275

Feingold, KR., Marshall, M., Gulli, R., Moser, AH., & Grunfeld, C. (1994). Effect of endotoxin and cytokines on lipoprotein lipase activity in mice. *Arterioscler. Thromb.*, Vol.14, No.11, pp. 1866-1872, ISSN 1049-8834

Feingold, KR., Soued, M., Adi, S., Staprans, I., Neese, R., Shigenaga, J., Doerrler, W., Moser, A., Dinarello, CA., & Grunfeld, C. (1991). Effect of interleukin-1 on lipid metabolism in the rat. Similarities to and differences from tumor necrosis factor. *Arterioscler. Thromb.*, Vol.11, No.3, pp. 495-500, ISSN 1049-8834

Feingold, KR., Soued, M., Serio, MK., Moser, AH., Dinarello, CA., & Grunfeld, C. (1989). Multiple cytokines stimulate hepatic lipid synthesis in vivo. *Endocrinology*, Vol.125, No.1, pp. 267-274, ISSN 0013-7227

Feingold, KR., Staprans, I., Memon, RA., Moser, AH., Shigenaga, JK., Doerrler, W., Dinarello, CA., & Grunfeld, C. (1992). Endotoxin rapidly induces changes in lipid metabolism that produce hypertriglyceridemia: low doses stimulate hepatic triglyceride production while high doses inhibit clearance. *J. Lipid Res*, Vol.33, No.12, pp. 1765-1776, ISSN 0022-2275

Fisher, EA&Ginsberg, HN. (2002). Complexity in the secretory pathway: the assembly and secretion of apolipoprotein B-containing lipoproteins. *J Biol Chem.*, Vol.277, No.20, pp. 17377-17380, ISSN 0021-9258

Fisher, EA., Pan, M., Chen, X., Wu, X., Wang, H., Jamil, H., Sparks, JD., & Williams, KJ. (2001). The triple threat to nascent apolipoprotein B. Evidence for multiple, distinct degradative pathways. *J. Biol. Chem.*, Vol.276, No.30, pp. 27855-27863, ISSN 0021-9258

Gianturco, SH., Ramprasad, MP., Song, R., Li, R., Brown, ML., & Bradley, WA. (1998). Apolipoprotein B-48 or its apolipoprotein B-100 equivalent mediates the binding of triglyceride-rich lipoproteins to their unique human monocyte-macrophage receptor. *Arterioscler. Thromb. Vasc. Biol.*, Vol.18, No.6, pp. 968-976, ISSN 1079-5642

Gibbons, GF&Burnham, FJ. (1991). Effect of nutritional state on the utilization of fatty acids for hepatitic triacylglycerol synthesis and secretion as very-low-density lipoprotein. *Biochem. J.*, Vol.275 (Pt 1)pp. 87-92, ISSN 0264-6021

Ginsberg, HN (2002). New perspectives on atherogenesis: role of abnormal triglyceride-rich lipoprotein metabolism. *Circulation*, Vol.106, No.16, pp. 2137-2142, ISSN 0009-7322

Ginsberg, HN&Fisher, EA. (2009). The ever-expanding role of degradation in the regulation of apolipoprotein B metabolism. *J. Lipid Res.*, Vol.50 Supplpp. S162-S166, ISSN 0022-2275

Gordon, DA&Jamil, H. (2000). Progress towards understanding the role of microsomal triglyceride transfer protein in apolipoprotein-B lipoprotein assembly. *Biochim. Biophys. Acta*, Vol.1486, No.1, pp. 72-83, ISSN 0006-3002

Grunfeld, C., Zhao, C., Fuller, J., Pollack, A., Moser, A., Friedman, J., & Feingold, KR. (1996). Endotoxin and cytokines induce expression of leptin, the ob gene product, in hamsters. *J. Clin. Invest.*, Vol.97, No.9, pp. 2152-2157, ISSN 0021-9738

Gusarova, V., Brodsky, JL., & Fisher, EA. (2003). Apolipoprotein B100 exit from the endoplasmic reticulum (ER) is COPII-dependent, and its lipidation to very low density lipoprotein occurs post-ER. *J. Biol. Chem.*, Vol.278, No.48, pp. 48051-48058, ISSN 0021-9258

Guzman, M&Castro, J. (1989). Zonation of fatty acid metabolism in rat liver. *Biochem. J.*, Vol.264, No.1, pp. 107-113, ISSN 0264-6021

Hardardottir, I., Grunfeld, C., & Feingold, KR. (1994). Effects of endotoxin and cytokines on lipid metabolism. *Curr. Opin. Lipidol.*, Vol.5, No.3, pp. 207-215, ISSN 0957-9672

Harris, HW., Gosnell, JE., & Kumwenda, ZL. (2000). The lipemia of sepsis: triglyceride-rich lipoproteins as agents of innate immunity. *J Endotoxin. Res.*, Vol.6, No.6, pp. 421-430, ISSN 0968-0519

Harris, HW., Johnson, JA., & Wigmore, SJ. (2002). Endogenous lipoproteins impact the response to endotoxin in humans. *Crit Care Med.*, Vol.30, No.1, pp. 23-31, ISSN 0090-3493

Hussain, MM., Rava, P., Pan, X., Dai, K., Dougan, SK., Iqbal, J., Lazare, F., & Khatun, I. (2008). Microsomal triglyceride transfer protein in plasma and cellular lipid metabolism. *Curr. Opin. Lipidol.*, Vol.19, No.3, pp. 277-284, ISSN 0957-9672

Hussain, MM., Shi, J., & Dreizen, P. (2003). Microsomal triglyceride transfer protein and its role in apoB-lipoprotein assembly. *J Lipid. Res.*, Vol.44, No.1, pp. 22-32, ISSN 0957-9672

Jungermann, K&Katz, N. (1989). Functional specialization of different hepatocyte populations. *Physiol. Rev.*, Vol.69, No.3, pp. 708-764, ISSN 0031-9333

Jura, J., Wegrzyn, P., Zarebski, A., Wladyka, B., & Koj, A. (2004). Identification of changes in the transcriptome profile of human hepatoma HepG2 cells stimulated with interleukin-1 beta. *Biochim. Biophys. Acta*, Vol.1689, No.2, pp. 120-133, ISSN 0006-3002

Kang, S&Davis, RA. (2000). Cholesterol and hepatic lipoprotein assembly and secretion. *Biochim. Biophys. Acta*, Vol.1529, No.1-3, pp. 223-230, ISSN 0006-3002

Khovidhunkit, W., Kim, MS., Memon, RA., Shigenaga, JK., Moser, AH., Feingold, KR., & Grunfeld, C. (2004). Effects of infection and inflammation on lipid and lipoprotein metabolism: mechanisms and consequences to the host. *J. Lipid Res*, Vol.45, No.7, pp. 1169-1196, ISSN 0022-2275

Kitchens, RL&Thompson, PA. (2003). Impact of sepsis-induced changes in plasma on LPS interactions with monocytes and plasma lipoproteins: roles of soluble CD14, LBP, and acute phase lipoproteins. *J. Endotoxin. Res*, Vol.9, No.2, pp. 113-118, ISSN 0968-0519

Kitchens, RL., Thompson, PA., Munford, RS., & O'Keefe, GE. (2003). Acute inflammation and infection maintain circulating phospholipid levels and enhance lipopolysaccharide binding to plasma lipoproteins. *J. Lipid Res*, Vol.44, No.12, pp. 2339-2348, ISSN 0022-2275

Kulinski, A., Rustaeus, S., & Vance, JE. (2002). Microsomal triacylglycerol transfer protein is required for lumenal accretion of triacylglycerol not associated with ApoB, as well as for ApoB lipidation. *J Biol Chem.*, Vol.277, No.35, pp. 31516-31525, ISSN 0021-9258

Lanza-Jacoby, S., Phetteplace, H., Sedkova, N., & Knee, G. (1998). Sequential alterations in tissue lipoprotein lipase, triglyceride secretion rates, and serum tumor necrosis factor alpha during Escherichia coli bacteremic sepsis in relation to the development of hypertriglyceridemia. *Shock*, Vol.9, No.1, pp. 46-51, ISSN 1073-2322

Lanza-Jacoby, S., Sedkova, N., Phetteplace, H., & Perrotti, D. (1997). Sepsis-induced regulation of lipoprotein lipase expression in rat adipose tissue and soleus muscle. *J. Lipid Res.*, Vol.38, No.4, pp. 701-710, ISSN 0022-2275

Lanza-Jacoby, S&Tabares, A. (1990). Triglyceride kinetics, tissue lipoprotein lipase, and liver lipogenesis in septic rats. *Am. J. Physiol.*, Vol.258, No.4 Pt 1, pp. E678-E685, ISSN 0002-9513

Levels, JH., Abraham, PR., van den, EA., & van Deventer, SJ. (2001). Distribution and kinetics of lipoprotein-bound endotoxin. *Infect. Immun.*, Vol.69, No.5, pp. 2821-2828, ISSN 1098-5522

Liang, J&Ginsberg, HN. (2001). Microsomal triglyceride transfer protein binding and lipid transfer activities are independent of each other, but both are required for secretion of apolipoprotein B lipoproteins from liver cells. *J. Biol. Chem.*, Vol.276, No.30, pp. 28606-28612, ISSN 0021-9258

McGuinness, OP (2005). Defective glucose homeostasis during infection. *Annu. Rev. Nutr.*, Vol.25pp. 9-35, ISSN 0199-9885

Memon, RA., Feingold, KR., Moser, AH., Fuller, J., & Grunfeld, C. (1998a). Regulation of fatty acid transport protein and fatty acid translocase mRNA levels by endotoxin and cytokines. *Am. J. Physiol*, Vol.274, No.2 Pt 1, pp. E210-E217, ISSN 0002-9513

Memon, RA., Fuller, J., Moser, AH., Smith, PJ., Feingold, KR., & Grunfeld, C. (1998b). In vivo regulation of acyl-CoA synthetase mRNA and activity by endotoxin and cytokines. *Am. J. Physiol*, Vol.275, No.1 Pt 1, pp. E64-E72, ISSN 0002-9513

Memon, RA., Staprans, I., Noor, M., Holleran, WM., Uchida, Y., Moser, AH., Feingold, KR., & Grunfeld, C. (2000). Infection and inflammation induce LDL oxidation in vivo. *Arterioscler. Thromb. Vasc. Biol.*, Vol.20, No.6, pp. 1536-1542, ISSN 1079-5642

Nonogaki, K., Fuller, GM., Fuentes, NL., Moser, AH., Staprans, I., Grunfeld, C., & Feingold, KR. (1995). Interleukin-6 stimulates hepatic triglyceride secretion in rats. *Endocrinology*, Vol.136, No.5, pp. 2143-2149, ISSN 0013-7227

Perez, S., Aspichueta, P., Ochoa, B., & Chico, Y. (2006). The 2-series prostaglandins suppress VLDL secretion in an inflammatory condition-dependent manner in primary rat hepatocytes. *Biochim. Biophys. Acta*, Vol.1761, No.2, pp. 160-171, ISSN 0006-3002

Phetteplace, HW., Sedkova, N., Hirano, KI., Davidson, NO., & Lanza-Jacoby, SP. (2000). Escherichia coli sepsis increases hepatic apolipoprotein B secretion by inhibiting degradation. *Lipids*, Vol.35, No.10, pp. 1079-1085, ISSN 0024-4201

Popa, C., Netea, MG., van Riel, PL., van der Meer, JW., & Stalenhoef, AF. (2007). The role of TNF-alpha in chronic inflammatory conditions, intermediary metabolism, and cardiovascular risk. J. Lipid Res., Vol.48, No.4, pp. 751-762, ISSN 0022-2275

Pullinger, CR., North, JD., Teng, BB., Rifici, VA., Ronhild de Brito, AE., & Scott, J. (1989). The apolipoprotein B gene is constitutively expressed in HepG2 cells: regulation of secretion by oleic acid, albumin, and insulin, and measurement of the mRNA half-life. *J Lipid Res*, Vol.30, No.7, pp. 1065-1077, ISSN 0022-2275

Singer, II., Kawka, DW., Kazazis, DM., Alberts, AW., Chen, JS., Huff, JW., & Ness, GC. (1984). Hydroxymethylglutaryl-coenzyme A reductase-containing hepatocytes are distributed periportally in normal and mevinolin-treated rat livers. *Proc. Natl. Acad. Sci. U S. A.*, Vol.81, No.17, pp. 5556-5560, ISSN 0027-8424

Sparks, JD., Cianci, J., Jokinen, J., Chen, LS., & Sparks, CE. (2010). Interleukin-6 mediates hepatic hypersecretion of apolipoprotein B. *Am. J. Physiol Gastrointest. Liver Physiol*, Vol.299, No.4, pp. G980-G989, ISSN 0193-1857

Takeyama, N., Itoh, Y., Kitazawa, Y., & Tanaka, T. (1990). Altered hepatic mitochondrial fatty acid oxidation and ketogenesis in endotoxic rats. *Am. J. Physiol*, Vol.259, No.4 Pt 1, pp. E498-E505, ISSN 0002-9513

Taskinen, MR (2003). Diabetic dyslipidaemia: from basic research to clinical practice. *Diabetologia*, Vol.46, No.6, pp. 733-749, ISSN 0012-186X

Triantafilou, M&Triantafilou, K. (2005). The dynamics of LPS recognition: complex orchestration of multiple receptors. *J Endotoxin. Res.*, Vol.11, No.1, pp. 5-11, ISSN 0968-0519

Van Lenten, BJ., Fogelman, AM., Haberland, ME., & Edwards, PA. (1986). The role of lipoproteins and receptor-mediated endocytosis in the transport of bacterial lipopolysaccharide. *Proc. Natl. Acad. Sci. U. S. A*, Vol.83, No.8, pp. 2704-2708, ISSN 0027-8424

Vreugdenhil, AC., Snoek, AM., van, ', V., Greve, JW., & Buurman, WA. (2001). LPS-binding protein circulates in association with apoB-containing lipoproteins and enhances endotoxin-LDL/VLDL interaction. *J. Clin. Invest*, Vol.107, No.2, pp. 225-234, ISSN 0021-9738

Yokoyama, K., Ishibashi, T., Yi-qiang, L., Nagayoshi, A., Teramoto, T., & Maruyama, Y. (1998). Interleukin-1beta and interleukin-6 increase levels of apolipoprotein B mRNA and decrease accumulation of its protein in culture medium of HepG2 cells. *J. Lipid Res*, Vol.39, No.1, pp. 103-113, ISSN 0022-2275

Zu, L., He, J., Jiang, H., Xu, C., Pu, S., & Xu, G. (2009). Bacterial endotoxin stimulates adipose lipolysis via toll-like receptor 4 and extracellular signal-regulated kinase pathway. *J Biol. Chem.*, Vol.284, No.9, pp. 5915-5926, ISSN 0021-9285

10

Pleiotropic Functions of HDL Lead to Protection from Atherosclerosis and Other Diseases

Vassilis Zannis[1,2], Andreas Kateifides[1,2], Panagiotis Fotakis[1,2],
Eleni Zanni[1] and Dimitris Kardassis[2]
[1]Molecular Genetics, Boston University School of Medicine Boston, MA,
[2]University of Crete Medical School, Greece,
[1]USA
[2]Greece

1. Introduction

High density lipoprotein (HDL) is a macromolecular complex of proteins and lipids that is produced primarily by the liver through a complex pathway that requires initially the functions of apolipoprotein A-I (apoA-I), ATP binding cassette transporter A1 (ABCA1) and lecithin:cholesterol acetyl transferase (LCAT) (Zannis et al., 2006b). Following synthesis, HDL affects the functions of the arterial wall cells through signaling mechanisms mediated by scavenger receptor class B type-I (SR-BI) and other cell surface proteins. The impetus for studying HDL has been the inverse correlation that exists between plasma HDL levels and the risk for coronary artery disease (CAD) (Gordon et al., 1989). HDL promotes cholesterol efflux (Gu et al., 2000; Nakamura et al., 2004), prevents oxidation of low density lipoprotein (LDL) (Navab et al., 2000a; Navab et al., 2000b), inhibits expression of proinflammatory cytokines by macrophages (Okura et al., 2010) as well as expression of adhesion molecules by endothelial cells (Cockerill et al., 1995; Nicholls et al,. 2005b). HDL inhibits cell apoptosis (Nofer et al., 2001) and promotes endothelial cell proliferation and migration (Seetharam et al., 2006). HDL stimulates release of nitric oxide (NO) from endothelial cells thus promoting vasodilation (Mineo et al., 2003). HDL also inhibits platelet aggregation and thrombosis (Dole et al., 2008) and has antibacterial, antiparasitic and antiviral activities (Parker et al., 1995; Singh et al., 1999; Vanhollebeke and Pays, 2010). Due to these properties HDL is thought to protect the endothelium and inhibit several steps in the cascade of events that lead to the pathogenesis of atherosclerosis and various other human diseases.

This review focuses on two important aspects of contemporary HDL research. The first part considers briefly the structure of apoA-I and HDL and the key proteins that participate in the pathway of the biogenesis of HDL as well as clinical phenotypes associated with HDL abnormalities. The second part considers various physiological functions of HDL and apoA-I and the protective role of HDL against atherosclerosis and other diseases.

2. Biogenesis of HDL

HDL is synthesized through a complex pathway (Zannis et al., 2004a). The first step involves an ABCA1 mediated transfer of cellular phospholipids and cholesterol to lipid poor apoA-I extracellularly. The lipidated apoA-I is gradually converted to discoidal particles that are remodelled in the plasma compartment by the esterification of cholesterol by the enzyme LCAT (Zannis et al., 2006a) and are converted to spherical HDL particles. The cholesteryl esters formed are transferred to very low-density lipoproteins/intermediate-density lipoproteins/low density lipoproteins (VLDL/IDL/LDL) by the cholesteryl ester transfer protein (CETP) (Barter et al., 2003). Additional remodelling of HDL involves transfer of phospholipids from VLDL/LDL to HDL by the phospholipid transfer protein (PLTP) (Lusa et al., 1996), cholesterol efflux from cells or delivery of cholesteryl esters to cells mediated by the SR-BI (Krieger, 2001) as well as cholesterol efflux mediated by the cell surface transporter ATP binding cassette transporter G1 (ABCG1) (Wang et al., 2004). Finally hydrolysis of lipids of HDL is mediated by various lipases [lipoprotein lipase (LpL), hepatic lipase (HL), endothelial lipase (EL)] (Breckenridge et al., 1982; Brunzell and Deeb, 2001; Ishida et al., 2003; Krauss et al., 1974). Mutations in any of these proteins may affect the biogenesis, maturation and the functions of HDL (Fig. 1).

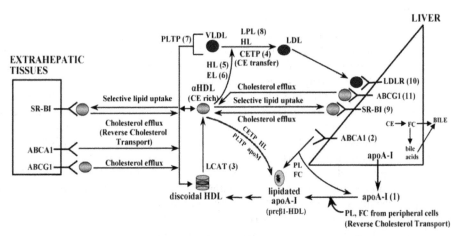

Fig. 1. Schematic representation of the pathway of the biogenesis and catabolism of HDL Numbers 1-11 indicate key cell membrane or plasma proteins shown to influence HDL levels or composition as follows: 1) apoA-I; 2) ABCA1; 3) LCAT; 4) CETP; 5) HL; 6) EL; 7) PLTP; 8) lipoproteins lipase; 9) SR-BI; 10) LDL receptor; 11) ABCG1. The figure is modified from ref. (Zannis et al., 2004b; Zannis et al., 2006b).

3. Proteins involved in the biogenesis, remodeling and signaling of HDL

3.1 Apolipoprotein A-I and its structure in solution and in discoidal and spherical HDL

ApoA-I is synthesized by the liver and the intestine in humans (Williamson et al., 1992) and it is the major protein component of the HDL. ApoA-I along with several other proteins participate in the biogenesis and remodeling of HDL as well as in signaling pathways induced by apoA-I and HDL (Yuhanna et al., 2001; Zannis et al., 2004a). ApoA-I contains 22 or 11 amino acid repeats which are organized in amphipathic a-helices (Nolte and Atkinson, 1992). Based on the crystal structure of apoA-I in solution (Borhani et al., 1997) a belt model was proposed to explain the structure of apoA-I on discoidal HDL particles. In this model, two antiparallel molecules of apoA-I are wrapped like a belt around a discoidal bilayer containing 160 phospholipid molecules and shields the hydrophobic fatty acid chains of the phospholipids. Analysis of the 93 Å spherical HDL in solution by small angle neutron scattering (SANS) showed that three molecules of apoA-I fold around a central lipid core that has 88.4 Å x 62.8 Å dimensions to form a spheroidal HDL (sHDL) particle (Wu et al., 2011).

3.2 Interactions of ApoA-I with ABCA1 are the first step in the biogenesis of HDL
ABCA1 is a ubiquitous protein that belongs to the ABC family of transporters and is expressed abundantly in the liver, macrophages, brain and various other tissues (Kielar et al., 2001). ABCA1 was shown to promote the efflux of cellular phospholipids and cholesterol to lipid free or minimally lipidated apoA-I and other apolipoproteins and amphipathic peptides, but it does not promote efflux to spherical HDL particles (Remaley et al., 2001; Wang et al., 2000). The functional interactions between apoA-I and ABCA-1 are important for the biogenesis of HDL. In the absence of either apoA-I (Matsunaga et al., 1991) or ABCA-1 (Brunham et al., 2006) HDL is not formed. Adenovirus mediated gene transfer of apoA-I mutants in apoA-I⁻/⁻ mice showed that deletion of the C-terminal region of apoA-I prevented the formation of HDL (Chroni et al., 2007). The ability of ABCA1 to promote cholesterol efflux from macrophages is very important for the prevention of formation of foam cells in the atherosclerotic lesions (Van Eck et al., 2002). Mutations resulting in inactivation of ABCA1 are present in patients with Tangier disease (Brunham et al., 2006). The deficiency is associated with very low levels of total plasma and HDL cholesterol and abnormal lipid deposition in various tissues (Christiansen-Weber et al., 2000; McNeish et al., 2000). The ABCA1 deficiency in humans or experimental animals may contribute to accelerated atherosclerosis (Joyce et al., 2002; Singaraja et al., 2003). Inactivation of the ABCA1 gene in macrophages increases the susceptibility to atherosclerosis (Van Eck et al., 2002; Van Eck et al., 2006). Specific amino acid substitutions found in the Danish general population were predictors of ischemic heart disease and reduced life expectancy (Frikke-Schmidt et al., 2008).

3.3 Interactions of lipid-bound ApoA-I with LCAT stabilize the nascent HDL
Plasma LCAT is a 416 amino acid long enzyme that is synthesized and secreted by the liver and esterifies the free cholesterol of HDL and LDL. ApoA-I is a potent activator of LCAT (Fielding et al., 1972). Following esterification, the cholesteryl esters formed become part of the lipid core and the discoidal HDL is converted to mature spherical HDL (Chroni et al., 2005a).
Mutations in LCAT are associated with two phenotypes in humans. The familiar LCAT deficiency (FLD) is characterized by the inability of the mutant LCAT to esterify cholesterol on HDL and LDL and causes accumulation of discoidal HDL in the plasma. The fish eye disease (FED) is characterized by the inability of mutant LCAT to esterify cholesterol on HDL only. Both diseases are characterized by low HDL levels due to the inability of LCAT to convert the nascent immature pre-β and discoidal particles to mature spherical HDL (Santamarina-Fojo et al., 2001).

3.4 Interactions of lipid-bound ApoA-I with SR-BI

SR-BI is an 82 kDa membrane glycoprotein primarily expressed in the liver, steroidogenic tissues and endothelial cells but is also found in other tissues. The most important property of SR-BI is considered to be its ability to act as the HDL receptor (Acton et al., 1996). SR-BI mediates both selective uptake of cholesteryl esters and other lipids from HDL to cells (Acton et al., 1996; Stangl et al., 1999; Thuahnai et al., 2001), as well as efflux of unesterified cholesterol (Gu et al., 2000). Transgenic mice expressing SR-BI in the liver had greatly decreased apoA-I and HDL levels as well as increased clearance of VLDL and LDL (Ueda et al., 1999) and were protected from atherosclerosis (Arai et al., 1999). SR-BI deficient mice had decreased HDL cholesterol clearance (Out et al., 2004), two fold increased plasma cholesterol and presence of large size abnormal apolipoprotein E (apoE) enriched particles that were distributed in the HDL/IDL/LDL region (Rigotti et al., 1997). The SR-BI deficiency in the background of LDL receptor (LDLr) deficient or apoE deficient mice accelerated dramatically the development of atherosclerosis (Huszar et al., 2000; Trigatti et al., 1999). The double deficient mice for apoE and SR-BI developed occlusive coronary atherosclerosis, cardiac hypertrophy, myocardial infarctions, cardiac dysfunction and died prematurely (mean age of death ~6 weeks) (Braun et al., 2002; Trigatti et al., 1999). The SR-BI deficiency reduced greatly cholesteryl ester levels in the steroidogenic tissues that utilize HDL cholesterol for synthesis of steroid hormones (Ji et al., 1999). It also decreased secretion of biliary cholesterol by approximately 50% (Mardones et al., 2001; Rigotti et al., 1997). The SR-BI deficiency also caused defective maturation of oocytes and red blood cells due to accumulation of cholesterol in the plasma membrane of progenitor cells (Holm et al., 2002; Trigatti et al., 1999) and caused infertility in the female but not the male mice (Trigatti et al., 1999; Yesilaltay et al., 2006). Interactions of HDL with SR-BI in endothelial cells triggers signaling mechanisms discussed below that involve activation of endothelial nitric oxide synthase (eNOS) and release of NO that causes vasodilation (Mineo et al., 2003; Yuhanna et al., 2001). Human subjects have been identified with a P297S substitution in SR-BI. Heterozygote carriers for this mutation had increased HDL levels, decreased adrenal stereoidogenesis and dysfunctional platelets but did not develop atherosclerosis (Vergeer et al., 2011).

A [Gly2Ser]SR-BI substitution in humans is associated with decreased follicular progesterone levels in Caucasian women and non viable fetuses 42 days post embryo transfer. Another single nucleotide polymorphism (SNP) (rs10846744) was associated with gestational sacs and fetal heart beats and with poor fetal viability in African-American women (Yates et al., 2011).

3.5 Interactions of HDL with ABCG1

ABCG1 is a 67 kDa protein which is a member of ABC family of half transporters. ABCG1 is expressed in the spleen, thymus, lung, brain, endothelial cells and other tissues (Savary et al., 1996) and promotes cholesterol efflux from cells to HDL but not to lipid free apoA-I (Nakamura et al., 2004; Vaughan and Oram, 2005). The absence of ABCG1 in mice causes cholesterol accumulation in various tissues (Kennedy et al., 2005) and selective deletion of both ABCA1 and ABCG1 genes in macrophages further increases cholesterol accumulation and results in severe atherosclerosis (Out et al., 2008; Yvan-Charvet et al., 2007).

4. Phenotypes of humans and experimental animals having apoA-I mutations

4.1 Natural apoA-I mutations

Several apoA-I mutations have been described in the general population that are associated with low plasma HDL levels. Most of the mutations affect the interaction of apoA-I with LCAT. Eight mutations between residues 26 and 107 and one on residue 173, have been associated with amyloidosis and low HDL levels (Sorci-Thomas and Thomas, 2002; Zannis et al., 1993) and one mutation on residue 164 is associated with increased risk for ischemic heart disease and reduced life expectancy (Haase et al., 2011). The in vivo interactions of representative naturally occurring apoA-I mutants with LCAT were studied by adenovirus-mediated gene transfer in apoA-I deficient mice. The mutants apoA-I(Leu141Arg)$_{Pisa}$ and apoA-I(Leu159Arg)$_{FIN}$ produced only small amounts of HDL that formed mostly preβ1 and small size α4 HDL particles. The apoA-I(Arg151Cys)$_{Paris}$ and apoA-I(arg160Leu)$_{Oslo}$ formed discoidal HDL particles. These studies indicated that apoA-I(Leu141Arg)$_{Pisa}$ and apoA-I(Leu159Arg)$_{FIN}$ mutation may inhibit an early step in the biogenesis of HDL due to insufficient esterification of the cholesterol of the preβ1-HDL particles by the endogenous LCAT. The LCAT insufficiency appears to result from depletion of the plasma LCAT mass (Koukos et al., 2007). A remarkable finding of these studies was that all the aberrant phenotypes were corrected by treatment with exogenous LCAT. This indicates that LCAT administration could be a potential therapeutic intervention to correct low-HDL conditions in humans that are caused by these and other unidentified mutations (Amar et al., 2009).

4.2 Specific bioengineered mutations in ApoA-I may cause dyslipidemia

Four bioengineered mutations in apoA-I have been studied by adenovirus-mediated gene transfer in apoA-I deficient mice. Mutants apoA-I[Δ(62-78)], apoA-I [Glu110Ala/Glu111Ala] and apoA-I[Asp89Ala/Glu90Ala/Glu92Ala], caused combined hyperlipidemia, characterized by elevated plasma cholesterol and severe hypertriglyceridemia (Chroni et al., 2004; Chroni et al., 2005b; Kateifides et al., 2011). An apoA-I[Δ89-99] mutant induced high plasma cholesterol, but did not affect plasma triglyceride levels (Chroni et al., 2005b).

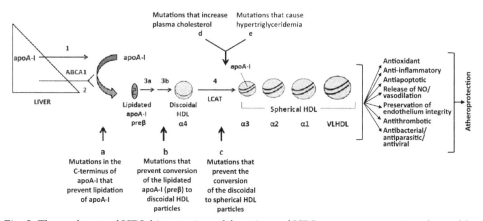

Fig. 2. The pathway of HDL biogenesis and functions of HDL. a-e represent sites of possible disruption of the HDL biogenesis pathway. Different subpopulations of HDL that have been generated due to these defects may have different functions.

The systematic study of the functions of apoA-I by adenovirus mediated gene transfer as well as the phenotypes of naturally occurring apoA-I mutants identified the following five steps where the pathway of biogenesis and/or catabolism of HDL can be disrupted: a) Lack of synthesis of HDL due to mutations in ABCA1 or mutations in apoA-I that affect the ABCA1/apoA-I interaction, b) Failure to convert efficiently the lipidated pre-β HDL to discoidal HDL. This defect most likely results from fast catabolism of apoA-I following its lipidation by ABCA1, c) Accumulation of discoidal HDL. This phenotype has been generated by the mutations in the 149-160 region of apoA-I that affect LCAT activation, d) Accumulation of discoidal HDL and induction of hypercholesterolemia. This condition has been observed in the case of the apoA-I[Δ(89-99)] mutant, e) Induction of hypertriglyceridemia. This defect has been observed in the case of apoA-I[Δ(62-78)], apoA-I[Glu110Ala/Glu111Ala] and apoA-I[Asp89Ala/Glu90Ala/Glu92Ala] mutants (Fig. 2).

5. Physiological functions of ApoA-I and HDL that may be relevant to its atheroprotective properties

5.1 Cell signaling pathways mediated by HDL and apoA-I

Various studies have shown that increased HDL levels are associated with greater vasodilator effects in humans and this effect is impaired in patients with coronary heart disease (CHD) (Li et al., 2000; Zeiher et al., 1994). Treatment with HDL increased eNOS protein levels in cultured human aortic endothelial cells (HAECs) (Ramet et al., 2003). Other studies in endothelial cells and Chinese hamster ovary (CHO) cells that express SR-BI, showed that SR-BI-HDL interactions lead to the phosphorylation and activation of eNOS. The HDL-induced eNOS activation occurs in the caveolae. The HDL-mediated NO-dependent relaxation is lost in aortic rings of SR-BI$^{-/-}$ mice (Yuhanna et al., 2001). Experiments in cultures of endothelial cells and COS M6 cells transfected with eNOS and SR-BI showed that interaction of HDL with SR-BI triggered signalling mechanisms which led to phosphorylation of eNOS at Ser1179 and increased its activity. On the other hand phosphorylation of Thr 497 of eNOS attenuated its activity. The signalling cascade initially involves the nonreceptor tyrosine kinase Src which phosphorylated PI3 kinase (PI3K). Inhibition of Src by specific inhibitors prevented eNOS phosphorylation. PI3K activation led to phosphorylation of Akt and mitogen-activated protein kinase (MAPK) which independently phosphorylated eNOS. Inhibitors of MAPK did not affect HDL-mediated Akt activation and a dominant negative Akt did not affect HDL-mediated MAPK activation and eNOS phosphorylation (Mineo et al., 2003) (figure 3A).

The mechanism of the SR-BI mediated activation of eNOS was studied in detail (Assanasen et al., 2005). HDL and cholesterol-free reconstituted HDL (rHDL) particles containing apoA-I and phosphatidylocholine (Lp2A-I) as well as cyclodextrin stimulated eNOS activity whereas rHDL particles that contain cholesterol did not. Blocking of cholesterol efflux with a monoclonal antibody to SR-BI abolished the activation of eNOS. Experiments were performed using SR-BII, a splice variant of SR-BI as well as a SR-BI mutant that lacks the carboxyterminal amino acid 509 [SR-BI(Δ509)] and chimeric receptors where the transmembrane and the C-terminal domains of SR-BI were replaced by the corresponding domains of CD36. These studies established that the C-terminal cytoplasmic PDZ-interacting domain and the C-terminal transmembrane domain of SR-BI were both required for eNOS activation (Assanasen et al., 2005). The cytoplasmic PDZK1 interacting domain of SR-BI binds adaptor proteins such as PDZK1 that may participate in cell signalling (Kocher et al., 2003). A photoactive derivative of cholesterol binds in the transmembrane region of SR-BI indicating that this region serves as a cholesterol sensor on the plasma membrane (Assanasen et al., 2005). HDL and lysophospholipids that are components of HDL including sphingosylphosphorylcholine, sphingosine-1-phospate (S1P) and lysosulphatide cause eNOS dependent relaxation of mouse aortic rings via intracellular Ca^{2+} mobilization and eNOS phosphorylation mediated by Akt (Nofer et al., 2004). Another study however, indicated that interactions of HDL with SR-BI stimulate eNOS by increasing intracellular ceramide levels without affecting intracellular calcium levels and Akt phosphorylation (Li et al., 2002). The proposed role of HDL-associated estradiol in the stimulation of eNOS activity is unclear (Gong et al., 2003). 5' AMP-activated protein kinase (AMPK) may also play a role in the HDL-mediated phosphorylation of eNOS at multiple sites (Ser116, Ser635, and Ser1179) (Drew et al., 2004). It was suggested that activation by AMPK may involve physical interactions between the apoA-I component of HDL and eNOS. Such interactions may be possible following SR-BI mediated endocytosis of HDL (Silver et al., 2001). HDL also affected the signaling in endothelial cells by the bone morphogenetic protein 4 (BMP4) and increased expression of the activin-like kinase receptor 1 and 2 (Yao et al., 2008). This resulted in increased expression of vascular endothelial growth factor (VEGF) and matrix gla protein (MGP). VEGF promotes endothelial cell survival and MGP prevents vascular calcification and thus contribute to the maintenance, the integrity and the preservation of the functions of the endothelium (Yao et al., 2008).

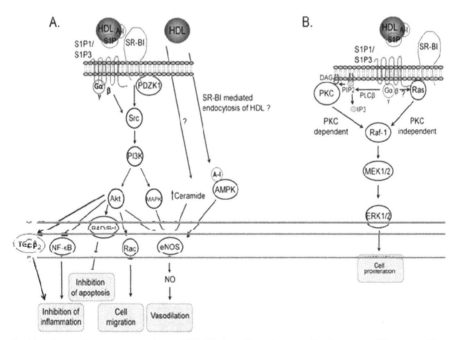

Fig. 3. A) Schematic representation of SR-BI signaling that can lead to vasodilation, cell migration and inhibition of inflammation and apoptosis. B) Schematic representation of PKC-dependent SR-BI-dependent signalling pathway that promote cell proliferation (Drew et al., 2004; Grewal et al., 2003; Kimura et al., 2003; Mineo et al., 2003).

5.2 Effect of HDL and apoA-I on inflammation

An initial step in the pathogenesis of atherosclerosis is the association of the monocytes to adhesion molecules of the endothelial cells that facilitates their entry in the sub-endothelial space (Zannis et al., 2004b). Induction of adhesion molecules is promoted by pro-inflammatory stimuli (Cybulsky and Gimbrone, Jr., 1991). Recruitment and migration of monocytes into sub-endothelial space is promoted by the monocyte chemoattractant factor (MCP-1) as well as by oxidized LDL (Peters and Charo, 2001). HDL has anti-oxidant properties and can prevent the oxidation of LDL (Navab et al., 2000a; Navab et al., 2000b). Interactions of HDL or apoA-I with cells of the vascular wall were shown to prevent the expression of pro-inflammatory cytokines and chemokines that induce the expression of adhesion molecules (Bursill et al., 2010; Cockerill et al., 1995; Nobecourt et al., 2010). The anti-inflammatory functions of HDL were manifested in several ways. HDL binds via its apoA-I moiety to progranulin produced by macrophages. This prevents conversion of progranulin to inflammatory granulins which were shown to induce expression of tumor necrosis factor α (TNFα) and interleukin (IL) 1β in monocyte macrophages (Okura et al., 2010). HDL and rHDL were shown to inhibit the cytokine induced expression of vascular cell adhesion molecule-1 (VCAM-1) and inter-cellular adhesion molecule-1 (ICAM-1) by endothelial cells (Cockerill et al., 1995). In addition, HDL promoted the expression of anti-inflammatory cytokines in endothelial cells. Thus treatment of endothelial cells (HUVEC) with HDL and lysosphingolipids present in HDL, increased the expression of TGF-β2 through mechanisms that involve the activation of Akt and extracellular signal regulated kinases (ERK) 1/2. Consistent with cell culture studies, the expression of transforming growth factor-β2 (TGF-β2) and the phosphorylation of ERK1/2, Akt and Smad2/3 were increased in apoA-I transgenic mice and diminished in apoA-I deficient mice (Norata et al., 2005). In vivo studies also showed that infusion of rHDL inhibited the pro-oxidant and pro-inflammatory events that occurred following implantation of non occlusive periarteral collars in rabbits that induce acute arterial inflammation. In these studies the rHDL inhibited neutrofil infiltration, production of reactive oxygen species (ROS) and the expression of VCAM-1, ICAM-1, MCP-1 and E-selectin (Nicholls et al., 2005b). The carotid vascular inflammation and neutrofil infiltration could be inhibited by rHDL containing normal apoA-I but not by apoA-I obtained from diabetic patients (Nobecourt et al., 2010). The beneficial effects of rHDL containing apoA-I in vivo and in cell cultures could be duplicated using synthetic apoA-I mimetics such as 5A, L37pA and D37pA (Gomaraschi et al., 2008; Tabet et al., 2010). The 5A/PLPC complexes reduced the vascular inflammation that is associated with collar insertion in a rabbit model by reducing the ICAM-1 and VCAM-1 expression, the infiltration of neutrofils and the Nox4 activity. In cultures of human carotid endothelial cells (HCEC) 5A/PLPC and rHDL containing apoA-I inhibited the TNF-α induced VCAM-1 and ICAM-1 expression as well as the activation of nuclear factor κB (NF-κB) pathway and these effects were abolished by ABCA1 silencing (Tabet et al., 2010). Complexes of L37pA or D37pA with β-oleoyl-γ-palmitoyl-L-α-phosphatidylcholine reduced the postischemic cardiac contractile dysfunction in a rat heart model of ischemia/reperfusion. They also reduced TNF-α levels and increased prostacyclin levels in the perfusate and inhibited the TNF-α mediated VCAM-1 expression in endothelial cell cultures (Gomaraschi et al., 2008). In monocyte and endothelial cell cultures HDL also suppressed expression of chemokines CCL2, CCL5 and CX3CL1 and chemokine receptors CCR2, CCR5 and CX3CR1 (Bursill et al., 2010). This effect was mediated by inhibition of Iκ-

Bα phosphorylation and NF-κB(p65) expression and in some cases by peroxisome proliferator-activated receptor γ (PPARγ) activation. Consistent with cell culture studies, in vivo infusion of apoA-I in cholesterol fed apoE deficient mice reduced expression of chemokines and chemokine receptors (Bursill et al., 2010). HDL and its protein moiety apoA-I have been shown to inhibit the expression of CD11b of human monocytes that is induced by phorbol myristate acetate (PMA) and promote cell adhesion. Inhibition of the ABCA1-mediated and to a lesser extent SR-BI mediated cholesterol efflux by monoclonal antibodies attenuated the inhibitory effect of apoA-I and HDL respectively. Expression of CD11b was also affected by depletion of the membrane cholesterol by treatment of the cells with cyclodextrin (Murphy et al., 2008), pointing out to a potential role of cholesterol efflux in the inhibition of inflammation. Consistent with the ex vivo studies infusion of rHDL in patients with type 2 diabetes mellitus, reduced the expression of CD11b of the peripheral monocytes and reduced the adhesion of the patients' neutrophils to a fibrinogen matrix. Plasma HDL isolated 4 to 72 hours post rHDL infusion suppressed the expression of VCAM-1 in cultures of HAECs and had increased ability to promote cholesterol efflux from THP-1 macrophages (Patel et al., 2009). In cultures of smooth muscle cells, HDL downregulated the NADPH-oxidase mediated generation of reactive oxygen species (ROS) and inhibited production of MCP-1. The inhibitory effect was attenuated by antagonists of $S1P_1$ and $S1P_3$ receptors. The data showed that free S1P or S3P alone or as components of HDL could attenuate production of MCP-1. Consistent with these findings, MCP-1 production and ROS generation in the aortas of $S1P_3^{-/-}$ receptor and $SR-BI^{-/-}$ mice were not affected by treatment with HDL, S1P and sphingosylphosphorylcholine (SPC) (Tolle et al., 2008). ApoA-I induced the expression of the adhesion molecule CD31, and changed the morphology and size distribution of lineage negative bone marrow cells. The treatment also increased the ability of the cells to bind to fibronectin and to cultured endothelial cells. Deletion of the C-terminal helix 10 of apoA-I abolished the effects of apoA-I on bone marrow cells (Mythreye et al., 2008).

5.3 Effect of HDL and apoA-I on endothelial cell apoptosis

Exposure of endothelial cells to inflammatory stimuli may disturb the endothelial monolayer integrity (Dimmeler et al., 2002). Numerous factors that promote endothelial apoptosis have been described and include OxLDL (Li et al., 1998), TNF-a (Dimmeler et al., 1999), homocysteine (Welch and Loscalzo, 1998), and angiotensin II (Strawn and Ferrario, 2002). HDL also can reverse the TNF-a induced and growth deprivation induced endothelial cell apoptosis (Nofer et al., 2001; Sugano et al., 2000). OxLDL increased intracellular calcium and resulted in apoptosis that could be inhibited by HDL and apoA-I (Suc et al., 1997). ApoA-I interacts with ABCA1 and F1-ATPase (Chroni et al., 2003; Vantourout et al., 2010), whereas HDL interacts with SR-BI and ABCG1 (Liadaki et al., 2000; Wang et al., 2004) respectively and the sphingolipid components of HDL interact with the S1P receptors (Kimura et al., 2003; Okajima et al., 2009). HDL protected endothelial cells from apoptosis induced by oxLDL by preventing the generation of intracellular ROS. The anti-apoptotic activity was highest for HDL_3 and diminished as the size of HDL increased. It was suggested that approximately 70% of the anti-apoptotic activity of HDL was attributed to apoA-I which has the capacity to accept through its methionine residues the phospholipid hydroperoxides (PLOOH) of oxLDL (de Souza et al., 2010). The anti-apoptotic functions of small size HDL_3 was reduced by 35% in subjects with metabolic syndrome and this reduction was correlated with the clinical phenotype of the human subjects. Compared to normal HDL the HDL$_3$ fractions of the diabetic subjects had increased total triglyceride levels and decreased cholesteryl esters/triglycerides ratio suggesting that the lipid core of HDL$_3$ was enriched with triglycerides (de Souza et al., 2008). HDL$_3$ also inhibited apoptotic cell death induced by oxLDL and preserved lysosomal integrity of an osteoblastic cell line (Brodeur et al., 2008). The anti-apoptotic effects were attributed to the increased expression of SR-BI that is mediated by HDL$_3$, combined with the ability of HDL to compete for the binding of oxLDL to osteoblasts as well as increased selective uptake of the cholesterol of the oxLDL by these cells (Brodeur et al., 2008).

Interactions of apoA-I with cell surface F1-ATPase inhibited apoptosis of HUVEC and stimulated cell proliferation (Radojkovic et al., 2009). In the absence of apoA-I, specific inhibitors for F1-ATPase (IF$_1$-H49K) and angiostatin or specific antibodies to F1-ATPase promoted apoptosis and inhibited cell proliferation. In the presence of apoA-I, F1-ATPase inhibitors and antibodies diminished its anti-apoptotic and anti-proliferative effects. Down-regulation of the ABCA1 by siRNA did not affect the anti-apoptotic and proliferative functions of apoA-I whereas inhibition of SR-BI by a specific antibody diminished the anti-apoptotic and proliferative functions of HDL$_3$ (Radojkovic et al., 2009). The findings suggest that interactions of lipid free apoA-I with F1-ATPase and of HDL with SR-BI contribute to their anti-apoptotic and proliferative effects on endothelial cells. The antiapoptotic effects of HDL on endothelial cells could be mimicked by the lysosphingolipid components of HDL (Nofer et al., 2001). The SR-BI mediated signalling that leads to activation of eNOS, also promotes cell growth and migration and protects cells from apoptosis (Mineo et al., 2006; Noor et al., 2007). Activation of eNOS required its localization in the caveolae, where caveolin SR-BI and CD36 are also found (Uittenbogaard et al., 2000). It has been proposed that oxLDL acting through CD36 depletes the cholesterol content of caveolae and leads to eNOS redistribution to intracellular sites thus resulting in decreased eNOS activity (Blair et al., 1999; Uittenbogaard et al., 2000). HDL acting through SR-BI maintains the concentration of caveolae-associated cholesterol, inhibits the actions of oxLDL and maintains eNOS in the caveolae (Uittenbogaard et al., 2000). This interpretation implies that strong interactions between eNOS and caveolin-1 (Cav-1) stimulate eNOS activity. Other studies provided the opposite mechanism of modulation of eNOS activity by interactions of eNOS with Cav-1 (Terasaka et al., 2010). It was shown that these interactions were enhanced by loading cells with cholesterol or oxysterols and decreased by cholesterol depletion in endothelial cells as a result of ABCG1-mediated cholesterol efflux. Studies in murine lung endothelial cells (MLEC) also showed that HDL could reverse the inhibition of eNOS activity caused by cholesterol loading in the normal but not the Cav-1 deficient cells (Terasaka et al., 2010). It was proposed that diminished interactions between eNOS and Cav-1 caused by ABCG1-mediated efflux stimulated eNOS activity. It has been shown that oxidized phospholipids uncouple eNOS activity and lead to the generation of oxygen radicals which induces the expression of sterol regulatory element binding protein (SREBP) and IL-8 (Gharavi et al., 2006; Yeh et al., 2004). ApoA-I mimetic peptides also prevent LDL from uncoupling eNOS activity to favour O$_2^-$ anion production as opposed to normal production of NO (Ou et al., 2003). Finally it has been shown that SR-BI via a highly conserved redox motif CXXS between residues 323-326 can promote a ligand independent apoptosis via a caspase 8 pathway and this effect could be reversed by HDL and eNOS (Li et al., 2005). It was proposed that at low HDL levels oxitative stress causes relocation of eNOS away from the caveolae and this results in SR-BI induced apoptosis (Li et al., 2005). The picture that emerges from these studies is that HDL promotes survival and migration of endothelial cells by signalling mechanisms that originate from the interactions of HDL with SR-BI, the interactions of S1P with S1P1 and S1P3 receptors and the interactions of lipid-free apoA-I with F1-ATPase.

5.4 Effect of HDL on endothelial cell proliferation and migration

Damage of the endothelium is associated with vascular disease which can be blunted by re-endothelialization (Werner et al., 2003). HDL promoted proliferation of HUVEC via mechanisms that increased intracellular Ca^{2+} and upregulated the production of prostacyclin (Tamagaki et al., 1996). HDL also promoted endothelial cell migration (Murugesan et al., 1994). Migration was promoted by signalling cascades mediated by interaction of S1P with S1P1 and S1P3 receptors that led to the activation of PI3 kinase, p38MAP kinase and Rho kinases (Kimura et al., 2003). Other studies showed that HDL can activate the MAPK pathway either through processes that involve protein kinase C (PKC), Raf-1, MEK and ERK1/2 or PKC independent pathways. This latter pathway leads to the activation of Ras and can be inhibited by pertussis toxin and neutralizing antibodies against SR-BI (Grewal et al., 2003). The data suggest that interactions of HDL with SR-BI activate Ras in a PKC independent manner and this leads to subsequent activation of MAPK signalling cascade (Grewal et al., 2003) (Fig.3B). Another beneficial effect of HDL is its capacity to promote capillary tube formation in vitro. This function is pertussis toxin sensitive and requires p44/42MAP kinase which is downstream of Ras (Miura et al., 2003). Other studies showed that interaction of SR-BI with HDL or rHDL, activated Src kinases and Rac GTPases and stimulated endothelial cell migration. In vivo experiments have also shown that re-endothelialization of carotid artery following injury is promoted by apoA-I expression and is inhibited in apoA-I deficient in mice (Seetharam et al., 2006).

5.5 Effect of HDL on thrombosis

Increased HDL cholesterol levels are associated with decreased risk of venous thrombosis (Doggen et al., 2004). In contrast low HDL levels are associated with increased risk of venous thrombosis (Deguchi et al., 2005). The ability of HDL to inhibit endothelial cell apoptosis (Dimmeler et al., 2002; Mineo et al., 2006) prevents vessel denudation and formation of microparticles that may contribute to thrombosis (Durand et al., 2004). It has been shown that thrombogenic membrane microparticles that may originate from apoptotic endothelial cells are increased in the plasma of patients with acute coronary syndrome (ACS) (Mallat et al., 2000). Infusion of rHDL in volunteers that received low levels of endotoxin limited the prothrombotic and procoagulant effect of endotoxin (Pajkrt et al., 1997). Furthermore infusion of apoA-I$_{MILANO}$ in a rat model of acute arterial thrombosis increased the time of thrombus formation and decreased the weight of the thrombus (Li et al., 1999). HDL may affect thrombosis via a variety of mechanisms: Early studies showed that HDL causes increased synthesis of prostacyclin in cultured endothelial cells (Fleisher et al., 1983; Tamagaki et al., 1996). Prostacyclin in combination with NO promote smooth muscle cells relaxation, inhibit platelet activation and local smooth muscle cell proliferation (Vane and Botting, 1995). It has been reported that HDL$_3$ induced expression of cyclooxygenase-2 (Cox-2) by smooth muscle cells and promoted release of prostacyclin (PGI2) via a signalling pathway that involves p38MAP kinase and c-Jun N terminal kinase

(JNK-1) (Escudero et al., 2003; Vinals et al., 1997). PGI2 synthesis was enhanced by HMGCoA reductase inhibitors (Martinez-Gonzalez et al., 2004). It has been shown that there is a positive correlation between plasma HDL levels and anticoagulant response to activated protein C (APC)/protein S in vitro (Griffin et al., 1999) and negative correlation with the plasma thrombin activation markers such as prothrombin fragments F1.2 and D-dimer (MacCallum et al., 2000). APC inactivates, by proteolysis, factors Va and VIIIa in plasma and thus it can downregulate thrombin formation. Administration of HDL to cholesterol-fed rabbits also increased endothelial cell thrombomodulin levels, promoted generation of APC and inhibited formation of thrombin (Nicholls et al., 2005a). Glucosylceramide and glycosphingolipids which are present in HDL are lipid cofactors for the anticoagulant activity of APC and in a significant number of patients with venous thrombosis the levels of glucosylceramides are low (Deguchi et al., 2002; Deguchi et al., 2001). Shpingosine, another molecule present in HDL, has been shown to inhibit prothrombin activation on platelets' surface by disrupting procoagulant interactions between factors Xa and Va (Deguchi et al., 2004). HDL also downregulated expression of plasminogen activator inhibitor-1 (PAI-1) and upregulated tissue plasminogen activator (t-PA) in endothelial cell cultures (Eren et al., 2002). Transgenic mice expressing the human PAI-1 developed age-dependent coronary arterial thrombosis (Eren et al., 2002). In contrast oxidized HDL_3 induced the expression of PAI-1 in endothelial cells through signalling mechanisms that involve activation of ERK1/2 and p38MAPK and mRNA stabilization (Norata et al., 2004).

5.6 Effects of HDL on diabetes mellitus
In vivo and in vitro studies have provided evidence that HDL may have beneficial effects on glucose metabolism (Koseki et al., 2009; Rutti et al., 2009). Ex vivo studies showed that HDL and delipidated apoA-I or S1P decreased IL-1β and glucose-mediated apoptosis and thus increased the survival of human and murine islets. HDL treatment down-regulated the expression of iNOS and its downstream target Fas which is pro-apoptotic and up-regulated the expression of FLICE-like inhibitory protein (FLIP) which is anti-apoptotic (Rutti et al., 2009). HDL also reversed the toxic effects of oxidized LDL on beta cells that are associated with apoptosis and cJNK mediated transcriptional repression of the insulin gene caused cJNK mediated (Abderrahmani et al., 2007).

Oral glucose tolerance test in a limited number of patients with Tangier disease (that lack or have dysfunctional ABCA1) showed that they had glucose intolerance as compared to controls (Koseki et al., 2009), thus implicating ABCA1, apoA-I and HDL in glucose metabolism. Cell culture studies using primary pancreatic islets cells and a pancreatic β-cell line (Min6), showed that lipid free apoA-I or apoA-II or reconstituted HDL increased insulin secretion up to 5-fold in a Ca^{2+} dependant manner (Fryirs et al., 2010). The free apolipoproteins also increased insulin mRNA levels. HDL mediated insulin secretion has also been observed in cultures of mouse pancreatic β-cells (MIN6N8) (Drew et al., 2009). The increase in insulin secretion mediated by lipid-free apoproteins and rHDL required the functions of ABCA1 and SRBI or ABCG1 respectively. These functions may be different from those involved in cholesterol efflux. For high glucose concentrations enhanced insulin secretion required the action of K_{ATP} channel and glucose catabolism in the pancreatic cell, but this did not occur for low glucose concentrations (Fryirs et al., 2010).

Further insight on the role of ABCA1 in diabetes was obtained by studies in mice with selective deficiency of ABCA1 in the pancreas (ABCA1$^{-P/-P}$). These mice accumulated cholesterol in their islets and were characterized by impaired acute phase insulin secretion and glucose intolerance. The ABCA1$^{-P/-P}$ mice exhibited normal insulin sensitivity indicating normal response of the peripheral tissues to insulin. The impairment in insulin secretion was verified in cell culture experiments using islets isolated from the ABCA1$^{-P/-P}$ mice. In contrast, whole ABCA1 deficient mice had normal glucose tolerance and displayed only small impairment in the islet function and did not accumulate significant amount of cholesterol in the islets (Brunham et al., 2007). Pancreatic islets isolated from apoE deficient mice had increased cholesterol content and reduced insulin secretion as compared to islets obtained from WT mice. The reduced insulin secretion in the pancreatic islets or cultures of β-cells could be restored by depletion of the cellular cholesterol using mevastatin or methyl-β-cyclodextrin (MβCD) (Hao et al., 2007). Experiments in cell lines of pancreatic β-cell origin indicated that cholesterol loading or cholesterol depletion affect the activity of glucokinase (GK) which is known to regulate insulin secretion (Rizzo and Piston, 2003). The experiments showed that under normal cholesterol levels GK is associated with a dimeric form of nNOS on insulin containing granules in the cytoplasm and is inactive (Rizzo and Piston, 2003). Increase in plasma cholesterol enhanced dimerization of nNOS and its association with GK whereas reduction in the cholesterol levels or increase in the extracellular glucose levels promoted monomerization of nNOS and release of active GK in the cytoplasm (Hao et al., 2007). The role of the increase in the cholesterol content of β-cells in insulin secretion was tested in transgenic mice expressing SREBP-2 in β-cells under the control of insulin promoter. These mice had normal plasma cholesterol levels but developed severe diabetes characterized by 5-fold increase in gluco-hemoglobin and defects in glucose and potassium-stimulated insulin secretion and were characterized by glucose intolerance. The islets were fewer, smaller and deformed and had increased levels of total and esterified cholesterol (Ishikawa et al., 2008). It was proposed that the loss of β-cell mass could be related to the down regulation of genes such as PDX-1 and BETA2 that are involved in β-cell differentiation.

A recent comprehensive study has measured the properties of HDL isolated from patients with type 2 diabetes mellitus and their functions on endothelial cells in vitro and in vivo. HDL isolated from patients with low HDL and type 2 diabetes mellitus contained increased levels of lipid peroxides and increased myeloperoxidase activity. In endothelial cell cultures diabetic HDL had reduced production of NO and increased NADPH oxidase activity that resulted in increased oxidant stress. Diabetic HDL had diminished endothelium dependent relaxation of aortic rings and endothelial progenitor cells obtained from diabetic subjects had diminished capacity to promote reendothelialization in vivo. A remarkable finding in this study was that extended release niacin treatment of the diabetic patients restored the properties and functions of HDL. The HDL obtained after treatment had normal levels of peroxides and normal myeloperoxidase (MPO) activity. Studies with endothelial cultures showed that following treatment of the diabetic patients their HDL could induce normal NO production and NADPH oxidase activity and could promote normal relaxation of aortic rings. Endothelial progenitor cells obtained from diabetic patients following niacin treatment had normal ability to promote reendothelialization in vivo (Sorrentino et al., 2010). In another study intravenous infusion of rHDL (80 mg/kg over 4 hours) in type 2 diabetic human subjects decreased plasma glucose level, increased plasma insulin level and increased β-cell functions as compared to patients receiving placebo (Drew et al., 2009). HDL and apoA-I increased glucose uptake of primary human skeletal muscle cultures established from patients with type 2 diabetes mellitus. HDL induced glucose uptake and fatty acid oxidation and increased AMPKα2 activity and phosphorylation. These effects were modulated through a Ca^{2+} dependent pathway. Subsequent in vitro and in vivo studies showed that rHDL inhibited lipolysis in 3T3-L1 adipocytes partially via activation of AMPK pathway (Drew et al., 2011). Infusion of rHDL also inhibited fasting induced lipolysis and fatty acid oxidation but increased the circulating non essential fatty acids possibly due to the action of phospholipase on the rHDL phospholipids (Drew et al., 2011). The HDL dependent glucose uptake by the skeletal muscle cells was abrogated by inhibition of ABCA1 with a blocking antibody suggesting that ABCA1 functions not related to cholesterol efflux, may contribute to the increased glucose uptake and β-oxidation by skeletal muscle cells obtained from patients with type 2 diabetic mellitus (Drew et al., 2011). The effect of apoA-I on glucose metabolism was also studied in C2C12 myocytes and apoA-I deficient mice. Consistent with the studies with primary human skeletal muscle cultures, apoA-I stimulated AMPK and acetyl-CoA carboxylase (ACC) phosphorylation and glucose uptake and endocytosis into C2C12 cells. The apoA-I deficient mice had increased fat content decreased glucose tolerance and increased expression of gluconeogenic enzymes in the liver and decreased AMPK-dependent phosphorylation in skeletal muscle and the liver (Han et al., 2007).

5.7 Role of apoA-I and HDL in atheroprotection

Atherosclerosis is associated with lipid and lipoprotein abnormalities (Zannis et al., 2004b). Low HDL levels (Gordon et al., 1989) and decreased concentration of the largest size HDL subpopulations (Asztalos et al., 2004) are associated with increased risk of CAD. The anti-atherogenic functions of HDL and apoA-I have been, to a large extent, attributed to the beneficial effects that HDL exerts on cells of the arterial wall as well as their ability to promote efflux from macrophages and other cells of the arterial wall via ABCA1, ABCG1 and SR-BI (Wang et al., 2007). Hepatic overexpression of apoA-I gene in the background of apoE or LDL_r deficient mice reduced the atherosclerosis burden of these mice following an atherogenic diet (Tangirala et al., 1999). These findings demonstrate the importance of apoA-I and HDL for atheroprotection. In contrast, double deficient mice for apoA-I and the LDL_r fed an atherogenic diet developed atherosclerosis and had increased concentration of circulating auto-anibodies, increased population of T, B, dendritic cells and macrophages, as well as increased T cell proliferation and activation. The abnormal phenotype was corrected by adenovirus mediated gene expression of apoA-I (Wilhelm et al., 2010). Similarly apoA-I transgenic rabbits were resistant to diet induced atherosclerosis (Duverger et al., 1996). Two clinical trials showed that intravenous administration of 15 mg/kg of apoA-I_{MILANO}/phospholipid complexes in five weekly doses in patients with acute coronary syndrome resulted in significant regression of atherosclerosis as it was shown by intravascular ultrasound (Nicholls et al., 2006; Nissen et al., 2003). The epidemiological studies (Gordon et al., 1989), combined with studies of experimental animals (Duverger et al., 1996; Tangirala et al., 1999) and clinical intervention studies (Barter et al., 2007; Sorrentino et al., 2010) highlight the importance of increased HDL levels for atheroprotection. However, human subjects have been identified with high HDL levels and CAD (Ansell et al., 2003). In addition, increased HDL levels in humans treated with the CETP inhibitor torcetrapib, increased cardiovascular, and non-cardiovascular deaths (Barter et al., 2007). These findings suggest that high HDL levels are not always synonymous with atheroprotection. The concept that emerges from all the studies is that the most important factor for atheroprotection is the functionality of HDL. Understanding of the structure-function and the cell signaling associated with HDL and apoA-I will provide molecular explanations for their beneficial effects for atherosclerosis and other human diseases and apoA-I.

6. Conclusion

Numerous prospective epidemiological studies have established an inverse correlation between HDL cholesterol levels and the risk for CAD. However, the discovery of human subjects with high HDL cholesterol levels and CAD, combined with clinical intervention studies designed to raise HDL levels and studies of animal models, led to the realization that high levels of HDL cholesterol alone are not sufficient to prevent atherosclerosis. HDL via its protein and/or lipid components participates in numerous interactions with the endothelium, other cells of the vascular wall, as well as with β pancreatic cells, and has a protective effect against atherothrombosis and other diseases. The key proteins that participate in the biogenesis, remodeling and signaling of HDL are of great importance for the functionality of HDL. Mutations in apoA-I, ABCA1 and LCAT affect the biogenesis of HDL and either prevent formation of HDL or generate aberrant HDL subpopulations which may have altered functions. The ability of HDL to inhibit the oxidation of LDL, prevents the induction of pro-inflammatory and pro-apoptotic pathways that are detrimental to the endothelium. HDL interacts directly with the endothelial cells via SR-BI and the ABCG1. These interactions lead to NO release and vasodilatation, promote reendothelialization and suppress expression of adhesion molecules on endothelial cells in response to pro-inflammatory cytokines. As a result of these and other interactions of the sphingolipid components of HDL with S1P receptors, HDL protects from apoptosis and inflammation and promotes endothelial cell growth and migration. Understanding the complexity and the functions of HDL may facilitate in the near future the development of new HDL-based therapies to prevent or treat atherosclerosis and other human diseases.

7. Acknowledgments

This work was supported by National Institutes of Health Grants HL-48739 and HL-68216. A.K. Kateifides and P. Fotakis are students of the graduate program "The Molecular Basis of Human Disease" of the University of Crete, Medical School and were supported by the Greek Ministry of Education, General Secretariat for Research and Technology Grants PENED 03-780 and HRAKLEITOS II.

8. References

Abderrahmani, A., G. Niederhauser, D. Favre et al., 2007, Human high-density lipoprotein particles prevent activation of the JNK pathway induced by human oxidised low-density lipoprotein particles in pancreatic beta cells: Diabetologia, v. 50, no. 6, p. 1304-1314.

Acton, S., A. Rigotti, K. T. Landschulz et al., 1996, Identification of scavenger receptor SR-BI as a high density lipoprotein receptor: Science, v. 271, no. 5248, p. 518-520.

Amar, M. J., R. D. Shamburek, B. Vaisman et al., 2009, Adenoviral expression of human lecithin-cholesterol acyltransferase in nonhuman primates leads to an antiatherogenic lipoprotein phenotype by increasing high-density lipoprotein and lowering low-density lipoprotein: Metabolism, v. 58, no. 4, p. 568-575.

Ansell, B. J., M. Navab, S. Hama et al., 2003, Inflammatory/antiinflammatory properties of high-density lipoprotein distinguish patients from control subjects better than high-density lipoprotein cholesterol levels and are favorably affected by simvastatin treatment: Circulation, v. 108, no. 22, p. 2751-2756.

Arai, T., N. Wang, M. Bezouevski et al., 1999, Decreased atherosclerosis in heterozygous low
    density lipoprotein receptor-deficient mice expressing the scavenger receptor BI
    transgene: J.Biol.Chem., v. 274, no. 4, p. 2366-2371.
Assanasen, C., C. Mineo, D. Seetharam et al., 2005, Cholesterol binding, efflux, and a PDZ-
    interacting domain of scavenger receptor-BI mediate HDL-initiated signaling:
    J.Clin.Invest, v. 115, no. 4, p. 969-977.
Asztalos, B. F., L. A. Cupples, S. Demissie et al., 2004, High-density lipoprotein
    subpopulation profile and coronary heart disease prevalence in male participants
    of the Framingham Offspring Study: Arterioscler.Thromb.Vasc.Biol., v. 24, no. 11,
    p. 2181-2187.
Barter, P. J., H. B. Brewer, Jr., M. J. Chapman et al., 2003, Cholesteryl ester transfer protein: a
    novel   target   for   raising   HDL   and   inhibiting   atherosclerosis:
    Arterioscler.Thromb.Vasc.Biol., v. 23, no. 2, p. 160-167.
Barter, P. J., M. Caulfield, M. Eriksson et al., 2007, Effects of torcetrapib in patients at high
    risk for coronary events: N.Engl.J.Med., v. 357, no. 21, p. 2109-2122.
Blair, A., P. W. Shaul, I. S. Yuhanna et al., 1999, Oxidized low density lipoprotein displaces
    endothelial nitric-oxide synthase (eNOS) from plasmalemmal caveolae and impairs
    eNOS activation: J.Biol.Chem., v. 274, no. 45, p. 32512-32519.
Borhani, D. W., D. P. Rogers, J. A. Engler et al., 1997, Crystal structure of truncated human
    apolipoprotein A-I suggests a lipid-bound conformation: Proc.Natl.Acad.Sci.U.S.A,
    v. 94, no. 23, p. 12291-12296.
Braun, A., B. L. Trigatti, M. J. Post et al., 2002, Loss of SR-BI expression leads to the early
    onset of occlusive atherosclerotic coronary artery disease, spontaneous myocardial
    infarctions, severe cardiac dysfunction, and premature death in apolipoprotein E-
    deficient mice: Circ.Res., v. 90, no. 3, p. 270-276.
Breckenridge, W. C., J. A. Little, P. Alaupovic et al., 1982, Lipoprotein abnormalities
    associated with a familial deficiency of hepatic lipase: Atherosclerosis, v. 45, no. 2,
    p. 161-179.
Brodeur, M. R., L. Brissette, L. Falstrault et al., 2008, HDL3 reduces the association and
    modulates the metabolism of oxidized LDL by osteoblastic cells: a protection
    against cell death: J.Cell Biochem., v. 105, no. 6, p. 1374-1385.
Brunham, L. R., J. K. Kruit, T. D. Pape et al., 2007, Beta-cell ABCA1 influences insulin
    secretion, glucose homeostasis and response to thiazolidinedione treatment:
    Nat.Med., v. 13, no. 3, p. 340-347.
Brunham, L. R., R. R. Singaraja, and M. R. Hayden, 2006, Variations on a gene: rare and
    common variants in ABCA1 and their impact on HDL cholesterol levels and
    atherosclerosis: Annu.Rev.Nutr., v. 26, p. 105-129.
Brunzell, J. D., and S. S. Deeb, 2001, Familial lipoprotein lipase deficiency, apoC-II
    deficiency, and hepatic lipase deficiency, in CR Scriver, AL Beaudet, D Valle, and
    WS Sly eds., The Metabolic & Molecular Bases of Inherited Disease: New York,
    McGraw-Hill, p. 2789-2816.
Bursill, C. A., M. L. Castro, D. T. Beattie et al., 2010, High-density lipoproteins suppress
    chemokines   and   chemokine   receptors   in   vitro   and   in   vivo:
    Arterioscler.Thromb.Vasc.Biol., v. 30, no. 9, p. 1773-1778.
Christiansen-Weber, T. A., J. R. Voland, Y. Wu et al., 2000, Functional loss of ABCA1 in mice
    causes severe placental malformation, aberrant lipid distribution, and kidney
    glomerulonephritis as well as high-density lipoprotein cholesterol deficiency:
    Am.J.Pathol., v. 157, no. 3, p. 1017-1029.

Chroni, A., A. Duka, H. Y. Kan et al., 2005a, Point mutations in apolipoprotein a-I mimic the phenotype observed in patients with classical lecithin:cholesterol acyltransferase deficiency: Biochemistry, v. 44, no. 43, p. 14353-14366.

Chroni, A., H. Y. Kan, K. E. Kypreos et al., 2004, Substitutions of glutamate 110 and 111 in the middle helix 4 of human apolipoprotein A-I (apoA-I) by alanine affect the structure and in vitro functions of apoA-I and induce severe hypertriglyceridemia in apoA-I-deficient mice: Biochemistry, v. 43, no. 32, p. 10442-10457.

Chroni, A., H. Y. Kan, A. Shkodrani et al., 2005b, Deletions of helices 2 and 3 of human apoA-I are associated with severe dyslipidemia following adenovirus-mediated gene transfer in apoA-I-deficient mice: Biochemistry, v. 44, no. 10, p. 4108-4117.

Chroni, A., G. Koukos, A. Duka et al., 2007, The carboxy-terminal region of apoA-I is required for the ABCA1-dependent formation of alpha-HDL but not prebeta-HDL particles in vivo: Biochemistry, v. 46, no. 19, p. 5697-5708.

Chroni, A., T. Liu, I. Gorshkova et al., 2003, The central helices of apoA-I can promote ATP-binding cassette transporter A1 (ABCA1)-mediated lipid efflux. Amino acid residues 220-231 of the wild-type apoA-I are required for lipid efflux in vitro and high density lipoprotein formation in vivo: J.Biol.Chem., v. 278, no. 9, p. 6719-6730.

Cockerill, G. W., K. A. Rye, J. R. Gamble et al., 1995, High-density lipoproteins inhibit cytokine-induced expression of endothelial cell adhesion molecules: Arterioscler.Thromb.Vasc.Biol., v. 15, no. 11, p. 1987-1994.

Cybulsky, M. I., and M. A. Gimbrone, Jr., 1991, Endothelial expression of a mononuclear leukocyte adhesion molecule during atherogenesis: Science, v. 251, no. 4995, p. 788-791.

de Souza, J. A., C. Vindis, B. Hansel et al., 2008, Metabolic syndrome features small, apolipoprotein A-I-poor, triglyceride-rich HDL3 particles with defective anti-apoptotic activity: Atherosclerosis, v. 197, no. 1, p. 84-94.

de Souza, J. A., C. Vindis, A. Negre-Salvayre et al., 2010, Small, dense HDL 3 particles attenuate apoptosis in endothelial cells: pivotal role of apolipoprotein A-I: J.Cell Mol.Med., v. 14, no. 3, p. 608-620.

Deguchi, H., J. A. Fernandez, and J. H. Griffin, 2002, Neutral glycosphingolipid-dependent inactivation of coagulation factor Va by activated protein C and protein S: Journal of Biological Chemistry, v. 277, no. 11, p. 8861-8865.

Deguchi, H., J. A. Fernandez, I. Pabinger et al., 2001, Plasma glucosylceramide deficiency as potential risk factor for venous thrombosis and modulator of anticoagulant protein C pathway: Blood, v. 97, no. 7, p. 1907-1914.

Deguchi, H., N. M. Pecheniuk, D. J. Elias et al., 2005, High-density lipoprotein deficiency and dyslipoproteinemia associated with venous thrombosis in men: Circulation, v. 112, no. 6, p. 893-899.

Deguchi, H., S. Yegneswaran, and J. H. Griffin, 2004, Sphingolipids as bioactive regulators of thrombin generation: Journal of Biological Chemistry, v. 279, no. 13, p. 12036-12042.

Dimmeler, S., K. Breitschopf, J. Haendeler et al., 1999, Dephosphorylation targets Bcl-2 for ubiquitin-dependent degradation: a link between the apoptosome and the proteasome pathway: J.Exp.Med., v. 189, no. 11, p. 1815-1822.

Dimmeler, S., J. Haendeler, and A. M. Zeiher, 2002, Regulation of endothelial cell apoptosis in atherothrombosis: Curr.Opin.Lipidol., v. 13, no. 5, p. 531-536.

Doggen, C. J. M., N. L. Smith, R. N. Lemaitre et al., 2004, Serum lipid levels and the risk of venous thrombosis: Arteriosclerosis Thrombosis and Vascular Biology, v. 24, no. 10, p. 1970-1975.

Dole, V. S., J. Matuskova, E. Vasile et al., 2008, Thrombocytopenia and platelet abnormalities in high-density lipoprotein receptor-deficient mice: Arterioscler.Thromb.Vasc.Biol., v. 28, no. 6, p. 1111-1116.

Drew, B. G., A. L. Carey, A. K. Natoli et al., 2011, Reconstituted high-density lipoprotein infusion modulates fatty acid metabolism in patients with type 2 diabetes mellitus: Journal of Lipid Research, v. 52, no. 3, p. 572-581.

Drew, B. G., S. J. Duffy, M. F. Formosa et al., 2009, High-Density Lipoprotein Modulates Glucose Metabolism in Patients With Type 2 Diabetes Mellitus: Circulation, v. 119, no. 15, p. 2103-U134.

Drew, B. G., N. H. Fidge, G. Gallon-Beaumier et al., 2004, High-density lipoprotein and apolipoprotein AI increase endothelial NO synthase activity by protein association and multisite phosphorylation: Proc.Natl.Acad.Sci.U.S.A, v. 101, no. 18, p. 6999-7004.

Durand, E., A. Scoazec, A. Lafont et al., 2004, In vivo induction of endothelial apoptosis leads to vessel thrombosis and endothelial denudation - A clue to the understanding of the mechanisms of thrombotic plaque erosion: Circulation, v. 109, no. 21, p. 2503-2506.

Duverger, N., H. Kruth, F. Emmanuel et al., 1996, Inhibition of atherosclerosis development in cholesterol-fed human apolipoprotein A-I-transgenic rabbits: Circulation, v. 94, no. 4, p. 713-717.

Eren, M., C. A. Painter, J. B. Atkinson et al., 2002, Age-dependent spontaneous coronary arterial thrombosis in transgenic mice that express a stable form of human plasminogen activator inhibitor-1: Circulation, v. 106, no. 4, p. 491-496.

Escudero, I., J. Martinez-Gonzalez, R. Alonso et al., 2003, Experimental and interventional dietary study in humans on the role of HDL fatty acid composition in PGI(2) release and Cox-2 expression by VSMC: European Journal of Clinical Investigation, v. 33, no. 9, p. 779-786.

Fielding, C. J., V. G. Shore, and P. E. Fielding, 1972, A protein cofactor of lecithin:cholesterol acyltransferase: Biochem.Biophys.Res.Commun., v. 46, no. 4, p. 1493-1498.

Fleisher, L. N., A. R. Tall, L. D. Witte et al., 1983, Effects of high-density lipoprotein and the apoprotein of high-density lipoprotein on Prostacyclin synthesis by endothelial cells: Advances in Prostaglandin Thromboxane and Leukotriene Research, v. 11, p. 475-480.

Frikke-Schmidt, R., B. G. Nordestgaard, G. B. Jensen et al., 2008, Genetic variation in ABCA1 predicts ischemic heart disease in the general population: Arterioscler.Thromb.Vasc.Biol., v. 28, no. 1, p. 180-186.

Fryirs, M. A., P. J. Barter, M. Appavoo et al., 2010, Effects of High-Density Lipoproteins on Pancreatic beta-Cell Insulin Secretion: Arteriosclerosis Thrombosis and Vascular Biology, v. 30, no. 8, p. 1642-U296.

Gharavi, N. M., N. A. Baker, K. P. Mouillesseaux et al., 2006, Role of endothelial nitric oxide synthase in the regulation of SREBP activation by oxidized phospholipids: Circ.Res., v. 98, no. 6, p. 768-776.

Gomaraschi, M., L. Calabresi, G. Rossoni et al., 2008, Anti-inflammatory and cardioprotective activities of synthetic high-density lipoprotein containing apolipoprotein A-I mimetic peptides: J.Pharmacol.Exp.Ther., v. 324, no. 2, p. 776-783.

Gong, M., M. Wilson, T. Kelly et al., 2003, HDL-associated estradiol stimulates endothelial NO synthase and vasodilation in an SR-BI-dependent manner: J.Clin.Invest, v. 111, no. 10, p. 1579-1587.

Gordon, D. J., J. L. Probstfield, R. J. Garrison et al., 1989, High-density lipoprotein cholesterol and cardiovascular disease. Four prospective American studies: Circulation, v. 79, no. 1, p. 8-15.

Grewal, T., D. de, I, M. F. Kirchhoff et al., 2003, High density lipoprotein-induced signaling of the MAPK pathway involves scavenger receptor type BI-mediated activation of Ras: J.Biol.Chem., v. 278, no. 19, p. 16478-16481.

Griffin, J. H., K. Kojima, C. L. Banka et al., 1999, High-density lipoprotein enhancement of anticoagulant activities of plasma protein S and activated protein C: Journal of Clinical Investigation, v. 103, no. 2, p. 219-227.

Gu, X., K. Kozarsky, and M. Krieger, 2000, Scavenger receptor class B, type I-mediated [3H]cholesterol efflux to high and low density lipoproteins is dependent on lipoprotein binding to the receptor: J.Biol.Chem., v. 275, no. 39, p. 29993-30001.

Haase, C. L., R. Frikke-Schmidt, B. G. Nordestgaard et al., 2011, Mutation in APOA1 predicts increased risk of ischaemic heart disease and total mortality without low HDL cholesterol levels: J.Intern.Med..

Han, R., R. Lai, Q. Ding et al., 2007, Apolipoprotein A-I stimulates AMP-activated protein kinase and improves glucose metabolism: Diabetologia, v. 50, no. 9, p. 1960-1968.

Hao, M., W. S. Head, S. C. Gunawardana et al., 2007, Direct effect of cholesterol on insulin secretion - A novel mechanism for pancreatic beta-cell dysfunction: Diabetes, v. 56, no. 9, p. 2328-2338.

Holm, T. M., A. Braun, B. L. Trigatti et al., 2002, Failure of red blood cell maturation in mice with defects in the high-density lipoprotein receptor SR-BI: Blood, v. 99, no. 5, p. 1817-1824.

Huszar, D., M. L. Varban, F. Rinninger et al., 2000, Increased LDL cholesterol and atherosclerosis in LDL receptor-deficient mice with attenuated expression of scavenger receptor B1: Arterioscler.Thromb.Vasc.Biol., v. 20, no. 4, p. 1068-1073.

Ishida, T., S. Choi, R. K. Kundu et al., 2003, Endothelial lipase is a major determinant of HDL level: J.Clin.Invest, v. 111, no. 3, p. 347-355.

Ishikawa, M., Y. Iwasaki, S. Yatoh et al., 2008, Cholesterol accumulation and diabetes in pancreatic beta-cell-specific SREBP-2 transgenic mice: a new model for lipotoxicity: Journal of Lipid Research, v. 49, no. 12, p. 2524-2534.

Ji, Y., N. Wang, R. Ramakrishnan et al., 1999, Hepatic scavenger receptor BI promotes rapid clearance of high density lipoprotein free cholesterol and its transport into bile: J.Biol.Chem., v. 274, no. 47, p. 33398-33402.

Joyce, C. W., M. J. Amar, G. Lambert et al., 2002, The ATP binding cassette transporter A1 (ABCA1) modulates the development of aortic atherosclerosis in C57BL/6 and apoE-knockout mice: Proc.Natl.Acad.Sci.U.S.A, v. 99, no. 1, p. 407-412.

Kateifides, A. K., I. N. Gorshkova, A. Duka et al., 2011, Alteration of negatively charged residues in the 89 to 99 domain of apoA-I affects lipid homeostasis and maturation of HDL: J.Lipid Res., v. 52, no. 7, p. 1363-1372.

Kennedy, M. A., G. C. Barrera, K. Nakamura et al., 2005, ABCG1 has a critical role in mediating cholesterol efflux to HDL and preventing cellular lipid accumulation: Cell Metab, v. 1, no. 2, p. 121-131.

Kielar, D., W. Dietmaier, T. Langmann et al., 2001, Rapid quantification of human ABCA1 mRNA in various cell types and tissues by real-time reverse transcription-PCR: Clin.Chem., v. 47, no. 12, p. 2089-2097.

Kimura, T., K. Sato, E. Malchinkhuu et al., 2003, High-density lipoprotein stimulates endothelial cell migration and survival through sphingosine 1-phosphate and its receptors: Arterioscler.Thromb.Vasc.Biol., v. 23, no. 7, p. 1283-1288.

Kocher, O., A. Yesilaltay, C. Cirovic et al., 2003, Targeted disruption of the PDZK1 gene in mice causes tissue-specific depletion of the HDL Receptor SR-BI and altered lipoprotein metabolism: J.Biol.Chem., v. 278, p. 52820-52825.

Koseki, M., A. Matsuyama, K. Nakatani et al., 2009, Impaired Insulin Secretion in Four Tangier Disease Patients with ABCA1 Mutations: Journal of Atherosclerosis and Thrombosis, v. 16, no. 3, p. 292-296.

Koukos, G., A. Chroni, A. Duka et al., 2007, LCAT can rescue the abnormal phenotype produced by the natural ApoA-I mutations (Leu141Arg)Pisa and (Leu159Arg)FIN: Biochemistry, v. 46, no. 37, p. 10713-10721.

Krauss, R. M., R. I. Levy, and D. S. Fredrickson, 1974, Selective measurement of two lipase activities in postheparin plasma from normal subjects and patients with hyperlipoproteinemia: J.Clin.Invest, v. 54, no. 5, p. 1107-1124.

Krieger, M., 2001, Scavenger receptor class B type I is a multiligand HDL receptor that influences diverse physiologic systems: J.Clin.Invest, v. 108, no. 6, p. 793-797.

Li, D., B. Yang, and J. L. Mehta, 1998, Ox-LDL induces apoptosis in human coronary artery endothelial cells: role of PKC, PTK, bcl-2, and Fas: Am.J.Physiol, v. 275, no. 2 Pt 2, p. H568-H576.

Li, D. Y., S. Weng, B. C. Yang et al., 1999, Inhibition of arterial thrombus formation by apoA1 Milano: Arteriosclerosis Thrombosis and Vascular Biology, v. 19, no. 2, p. 378-383.

Li, X. A., L. Guo, J. L. Dressman et al., 2005, A novel ligand-independent apoptotic pathway induced by SR-BI and suppressed by eNOS and HDL: J.Biol.Chem., v. 280, p. 19087-19096.

Li, X. A., W. B. Titlow, B. A. Jackson et al., 2002, High density lipoprotein binding to scavenger receptor, Class B, type I activates endothelial nitric-oxide synthase in a ceramide-dependent manner: J.Biol.Chem., v. 277, no. 13, p. 11058-11063.

Li, X. P., S. P. Zhao, X. Y. Zhang et al., 2000, Protective effect of high density lipoprotein on endothelium-dependent vasodilatation: Int.J.Cardiol., v. 73, no. 3, p. 231-236.

Liadaki, K. N., T. Liu, S. Xu et al., 2000, Binding of high density lipoprotein (HDL) and discoidal reconstituted HDL to the HDL receptor scavenger receptor class B type I. Effect of lipid association and APOA-I mutations on receptor binding: J.Biol.Chem., v. 275, no. 28, p. 21262-21271.

Lusa, S., M. Jauhiainen, J. Metso et al., 1996, The mechanism of human plasma phospholipid transfer protein-induced enlargement of high-density lipoprotein particles: evidence for particle fusion: Biochem.J., v. 313 (Pt 1), p. 275-282.

MacCallum, P. K., J. A. Cooper, J. Martin et al., 2000, Haemostatic and lipid determinants of prothrombin fragment F1.2 and D-dimer in plasma: Thrombosis and Haemostasis, v. 83, no. 3, p. 421-426.

Mallat, Z., H. Benamer, B. Hugel et al., 2000, Elevated levels of shed membrane microparticles with procoagulant potential in the peripheral circulating blood of patients with acute coronary syndromes: Circulation, v. 101, no. 8, p. 841-843.

Mardones, P., V. Quinones, L. Amigo et al., 2001, Hepatic cholesterol and bile acid metabolism and intestinal cholesterol absorption in scavenger receptor class B type I-deficient mice: J.Lipid Res., v. 42, no. 2, p. 170-180.

Martinez-Gonzalez, J., I. Escudero, and L. Badimon, 2004, Simvastatin potenciates PGI(2) release induced by HDL in human VSMC: effect on Cox-2 up-regulation and MAPK signalling pathways activated by HDL: Atherosclerosis, v. 174, no. 2, p. 305-313.

Matsunaga, T., Y. Hiasa, H. Yanagi et al., 1991, Apolipoprotein A-I deficiency due to a codon 84 nonsense mutation of the apolipoprotein A-I gene: Proc.Natl.Acad.Sci.U.S.A, v. 88, no. 7, p. 2793-2797.

McNeish, J., R. J. Aiello, D. Guyot et al., 2000, High density lipoprotein deficiency and foam cell accumulation in mice with targeted disruption of ATP-binding cassette transporter-1: Proc.Natl.Acad.Sci.U.S.A, v. 97, no. 8, p. 4245-4250.

Mineo, C., H. Deguchi, J. H. Griffin et al., 2006, Endothelial and antithrombotic actions of HDL: Circ.Res., v. 98, no. 11, p. 1352-1364.

Mineo, C., I. S. Yuhanna, M. J. Quon et al., 2003, High density lipoprotein-induced endothelial nitric-oxide synthase activation is mediated by Akt and MAP kinases: J.Biol.Chem., v. 278, no. 11, p. 9142-9149.

Miura, S., M. Fujino, Y. Matsuo et al., 2003, High density lipoprotein-induced angiogenesis requires the activation of Ras/MAP kinase in human coronary artery endothelial cells: Arterioscler.Thromb.Vasc.Biol., v. 23, no. 5, p. 802-808.

Murphy, A. J., K. J. Woollard, A. Hoang et al., 2008, High-density lipoprotein reduces the human monocyte inflammatory response: Arterioscler.Thromb.Vasc.Biol., v. 28, no. 11, p. 2071-2077.

Murugesan, G., G. Sa, and P. L. Fox, 1994, High-density lipoprotein stimulates endothelial cell movement by a mechanism distinct from basic fibroblast growth factor: Circ.Res., v. 74, no. 6, p. 1149-1156.

Mythreye, K., L. L. Satterwhite, W. S. Davidson et al., 2008, ApoA-I induced CD31 in bone marrow-derived vascular progenitor cells increases adhesion: implications for vascular repair: Biochim.Biophys.Acta, v. 1781, no. 11-12, p. 703-709.

Nakamura, K., M. A. Kennedy, A. Baldan et al., 2004, Expression and regulation of multiple murine ATP-binding cassette transporter G1 mRNAs/isoforms that stimulate cellular cholesterol efflux to high density lipoprotein: J.Biol.Chem., v. 279, no. 44, p. 45980-45989.

Navab, M., S. Y. Hama, G. M. Anantharamaiah et al., 2000a, Normal high density lipoprotein inhibits three steps in the formation of mildly oxidized low density lipoprotein: steps 2 and 3: J.Lipid Res., v. 41, no. 9, p. 1495-1508.

Navab, M., S. Y. Hama, C. J. Cooke et al., 2000b, Normal high density lipoprotein inhibits three steps in the formation of mildly oxidized low density lipoprotein: step 1: J.Lipid Res., v. 41, no. 9, p. 1481-1494.

Nicholls, S. J., B. Cutri, S. G. Worthley et al., 2005a, Impact of short-term administration of high-density lipoproteins and atorvastatin on atherosclerosis in rabbits: Arteriosclerosis Thrombosis and Vascular Biology, v. 25, no. 11, p. 2416-2421.

Nicholls, S. J., G. J. Dusting, B. Cutri et al., 2005b, Reconstituted high-density lipoproteins inhibit the acute pro-oxidant and proinflammatory vascular changes induced by a periarterial collar in normocholesterolemic rabbits: Circulation, v. 111, no. 12, p. 1543-1550.

Nicholls, S. J., E. M. Tuzcu, I. Sipahi et al., 2006, Relationship between atheroma regression and change in lumen size after infusion of apolipoprotein A-I Milano: J.Am.Coll.Cardiol., v. 47, no. 5, p. 992-997.

Nissen, S. E., T. Tsunoda, E. M. Tuzcu et al., 2003, Effect of recombinant ApoA-I Milano on coronary atherosclerosis in patients with acute coronary syndromes: a randomized controlled trial: JAMA, v. 290, no. 17, p. 2292-2300.

Nobecourt, E., F. Tabet, G. Lambert et al., 2010, Nonenzymatic glycation impairs the antiinflammatory properties of apolipoprotein A-I: Arterioscler.Thromb.Vasc.Biol., v. 30, no. 4, p. 766-772.

Nofer, J. R., B. Levkau, I. Wolinska et al., 2001, Suppression of endothelial cell apoptosis by high density lipoproteins (HDL) and HDL-associated lysosphingolipids: J.Biol.Chem., v. 276, no. 37, p. 34480-34485.

Nofer, J. R., G. M. van der, M. Tolle et al., 2004, HDL induces NO-dependent vasorelaxation via the lysophospholipid receptor S1P3: J.Clin.Invest, v. 113, no. 4, p. 569-581.

Nolte, R. T., and D. Atkinson, 1992, Conformational analysis of apolipoprotein A-I and E-3 based on primary sequence and circular dichroism: Biophys.J., v. 63, no. 5, p. 1221-1239.

Noor, R., U. Shuaib, C. X. Wang et al., 2007, High-density lipoprotein cholesterol regulates endothelial progenitor cells by increasing eNOS and preventing apoptosis: Atherosclerosis, v. 192, no. 1, p. 92-99.

Norata, G. D., C. Banfi, A. Pirillo et al., 2004, Oxidised-HDL3 induces the expression of PAI-1 in human endothelial cells. Role of p38MAPK activation and mRNA stabilization: British Journal of Haematology, v. 127, no. 1, p. 97-104.

Norata, G. D., E. Callegari, M. Marchesi et al., 2005, High-density lipoproteins induce transforming growth factor-beta2 expression in endothelial cells: Circulation, v. 111, no. 21, p. 2805-2811.

Okajima, F., K. Sato, and T. Kimura, 2009, Anti-atherogenic actions of high-density lipoprotein through sphingosine 1-phosphate receptors and scavenger receptor class B type I: Endocr.J., v. 56, no. 3, p. 317-334.

Okura, H., S. Yamashita, T. Ohama et al., 2010, HDL/Apolipoprotein A-I Binds to Macrophage-Derived Progranulin and Suppresses its Conversion into Proinflammatory Granulins: Journal of Atherosclerosis and Thrombosis, v. 17, no. 6, p. 568-577.

Ou, Z., J. Ou, A. W. Ackerman et al., 2003, L-4F, an apolipoprotein A-1 mimetic, restores nitric oxide and superoxide anion balance in low-density lipoprotein-treated endothelial cells: Circulation, v. 107, no. 11, p. 1520-1524.

Out, R., M. Hoekstra, J. A. Spijkers et al., 2004, Scavenger receptor class B type I is solely responsible for the selective uptake of cholesteryl esters from HDL by the liver and the adrenals in mice: J.Lipid Res., v. 45, no. 11, p. 2088-2095.

Out, R., W. Jessup, W. Le Goff et al., 2008, Coexistence of foam cells and hypocholesterolemia in mice lacking the ABC transporters A1 and G1: Circ.Res., v. 102, no. 1, p. 113-120.

Pajkrt, D., P. G. Lerch, T. vanderPoll et al., 1997, Differential effects of reconstituted high-density lipoprotein on coagulation, fibrinolysis and platelet activation during human endotoxemia: Thrombosis and Haemostasis, v. 77, no. 2, p. 303-307.

Parker, T. S., D. M. Levine, J. C. C. Chang et al., 1995, Reconstituted High-Density-Lipoprotein Neutralizes Gram-Negative Bacterial Lipopolysaccharides in Human Whole-Blood: Infection and Immunity, v. 63, no. 1, p. 253-258.

Patel, S., B. G. Drew, S. Nakhla et al., 2009, Reconstituted high-density lipoprotein increases plasma high-density lipoprotein anti-inflammatory properties and cholesterol efflux capacity in patients with type 2 diabetes: J.Am.Coll.Cardiol., v. 53, no. 11, p. 962-971.

Peters, W., and I. F. Charo, 2001, Involvement of chemokine receptor 2 and its ligand, monocyte chemoattractant protein-1, in the development of atherosclerosis: lessons from knockout mice: Curr Opin Lipidol., v. 12, no. 2, p. 175-180.

Radojkovic, C., A. Genoux, V. Pons et al., 2009, Stimulation of Cell Surface F-1-ATPase Activity by Apolipoprotein A-I Inhibits Endothelial Cell Apoptosis and Promotes Proliferation: Arteriosclerosis Thrombosis and Vascular Biology, v. 29, no. 7, p. 1125-U214.

Ramet, M. E., M. Ramet, Q. Lu et al., 2003, High-density lipoprotein increases the abundance of eNOS protein in human vascular endothelial cells by increasing its half-life: Journal of the American College of Cardiology, v. 41, no. 12, p. 2288-2297.

Remaley, A. T., J. A. Stonik, S. J. Demosky et al., 2001, Apolipoprotein specificity for lipid efflux by the human ABCAI transporter: Biochem.Biophys.Res.Commun., v. 280, no. 3, p. 818-823.

Rigotti, A., B. L. Trigatti, M. Penman et al., 1997, A targeted mutation in the murine gene encoding the high density lipoprotein (HDL) receptor scavenger receptor class B type I reveals its key role in HDL metabolism: Proc.Natl.Acad.Sci.U.S.A, v. 94, no. 23, p. 12610-12615.

Rizzo, M. A., and D. W. Piston, 2003, Regulation of beta cell glucokinase by S-nitrosylation and association with nitric oxide synthase: Journal of Cell Biology, v. 161, no. 2, p. 243-248.

Rutti, S., J. A. Ehses, R. A. Sibler et al., 2009, Low- and high-density lipoproteins modulate function, apoptosis, and proliferation of primary human and murine pancreatic beta-cells: Endocrinology, v. 150, no. 10, p. 4521-4530.

Santamarina-Fojo, S., J. M. Hoeg, G. Assmann, and H. B. Brewer, Jr., 2001, Lecithin cholesterol acyltransferase deficiency and fish eye disease, in CR Scriver, AL Beaudet, WS Sly, and D Valle eds., The Metabolic & Molecular Bases of Inherited Disease: New York, McGraw-Hill, p. 2817-2834.

Savary, S., F. Denizot, M. Luciani et al., 1996, Molecular cloning of a mammalian ABC transporter homologous to Drosophila white gene: Mamm.Genome, v. 7, no. 9, p. 673-676.

Seetharam, D., C. Mineo, A. K. Gormley et al., 2006, High-density lipoprotein promotes endothelial cell migration and reendothelialization via scavenger receptor-B type I: Circulation Research, v. 98, no. 1, p. 63-72.

Silver, D. L., N. Wang, X. Xiao et al., 2001, High density lipoprotein (HDL) particle uptake mediated by scavenger receptor class B type 1 results in selective sorting of HDL cholesterol from protein and polarized cholesterol secretion: J.Biol.Chem., v. 276, no. 27, p. 25287-25293.

Singaraja, R. R., L. R. Brunham, H. Visscher et al., 2003, Efflux and atherosclerosis: the clinical and biochemical impact of variations in the ABCA1 gene: Arterioscler.Thromb.Vasc.Biol., v. 23, no. 8, p. 1322-1332.

Singh, I. P., A. K. Chopra, D. H. Coppenhaver et al., 1999, Lipoproteins account for part of the broad non-specific antiviral activity of human serum: Antiviral Research, v. 42, no. 3, p. 211-218.

Sorci-Thomas, M. G., and M. J. Thomas, 2002, The effects of altered apolipoprotein A-I structure on plasma HDL concentration: Trends Cardiovasc.Med., v. 12, no. 3, p. 121-128.

Sorrentino, S. A., C. Besler, L. Rohrer et al., 2010, Endothelial-vasoprotective effects of high-density lipoprotein are impaired in patients with type 2 diabetes mellitus but are improved after extended-release niacin therapy: Circulation, v. 121, no. 1, p. 110-122.

Stangl, H., M. Hyatt, and H. H. Hobbs, 1999, Transport of lipids from high and low density lipoproteins via scavenger receptor-BI: J.Biol.Chem., v. 274, no. 46, p. 32692-32698.

Strawn, W. B., and C. M. Ferrario, 2002, Mechanisms linking angiotensin II and atherogenesis: Curr.Opin.Lipidol., v. 13, no. 5, p. 505-512.

Suc, I., I. Escargueil-Blanc, M. Troly et al., 1997, HDL and ApoA prevent cell death of endothelial cells induced by oxidized LDL: Arterioscler.Thromb.Vasc.Biol., v. 17, no. 10, p. 2158-2166.

Sugano, M., K. Tsuchida, and N. Makino, 2000, High-density lipoproteins protect endothelial cells from tumor necrosis factor-alpha-induced apoptosis: Biochem.Biophys.Res.Commun., v. 272, no. 3, p. 872-876.

Tabet, F., A. T. Remaley, A. I. Segaliny et al., 2010, The 5A apolipoprotein A-I mimetic peptide displays antiinflammatory and antioxidant properties in vivo and in vitro: Arterioscler.Thromb.Vasc.Biol., v. 30, no. 2, p. 246-252.

Tamagaki, T., S. Sawada, H. Imamura et al., 1996, Effects of high-density lipoproteins on intracellular pH and proliferation of human vascular endothelial cells: Atherosclerosis, v. 123, no. 1-2, p. 73-82.

Tangirala, R. K., K. Tsukamoto, S. H. Chun et al., 1999, Regression of atherosclerosis induced by liver-directed gene transfer of apolipoprotein A-I in mice: Circulation, v. 100, no. 17, p. 1816-1822.

Terasaka, N., M. Westerterp, J. Koetsveld et al., 2010, ATP-binding cassette transporter G1 and high-density lipoprotein promote endothelial NO synthesis through a decrease in the interaction of caveolin-1 and endothelial NO synthase: Arterioscler.Thromb.Vasc.Biol., v. 30, no. 11, p. 2219-2225.

Thuahnai, S. T., S. Lund-Katz, D. L. Williams et al., 2001, Scavenger receptor class B, type I-mediated uptake of various lipids into cells. Influence of the nature of the donor particle interaction with the receptor: J.Biol.Chem., v. 276, no. 47, p. 43801-43808.

Tolle, M., A. Pawlak, M. Schuchardt et al., 2008, HDL-associated lysosphingolipids inhibit NAD(P)H oxidase-dependent monocyte chemoattractant protein-1 production: Arteriosclerosis Thrombosis and Vascular Biology, v. 28, no. 8, p. 1542-1548.

Trigatti, B., H. Rayburn, M. Vinals et al., 1999, Influence of the high density lipoprotein receptor SR-BI on reproductive and cardiovascular pathophysiology: Proc.Natl.Acad.Sci.U.S.A, v. 96, no. 16, p. 9322-9327.

Ueda, Y., L. Royer, E. Gong et al., 1999, Lower plasma levels and accelerated clearance of high density lipoprotein (HDL) and non-HDL cholesterol in scavenger receptor class B type I transgenic mice: J.Biol.Chem., v. 274, no. 11, p. 7165-7171.

Uittenbogaard, A., P. W. Shaul, I. S. Yuhanna et al., 2000, High density lipoprotein prevents oxidized low density lipoprotein-induced inhibition of endothelial nitric-oxide synthase localization and activation in caveolae: Journal of Biological Chemistry, v. 275, no. 15, p. 11278-11283.

Van Eck, M., I. S. Bos, W. E. Kaminski et al., 2002, Leukocyte ABCA1 controls susceptibility to atherosclerosis and macrophage recruitment into tissues: Proc.Natl.Acad.Sci. U.S.A, v. 99, no. 9, p. 6298-6303.

Van Eck, M., R. R. Singaraja, D. Ye et al., 2006, Macrophage ATP-binding cassette transporter A1 overexpression inhibits atherosclerotic lesion progression in low-density lipoprotein receptor knockout mice: Arterioscler.Thromb.Vasc.Biol., v. 26, no. 4, p. 929-934.

Vane, J. R., and R. M. Botting, 1995, Pharmacodynamic Profile of Prostacyclin: American Journal of Cardiology, v. 75, no. 3, p. A3-A10.

Vanhollebeke, B., and E. Pays, 2010, The trypanolytic factor of human serum: many ways to enter the parasite, a single way to kill: Molecular Microbiology, v. 76, no. 4, p. 806-814.

Vantourout, P., C. Radojkovic, L. Lichtenstein et al., 2010, Ecto-F-ATPase: a moonlighting protein complex and an unexpected apoA-I receptor: World J.Gastroenterol., v. 16, no. 47, p. 5925-5935.

Vaughan, A. M., and J. F. Oram, 2005, ABCG1 redistributes cell cholesterol to domains removable by HDL but not by lipid-depleted apolipoproteins: J.Biol.Chem., v. 280, p. 30150-30157.

Vergeer, M., S. J. A. Korporaal, R. Franssen et al., 2011, Genetic Variant of the Scavenger Receptor BI in Humans: New England Journal of Medicine, v. 364, no. 2, p. 136-145.

Vinals, M., J. Martinez-Gonzalez, J. J. Badimon et al., 1997, HDL-induced prostacyclin release in smooth muscle cells is dependent on cyclooxygenase-2 (Cox-2): Arteriosclerosis Thrombosis and Vascular Biology, v. 17, no. 12, p. 3481-3488.

Wang, N., D. Lan, W. Chen et al., 2004, ATP-binding cassette transporters G1 and G4 mediate cellular cholesterol efflux to high-density lipoproteins: Proc.Natl.Acad.Sci. U.S.A, v. 101, no. 26, p. 9774-9779.

Wang, N., D. L. Silver, P. Costet et al., 2000, Specific binding of ApoA-I, enhanced cholesterol efflux, and altered plasma membrane morphology in cells expressing ABC1: J.Biol.Chem., v. 275, no. 42, p. 33053-33058.

Wang, X., H. L. Collins, M. Ranalletta et al., 2007, Macrophage ABCA1 and ABCG1, but not SR-BI, promote macrophage reverse cholesterol transport in vivo: J.Clin.Invest, v. 117, no. 8, p. 2216-2224.

Welch, G. N., and J. Loscalzo, 1998, Homocysteine and atherothrombosis: N.Engl.J.Med., v. 338, no. 15, p. 1042-1050.

Werner, N., S. Junk, U. Laufs et al., 2003, Intravenous transfusion of endothelial progenitor cells reduces neointima formation after vascular injury: Circ.Res., v. 93, p. e17-e24.

Wilhelm, A. J., M. Zabalawi, J. S. Owen et al., 2010, Apolipoprotein A-I modulates regulatory T cells in autoimmune LDLr-/-, ApoA-I-/- mice: J.Biol.Chem., v. 285, no. 46, p. 36158-36169.

Williamson, R., D. Lee, J. Hagaman et al., 1992, Marked reduction of high density lipoprotein cholesterol in mice genetically modified to lack apolipoprotein A-I: Proc.Natl.Acad.Sci.U.S.A, v. 89, no. 15, p. 7134-7138.

Wu, Z., V. Gogonea, X. Lee et al., 2011, The low resolution structure of ApoA1 in spherical high density lipoprotein revealed by small angle neutron scattering: J.Biol.Chem.

Yao, Y., E. S. Shao, M. Jumabay et al., 2008, High-density lipoproteins affect endothelial BMP-signaling by modulating expression of the activin-like kinase receptor 1 and 2: Arterioscler.Thromb.Vasc.Biol., v. 28, no. 12, p. 2266-2274.

Yates, M., A. Kolmakova, Y. Zhao et al., 2011, Clinical impact of scavenger receptor class B type I gene polymorphisms on human female fertility: Hum.Reprod..

Yeh, M., A. L. Cole, J. Choi et al., 2004, Role for sterol regulatory element-binding protein in activation of endothelial cells by phospholipid oxidation products: Circ.Res., v. 95, no. 8, p. 780-788.

Yesilaltay, A., M. G. Morales, L. Amigo et al., 2006, Effects of hepatic expression of the high-density lipoprotein receptor SR-BI on lipoprotein metabolism and female fertility: Endocrinology, v. 147, no. 4, p. 1577-1588.

Yuhanna, I. S., Y. Zhu, B. E. Cox et al., 2001, High-density lipoprotein binding to scavenger receptor-BI activates endothelial nitric oxide synthase: Nat.Med., v. 7, no. 7, p. 853-857.

Yvan-Charvet, L., M. Ranalletta, N. Wang et al., 2007, Combined deficiency of ABCA1 and ABCG1 promotes foam cell accumulation and accelerates atherosclerosis in mice: J.Clin.Invest, v. 117, no. 12, p. 3900-3908.

Zannis, V. I., A. Chroni, and M. Krieger, 2006a, Role of apoA-I, ABCA1, LCAT, and SR-BI in the biogenesis of HDL: J.Mol.Med., v. 84, no. 4, p. 276-294.

Zannis, V. I., A. Chroni, K. E. Kypreos et al., 2004a, Probing the pathways of chylomicron and HDL metabolism using adenovirus-mediated gene transfer: Curr Opin Lipidol., v. 15, no. 2, p. 151-166.

Zannis, V. I., D. Kardassis, and E. E. Zanni, 1993, Genetic mutations affecting human lipoproteins, their receptors, and their enzymes: Adv.Hum.Genet., v. 21, p. 145-319.

Zannis, V. I., K. E. Kypreos, A. Chroni, D. Kardassis, and E. E. Zanni, 2004b, Lipoproteins and atherogenesis, in J Loscalzo ed., Molecular Mechanisms of Atherosclerosis: New York, NY, Taylor & Francis, p. 111-174.

Zannis, V. I., E. E. Zanni, A. Papapanagiotou, D. Kardassis, and A. Chroni, 2006b, ApoA-I functions and synthesis of HDL: Insights from mouse models of human HDL metabolism, High-Density Lipoproteins. From Basic Biology to Clinical Aspects: Weinheim, Wiley-VCH, p. 237-265.

Zeiher, A. M., V. Schachlinger, S. H. Hohnloser et al., 1994, Coronary atherosclerotic wall thickening and vascular reactivity in humans. Elevated high-density lipoprotein levels ameliorate abnormal vasoconstriction in early atherosclerosis: Circulation, v. 89, no. 6, p. 2525-2532.

11

Peroxisome Proliferator-Activated Receptor β/δ (PPAR β/δ) as a Potential Therapeutic Target for Dyslipidemia

Emma Barroso, Lucía Serrano-Marco, Laia Salvadó,
Xavier Palomer and Manuel Vázquez-Carrera
Department of Pharmacology and Therapeutic Chemistry,
Spanish Biomedical Research Centre in Diabetes and Associated Metabolic
Disorders(CIBERDEM)-Instituto de SaludCarlos III and IBUB,
(Biomedicine Institute of the University of Barcelona),
Faculty of Pharmacy, University of Barcelona, Barcelona,
Spain

1. Introduction

Dyslipidemia is a powerful predictor of cardiovascular disease in patients at high risk (Turner et al., 1998), such as type 2 diabetic patients. Lowering of LDL-C is the prime target for treatment (2002), but even with intensification of statin therapy, a substantial residual cardiovascular risk remains (Barter et al., 2007; Miller et al., 2008; Fruchart et al., 2008; Shepherd et al., 2006). This may partly be due to atherogenic dyslipidemia. This term is commonly used to describe a condition of abnormally elevated plasma triglycerides and low high-density lipoprotein cholesterol (HDL-C), irrespective of the levels of LDL-C (Grundy, 1995). In addition to these key components, increased levels of small, dense LDL-C particles are also present, which in conjunction with the former components conform the also called "lipid triad" (Shepherd et al., 2005). Other abnormalities include accumulation in plasma of triglyceride-rich lipoproteins (TLRs), including chylomicron and very-low-density lipoprotein (VLDL) remnants. This is reflected by elevated plasma concentrations of non-HDL-C and apolipoprotein B-100 (apoB). Postprandially, there is also accumulation in plasma of TLRs and their remnants, as well as qualitative alterations in LDL and HDL particles. Thus, hypertriglyceridemia is associated with a wide spectrum of atherogenic lipoproteins not measured routinely (Taskinen, 2003). The presence of this lipid plasma profile with high triglyceride and low HDL-C levels have been shown to increase the risk of cardiovascular events independent of conventional risk factors (Bansal et al., 2007; Barter et al., 2007; deGoma et al., 2008). In fact, guidelines recommend modifying high triglyceride and low HDL-C as secondary therapeutic targets to provide additional vascular protection (2002). The presence of atherogenic dyslipidemia is seen in almost all patients with triglycerides > 2.2 mmol/l and HDL-C < 1.0 mmol/l, virtually all of whom have type 2 diabetes or abdominal obesity and insulin resistance (Taskinen, 2003). Most of these alterations are also characteristic of metabolic syndrome, which is defined as the clustering of multiple metabolic abnormalities, including abdominal obesity, dyslipidemia (high serum triglycerides and low serum HDL-C levels), glucose intolerance and hypertension (Eckel et al., 2005; Grundy et al., 2005).

2. Hypertriglyceridemia is crucial in the pathogenesis of atherogenic dyslipidemia

It is now recognized that the atherogenic dyslipidemia is mainly initiated by the hepatic overproduction of the plasma lipoproteins carrying triglycerides, the VLDL, which induce a sequence of lipoprotein changes leading to atherogenic lipid abnormalities in type 2 diabetes mellitus and metabolic syndrome (Adiels et al., 2008). Under these pathological conditions, the presence of insulin resistance at the level of adipose tissue leads to enhanced lypolisis and reduced free fatty acid (FFA) uptake and esterification which results in increased flux into the liver of FFA, which are either oxidized or esterified for triglyceride production, leading to hepatic steatosis and oversecretion into plasma of larger triglyceride-rich VLDL particles (Chan & Watts, 2011). These particles compete with chylomicrons and its remnants for clearance pathways regulated by lipoprotein lipase, an endothelial-bound enzyme, and by hepatic receptors, thereby exacerbating postprandial dyslipidemia. In addition, insulin resistance increases hepatic secretion of apoC-III, which is attached to VLDL delaying the catabolism of TRLs by inhibiting lipoprotein lipase and binding of remnant TRLs to hepatic clearance receptors (Chan & Watts, 2011). Finally, expansion of the VLDL triglyceride pool leads to cholesterol depletion and triglyceride enrichment of LDL and HDL through cholesteryl ester transfer protein, which facilitates the movement of cholesterol esters to VLDL, intermediate-density lipoprotein (IDL) and LDL from cholesterol ester rich HDL, leading to the accumulation in plasma of small, dense LDLs and a reduction in HDLs (Taskinen, 2003).

Since residual risk remains even after achieving an optimal LDL-C concentration with statins (Barter et al., 2007), probably due to other risk factors, such as high triglycerides, low HDL-C levels, defective glucose metabolism and other non-lipid-related risk factors (Kannel, 1983; Castelli, 1992; Lorenzo et al., 2010; Cederberg et al., 2010), the development of new drugs aimed at improving risk reduction is necessary. Among the new drugs for the treatment of the risk factors leading to the residual risk, PPARβ/δ activators might have a promising future. Interestingly, PPARβ/δ agonists have been demonstrated to be effective raising HDL-C and lowering triglyceride concentrations (Kersten, 2008). In addition to their lipid-modifying properties, PPARβ/δ agonists improve insulin resistance, which may also confer protection against the development of dyslipidemia (Coll et al., 2010a). This review summarizes the effects of PPARβ/δ on dyslipidemia identified during the last few years.

3. The PPAR family

PPARs are members of the nuclear receptor superfamily of ligand-activated transcription factors that regulate the expression of genes involved in fatty acid uptake and oxidation, lipid metabolism and inflammation (Kersten et al., 2000). To be transcriptionally active, PPARs need to heterodimerize with the 9-*cis* retinoic acid receptor (RXR) (NR2B) (Figure 1). PPAR-RXR heterodimers bind to DNA-specific sequences called peroxisome proliferator-response elements (PPREs), consisting of an imperfect direct repeat of the consensus binding site for nuclear hormone receptors (AGGTCA) separated by one nucleotide (DR-1). These sequences have been characterized within the promoter regions of PPAR target genes. The binding occurs in such a way that PPAR is always oriented to the DNA's 5'-end, while RXR is to the 3'-end. In the absence of ligand, high-affinity complexes are formed between PPAR-RXR heterodimers and nuclear receptor co-repressor proteins, which block transcriptional activation by sequestering the heterodimer from the promoter. Binding of the ligand to PPAR induces a conformational change resulting in dissociation of co-repressor proteins, so that the PPAR-RXR heterodimer can then bind to PPREs. Moreover, once activated by the ligand, the heterodimer recruits co-activator proteins that promote the initiation of transcription (Feige et al., 2006). As a consequence of these changes in transcriptional activity, binding of ligands to the receptor results in changes in the expression level of mRNAs encoded by PPAR target genes. In a specific cellular context, the activity of PPARs regulating the transcription of their target genes depends on many factors (relative expression of the PPARs, the promoter context of the target gene, the presence of co-activator and co-repressor proteins, etc.).

Thus, the transcriptional activity of PPARs is modulated by co-activators and co-repressors (Feige et al., 2006). One of the best described PPAR co-activators is PPARγ coactivator 1 α (PGC-1α). Silencing mediator for retinoic and thyroid hormone receptor (SMRT) and the nuclear receptor co-repressor (NCoR) are co-repressors that interact with the PPARs in the absence of ligands (Zamir et al., 1997). Receptor-interacting protein 140 (RIP140), an important metabolic regulator, is another ligand-dependent co-repressor which interacts with PPARs.

Finally, PPAR activity is also regulated at the post-transcriptional level by phosphorylation, ubiquitinylation, and sumoylation (for a detailed review see (Feige et al., 2006)).

However, the regulation of gene transcription by PPARs extends beyond their ability to trans-activate specific target genes in an agonist-dependent manner. PPARs also regulate gene expression independently of binding to PPREs. They cross-talk with other types of transcription factors and influence their function without binding to DNA, through a mechanism termed receptor-dependent trans-repression (Daynes & Jones, 2002). Most of the anti-inflammatory effects of PPARs are probably explained by this mechanism (Kamei et al., 1996; Li et al., 2000). Thus, through this DNA-binding independent mechanism, PPARs suppress the activities of several transcription factors, including nuclear factor κB (NF-κB), activator protein 1 (AP-1), signal transducers and activators of transcription (STATs) and nuclear factor of activated T cells (NFAT). There are three main trans-repression mechanisms by which ligand-activated PPAR-RXR complexes negatively regulate the activities of other transcription factors. First, trans-repression may result from competition for limiting amounts of shared co-activators. Under conditions in which the levels of specific co-activators are rate-limiting, activation of PPAR may suppress the activity of other transcription factors that use the same co-activators (Delerive et al., 1999; Delerive et al., 2002). In the second mechanism, activated PPAR-RXR heterodimers are believed to act through physical interaction with other transcription factors (for example AP-1, NF-κB, NFAT or STATs). This association prevents the transcription factor from binding to its response element and thereby inhibits its ability to induce gene transcription (Desreumaux et al., 2001). The third trans-repression mechanism relies on the ability of activated PPAR-RXR heterodimers to inhibit the phosphorylation and activation of certain members of the mitogen-activated protein kinase (MAPK) cascade (Johnson et al., 1997), preventing activation of downstream transcription factors.

The PPAR family consists of three members, PPARα (NR1C1 according to the unified nomenclature system for the nuclear receptor superfamily), PPARβ/δ (NR1C2) and PPARγ (NR1C3) (Auwerx et al., 1999). PPARα was the first PPAR to be identified and is the molecular target of the fibrate hypolipidemic class of drugs. This PPAR isotype is expressed primarily in tissues with a high level of fatty acid catabolism such as liver, brown fat, kidney, heart and skeletal muscle (Braissant et al., 1996). PPARγ has a restricted pattern of expression, mainly in white and brown adipose tissues and macrophages, whereas other tissues such as skeletal muscle and heart contain limited amounts. The γ isotype is the molecular target for the anti-diabetic drugs, thiazolidinediones. PPARβ/δ is ubiquitously expressed and, for this reason, was initially thought to be a "housekeeping gene" (Kliewer et al., 1994). However, studies with knockout mice (Barak et al., 2002; Peters et al., 2000; Tan et al., 2001) and the development of specific and high-affinity ligands for this receptor have shown that PPARβ/δ is a potential molecular target for prevention or treatment of several disorders. In this review we will highlight the role of PPARβ/δ in those metabolic processes with potential for treating dyslipidemia.

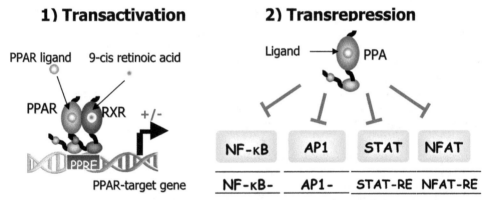

1) Transactivation   **2) Transrepression**

Fig. 1. Molecular mechanisms of Peroxisome Proliferator-Activated Receptors (PPARs). PPARs are ligand-activated transcription factors that regulate gene expression through two mechanisms: transactivation and transrepression. In transactivation PPAR-RXR heterodimers bind to DNA-specific sequences called peroxisome proliferator-response elements (PPREs), which are located in the promoter regions of genes involved in glucose and fatty acid metabolism. PPARs may also regulate gene expression through a DNA-independent mechanism called transrepression. Through this mechanism, PPARs inhibit the activity of several transcription factors such as NF-κB, which leads to anti-inflammatory effects. STAT denotes signal transducers and activators of transcription.

4. PPARβ/δ-specific features and ligands

The crystal structure of the ligand-binding domain of the PPARβ/δ isotype, which was first cloned in *Xenopus laevis* (Dreyer et al., 1992), revealed an exceptionally large pocket of approximately 1300 Å³. This pocket is similar to that of PPARγ, but much larger than the pockets of other nuclear receptors (Takada et al., 2000; Xu et al., 1999), which may explain, at least in part, the great variety of natural and synthetic ligands that bind to and activate this nuclear receptor. Saturated (14 to 18 carbons) and polyunsaturated (20 carbons in length) fatty acids have affinities for PPARβ/δ in the low micromolar range (Xu et al., 1999; Forman et al., 1997; Yu et al., 1995; Krey et al., 1997). In addition, all-trans-retinoic acid (vitamin A) (Shaw et al., 2003) and fatty acids derived from VLDL (Chawla et al., 2003) can activate PPARβ/δFinally, the availability of three synthetic ligands (GW501516, GW0742 and L-165041) that activate PPARβ/δ at very low concentrations both in vivo and in vitro with high selectivity over other PPAR isotypes (Sznaidman et al., 2003) led to a huge increase in experimental studies on the role of PPARβ/δ in cellular processes. The EC_{50} for these compounds assessed with recombinant human PPARβ/δ were 1.0 nM for GW0742, 1.1 nM for GW501516 and 50 nM for L-165041 (Berger et al., 1999; Sznaidman et al., 2003).

5. Role of PPARβ/δ in lipoprotein metabolism

Treatment of the atherogenic dyslipidemia associated with type 2 diabetes mellitus and metabolic syndrome requires lowering triglycerides, increasing HDL-C and increasing the size of the LDL-C particle. Studies using the PPARβ/δ agonist GW501516 have demonstrated that this drug increased HDL-C (79%), and decreased triglycerides (56%), LDL-C (29%) and fasting insulin levels (48%) in obese rhesus monkeys, a model for human obesity and its associated metabolic disorders (Oliver, Jr. et al., 2001). A decrease in small dense LDL was also observed in treated animals (Oliver, Jr. et al., 2001). It has been suggested that the increase in HDL-C levels after PPARβ/δ treatment is caused by enhanced cholesterol efflux stimulated by a higher expression of the reverse cholesterol transporter ATP-binding cassette A1 (ABCA1) in several tissues, including human and mouse macrophages and intestinal cells and fibroblasts (Leibowitz et al., 2000; van, V et al., 2005). Apart from these beneficial effects of PPARβ/δ activation on HDL levels, treatment with this compound also increased HDL particle size in primates (Wallace et al., 2005), an effect which is thought to be protective against the progression of coronary artery disease in humans (Rosenson et al., 2002). In addition, PPARβ/δ activation reduces cholesterol absorption through a mechanism that may involve, at least in part, reduced intestinal expression of Niemann-Pick C1-like 1 (Npc1l1), the proposed target for the inhibitor of cholesterol absorption ezetimibe (van, V et al., 2005). However, additional studies are necessary to clearly demonstrate that the effects of these drugs are mediated through PPARβ/δ activation.

In obese and diabetic db/db mice, administration of a PPARβ/δ agonist modestly increased HDL particles, without affecting triglyceride levels (Leibowitz et al., 2000), whereas in a shorter treatment with GW501516 a reduction in plasma free fatty acids and triglyceride levels was observed in db/db mice, but not in mice exposed to a high fat diet (Tanaka et al., 2003).

In mice, deletion of PPARβ/δ led to enhanced LDL and triglyceride levels (Akiyama et al., 2004). It has been proposed that the increase in triglycerides observed in these PPARβ/δ-null mice is caused by a combination of increased VLDL production and decreased plasma triglyceride clearance, as demonstrated by a decrease in postheparin LPL activity and increased hepatic expression of the LPL inhibitors Angptl3 and 4 (Akiyama et al., 2004). Recent findings obtained by our laboratory indicate that additional mechanisms can also contribute to the hypotriglyceridemic effect of PPARβ/δ (Barroso et al., 2011). Interestingly, the main factor influencing hepatic triglyceride secretion is fatty acid availability (Lewis, 1997). In liver, fatty acids are either incorporated into triglycerides or oxidized by mitochondrial β-oxidation. An increase in fatty acid oxidation in liver would thus reduce the availability of fatty acids and subsequent hepatic triglyceride secretion. However, it was unknown whether the hypotriglyceridemic effect observed following PPARβ/δ activation involved increased hepatic fatty acid oxidation and the mechanisms implicated. The rate-limiting step for mitochondrial β-oxidation is the transport of fatty acid into mitochondria by liver carnitine palmitoyltransferase-1 (CPT1a). This fatty acid transporter is under the control of both PPARs and AMP-activated protein kinase (AMPK), which detects low ATP levels and in turn increases oxidative metabolism (Zhang et al., 2009) by reducing the levels of malonyl-CoA. Interestingly, PPARβ/δ activation can increase the activity of AMPK and the increase in fatty acid oxidation in human skeletal muscle cells following GW501516 treatment is dependent on both PPARβ/δ and AMPK (Kramer et al., 2007). It is worth noting that a recent discovered protein, lipin 1, plays an important role in hepatic fatty acid oxidation since it determines whether fatty acids are incorporated into triglycerides or undergo mitochondrial β-oxidation. In addition, the expression and compartmentalization of lipin 1 controls the secretion of hepatic triglycerides (Bou et al., 2009). Thus, in the cytoplasm, lipin 1 promotes triglyceride accumulation and phospholipid synthesis by functioning as an Mg^{2+}-dependent phosphatidate phosphatase (phosphatidic acid phosphatase-1, PAP-1). In contrast, in the nucleus lipin 1 acts as a transcriptional co-activator linked to fatty acid oxidation by regulating the induction of PGC-1α-PPARα-target genes (Finck et al., 2006). Lipin 1 induces PPARα gene expression and forms a complex with PPARα and PGC-1α leading to the induction of genes involved in fatty acid oxidation, including *Cpt1a* and *Mcad* (medium chain acyl-CoA dehydrogenase) (Finck et al., 2006).

When we examined the effects a high-fat diet (HFD) on hypertriglyceridemia and on the hepatic fatty acid oxidation pathway, we observed that exposure to HFD caused hypertriglyceridemia that was accompanied by reduced hepatic mRNA levels of PGC-1α and lipin 1, reduced hepatic phospho-AMPK levels and increased activity of extracellular-signal-regulated kinase 1/2 (ERK1/2) (Figure 2). Interestingly, drug treatment reduced hypertriglyceridemia, and restored hepatic phosphorylated levels of AMPK and ERK1/2. GW501516 treatment increased nuclear lipin 1 protein levels, leading to amplification of the PGC-1α-PPARα signaling system, as demonstrated by the increase in PPARα levels and PPARα-DNA binding activity and the increased expression of PPARα-target genes involved in fatty acid oxidation. These effects of GW501516 were accompanied by an increase in plasma β-hydroxybutyrate levels, demonstrating enhanced hepatic fatty acid oxidation.

The maintenance of AMPK phosphorylation following GW501516 treatment was accompanied by the recovery in the expression levels of *Lipin 1* and *Pgc-1α* and the increase in the mRNA levels of the *Vldl receptor* (Figure 2). Although we cannot rule out direct transcriptional activation of these genes by PPARβ/δ since it has been suggested that *Lipin 1*, the *Vldl receptor* (Sanderson et al., 2010) and *Pgc-1α* (Hondares et al., 2007) might be PPARβ/δ-target genes, most effects of GW501516 might be the result of the increase in AMPK phosphorylation (Kramer et al., 2007). In fact, it has been reported that this kinase upregulates the expression of *Lipin 1* (Higashida et al., 2008), the *Vldl receptor* (Zenimaru et al., 2008) and *Pgc-1α* (Lee et al., 2006b). The increase in AMPK phosphorylation following GW501516 treatment might involve several mechanisms. Since inhibitory crosstalk between ERK1/2 and AMPK has been reported (Du et al., 2008), the increase in phospho-AMPK levels could be the result of the inhibition by GW501516 of the phosphorylation of ERK1/2 induced by the HFD, which is in agreement with our previous study reporting that

GW501516 prevents LPS-induced ERK1/2 phosphorylation in adipocytes (Rodriguez-Calvo et al., 2008). It is important to note that a previous study found that obesity leads to increased hepatic ERK1/2 activity and that caloric restriction blunts this increase and improves insulin sensitivity (Zheng et al., 2009). In our study, the improvement in glucose tolerance caused by GW501516 was also accompanied by the reduction in phospho-ERK1/2 levels. An additional mechanism could involve SIRT1, since it has recently been reported that pharmacological PPARβ/δ activation increases the expression of SIRT1 (Okazaki et al., 2010), a deacetylase which regulates AMPK activity (Ruderman et al., 2010) through LKB1 acetylation (Lan et al., 2008), and might be essential to the regulatory loop involving PPARα, PGC-1α and Lipin 1 (Sugden et al., 2010). However, our findings made this possibility unlikely given that the increase in SIRT1 levels induced by GW501516 did not modify the acetylation status of LKB1. Interestingly, we showed that GW501516 increased the AMP/ATP ratio in liver, indicating that, in line with a previous study in skeletal muscle cells (Kramer et al., 2007), the underlying mechanism responsible for the increase in AMPK phosphorylation induced by this drug could be a modification of the cellular energy status. Previous studies have suggested that the reduction in ATP levels caused by GW501516 can be the result of a specific inhibition of one or more complexes of the respiratory chain, an effect on the ATP synthase system, or to mitochondrial uncoupling (Kramer et al., 2007). These potential changes would reduce the yield of ATP synthesis by the mitochondria, leading to AMPK activation.

In agreement with the reported regulation of PGC-1α (Canto et al., 2009; Jeninga et al., 2010; Lee et al., 2006a) and Lipin 1 (Higashida et al., 2008) by AMPK, exposure to the HFD reduced both *Pgc-1α* and *Lipin 1* expression. The reduction in Lipin 1 was likely to be the result of the decrease of PGC-1α, since it has been reported that genetic reduction of hepatic PGC-1α decreases the expression of *Lipin 1* (Estall et al., 2009). In addition, it has been shown that physiological stimuli that increase mitochondrial fatty acid oxidation induce *Pgc-1α* gene expression, which in turn activates the expression of *Lipin 1* (Finck et al., 2006). Interestingly, it has been reported that upregulation of *Lipin 1* in liver increases PPARα activity by two mechanisms: transcriptional activation of the *Ppara* gene and direct coactivation of PPARα in cooperation with PGC-1α (Finck et al., 2006). Thus, Lipin 1 is considered to be an inducible "booster" that amplifies pathways downstream PGC-1α-PPARα, mainly mitochondrial fatty acid oxidation (Finck et al., 2006). In agreement with this, GW501516 treatment prevented the reduction in PGC-1α, increased the nuclear protein levels of Lipin 1 and amplified the PGC-1αPPARα pathway, as demonstrated by the increase in the transcriptional activation of *Ppara* and the increase in PPARα transcriptional activity. These effects subsequently enhanced hepatic fatty acid oxidation, as shown by the increase in β-hydroxybutyrate levels. The reduction in PGC-1α and Lipin 1 levels caused by the HFD and their restoration after GW501516 treatment observed in our study might also contribute to the changes of plasma triglyceride levels, since both proteins are involved in the control of hepatic triglyceride secretion and fatty acid oxidation (Zhang et al., 2004; Chen et al., 2008; Estall et al., 2009). Overall, these data implicated PGC-1α and Lipin 1 in the hypotriglyceridemic effect of PPARβ/δ and complemented the findings of a previous study reporting that elevated plasma triglyceride levels in PPARβ/δ-null mouse were related to a combination of increased VLDL production and decreased plasma triglyceride clearance (Akiyama et al., 2004).

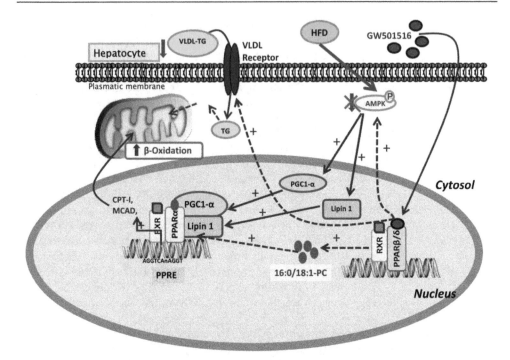

Fig. 2. A schematic of the potential effects of GW501516 (dashed lines) on liver metabolism is shown. Drug treatment with the PPARβ/δ agonist GW501516 prevents the reduction in phospho-AMPK levels and the subsequent increase in phospho-ERK1/2 levels caused by the HFD. In addition, GW501516 prevents the reduction in PGC-1α and increases Lipin 1 protein levels in the nucleus leading to amplification of the PPARα-PGC-1α pathway, which subsequently induces hepatic fatty acid oxidation. This pathway is additionally increased by GW501516 through the enhanced synthesis of the hepatic PPARα endogenous ligand 16:0/18:1-PC. As a result of the increase in this pathway the availability of fatty acids to be secreted as triglycerides might be compromised. The increase in the hepatic levels of the Vldl receptor can also contribute to reduce plasma triglyceride levels.

The data reported in our study also demonstrated that PPARβ/δ activation by GW501516 can amplify the PPARα pathway by an additional mechanism. Previous studies had demonstrated that hepatic fatty acid synthase (FAS) was necessary for the normal activation of PPARα target genes but did not identify the ligand involved in this process (Chakravarthy et al., 2005). Recently, this endogenous PPARα ligand was identified as 16:0/18:1-phosphatidilcholine (PC) (Chakravarthy et al., 2009). The synthesis of this ligand requires FAS activity, which yields palmitate (16:0), whereas 16:0/18:1-PC is generated through the enzymatic activity of CEPT1 (Chakravarthy et al., 2009). Subsequent binding of 16:0/18:1-PC to PPARα in the nucleus turns on PPARα-dependent genes and affects hepatic lipid metabolism. Interestingly, activation of PPARβ/δ by GW501516 induces FAS expression in liver as a result of increased glycolysis and the pentose phosphate shunt (Lee et al., 2006a). Our findings confirmed that GW501516 also increased *Cept1* expression and the levels of 16:0/18:1-PC, contributing to further amplification of the PPARα pathway.

The increase in fatty acid oxidation caused by GW501516 was apparently inconsistent with its lack of effects on hepatic triglyceride levels observed in our study. Several reasons may account for this. First, similar to the effects of GW501516, which restores Lipin 1 levels, hepatic *Lipin 1* overexpression leads to increased liver triglyceride content (Finck et al., 2006). This apparently conflicts with the effects of Lipin 1 on fatty acid oxidation, but it has been explained by hepatic triglyceride sequestration secondary to diminished triglyceride secretion, increased fatty acid uptake, or the PAP activity of Lipin 1 (Finck et al., 2006). Second, in our study we reported an additional possibility, the increase caused by GW501516 in the expression of the *Vldl receptor* in liver. The huge increase of this receptor observed in liver after GW501516 treatment might also reduce plasma triglyceride levels by increasing VLDL uptake by the liver. However, this can also lead to an increase in hepatic triglyceride content. Third, it has been reported that GW501516 improves hyperglycemia by increasing glucose flux through the pentose phosphate pathway and enhancing fatty acid synthesis in liver (Lee et al., 2006a). In that study, GW501516 increased liver triglyceride content but the authors reported that although this might raise concerns that long-term drug treatment might cause hepatic steatosis, they did not observe signs of fatty liver with treatment up to 6 months. In addition, long-term GW501516 treatment has been shown to reduce body weight and levels of circulating and liver triglycerides (Wang et al., 2004; Tanaka et al., 2003). In summary, our findings indicated that PPARβ/δ activation by GW501516 amplified the PPARα-PGC1-α pathway through the restoration of AMPK activity, contributing to the hypotriglyceridemic effect of this drug.

In humans, there are conflicting reports as to whether PPARβ/δ polymorphisms are associated with changes in plasma lipoproteins. Thus, while some studies found an association between a PPARβ/δ polymorphism and plasma lipids (Skogsberg et al., 2003), this was not confirmed in other studies (Gouni-Berthold et al., 2005). These discrepancies could be caused by differences in gender or the influence of gene-environment interactions, since a recent study reported that the association between the PPARβ/δ -87T>C polymorphism and plasma HDL-cholesterol might be sex-specific, women showing a stronger association, and that this association was only observed in subjects consuming a low-fat diet (Robitaille et al., 2007). The authors of this study concluded that the presence of the PPARβ/δ -87T>C polymorphism, which may result in enhanced PPARβ/δ activity, is associated with lower risk of suffering metabolic syndrome and that this association depends on the amount of fat consumed. In summary, the findings available at present on the effects of PPARβ/δ activation on lipoprotein metabolism are so promising that PPARβ/δ drugs are now in clinical trials for the treatment of human dyslipidemia.

6. Role of PPARβ/δ in insulin resistance

As stated above insulin resistance plays a crucial role in the development of hypertrigliceridemia, resulting in a sequence of lipoprotein changes leading to atherogenic dyslipidemia. Thus, those drugs, such as the PPARβ/δ ligands, which improve insulin resistance may also contribute to ameliorate the atherogenic dyslipidemia.

6.1 PPARβ/δ, inflammation and insulin resistance in adipose tissue

The expansion of adipose tissue, mainly in the form of visceral obesity, may contribute to enhanced inflammation in this tissue and insulin resistance through several processes. First, macrophages can infiltrate in adipose tissue, which contributes to the overproduction of inflammatory cytokines, such as tumor necrosis factor α (TNF-α and interleukin 6 (IL-6) (Gustafson et al., 2009). Indeed, the infiltration of macrophages into adipose tissue correlates with the degree of insulin resistance (Mathieu et al., 2010). Second, as visceral fat (which is very sensitive to lipolytic stimuli) increases, so does the rate of lipolysis. This leads to increased free fatty acid (FFA) mobilization and elevated levels of circulating FFA. Several studies have consistently demonstrated that elevations of plasma FFA produce insulin resistance in diabetic patients and in nondiabetic subjects (Boden et al., 1991; Boden, 1997). Saturated FFA are potent activators of the Toll-like receptor-4 (TLR4) (Mathieu et al., 2006) and recent evidence suggests that inflammatory processes induced by obesity and a high-fat diet cause systemic insulin resistance via a mechanism involving this receptor (Shi et al., 2006). TLR-4 is expressed in virtually all human cells and binds a wide spectrum of exogenous and endogenous ligands, including bacterial lipopolysaccharide (LPS) (Akira et al., 2006). In the presence of LPS, the TLR4 complex (including CD-14 and an accessory protein, MD-2), recruits the adaptor protein, myeloid differentiation factor-88 (MyD88), which in turn recruits interleukin-1 receptor-associated kinase (IRAK). This leads to the activation of the pro-inflammatory transcription factor NF-κB (Shoelson et al., 2006) and the subsequent enhanced expression of several inflammatory mediators (including IL-6 and monocyte chemoattractant protein-1 [MCP-1]). These observations indicate that saturated FFA derived from adipocytes and from high-fat diets activate TLR and the inflammatory pathway in adipocytes and macrophages, which contribute to the synthesis and production of cytokines such as TNF-α (Nguyen et al., 2007). In addition, high-fat diets raise plasma LPS to a concentration that is high enough to increase body weight, fasting glycemia and inflammation (Cani et al., 2007). Furthermore, LPS receptor-deleted mice (CD14 mutants) are hypersensitive to insulin, and the development of insulin resistance, obesity and diabetes in this animal model is delayed in response to a high-fat diet (Cani et al., 2007). Experiments performed in our laboratory have demonstrated that the PPARβ/δ agonist GW501516 inhibits LPS-induced cytokine expression and secretion by preventing NF-κB activation in adipocytes (Rodriguez-Calvo et al., 2008). Of note, NF-κB activation by LPS requires mitogen-activated protein kinase (MAPK)–extracellular signal–related kinase (ERK)1/2 (MEK1/2) activation, since inhibition of this pathway reduces LPS-induced cytokine production in adipocytes (Chung et al., 2006). In agreement with this role of ERK1/2 in inflammation in adipocytes, the expression of pro-inflammatory cytokines in these cells drops when they are exposed to LPS in the presence of the MAPK pathway inhibitor U0126. Interestingly, in white adipose tissue from PPARβ/δ-null mice we observed increased ERK1/2 phosphorylation and NF-κB activity and higher expression of IL-6 compared with wild-type mice (Rodriguez-Calvo et al., 2008). Moreover, in the white adipose tissue of a genetic model of obesity and diabetes, the Zucker diabetic fatty (ZDF) rat, the reduction in the expression of PPARβ/δ correlated with an increase in ERK1/2 phosphorylation and NF-κB activity. These findings suggest that PPARβ/δ activation prevents LPS-induced NF-κB activation via ERK1/2, thereby reducing the production of pro-inflammatory cytokines involved in the development of insulin resistance.

In addition, it has been suggested that IL-6 is another of the mediators linking obesity-derived chronic inflammation with insulin resistance through activation of signal transducer and activator of transcription 3 (STAT3), with subsequent up-regulation of suppressor of cytokine signaling 3 (SOCS3). Recently we have demonstrated that the PPARβ/δ agonist GW501516 prevents both IL-6-dependent reduction in insulin-stimulated Akt phosphorylation and glucose uptake in adipocytes (Serrano-Marco et al., 2011). In addition, this drug treatment abolished IL-6-induced SOCS3 expression in differentiated 3T3-L1 adipocytes. This effect was associated with the capacity of the drug to prevent IL-6-induced STAT3 phosphorylation on Tyr[705] and Ser[727] residues in vitro and in vivo. Moreover, GW501516 prevented IL-6-dependent induction of ERK1/2, a serine-threonine-protein kinase involved in serine STAT3 phosphorylation. Furthermore, in white adipose tissue from PPARβ/δ-null mice, STAT3 phosphorylation (Tyr[705] and Ser[727]), STAT3 DNA-binding activity and SOCS3 protein levels were higher than in wild-type mice. Several steps in STAT3 activation require its association with heat shock protein 90 (Hsp90), which was prevented by GW501516 as revealed in immunoprecipitation studies. Consistent with this finding, the STAT3-Hsp90 association was enhanced in white adipose tissue from PPARβ/δ-null mice compared to wild-type mice. Collectively, our findings indicate that PPARβ/δ activation prevents IL-6-induced STAT3 activation by inhibiting ERK1/2 and preventing the STAT3-Hsp90 association, an effect that may contribute to the prevention of cytokine-induced insulin resistance in adipocytes.

6.2 PPARβ/δ, inflammation and insulin resistance in skeletal muscle cells

FFAs may cause insulin resistance in skeletal muscle through several mechanisms, including effects on metabolism (Roden et al., 1996; Haber et al., 2003), signaling (Hirabara et al., 2007; Silveira et al., 2008) and mitochondrial function (Schrauwen et al., 2010; Hirabara et al., 2010). In addition, FFAs activate pro-inflammatory pathways, linking the development of this pathology to a chronic low-grade systemic inflammatory response (Wellen & Hotamisligil, 2005). In addition to FFA-induced inflammation through TLR, an additional pathway leads to FFA-mediated inflammation. This pathway involves intracellular accumulation of fatty acid derivatives. Once fatty acids are taken up by skeletal muscle cells they are either stored as fatty acid derivatives or undergo β-oxidation in the mitochondria. In the presence of high plasma FFA, fatty acid flux in skeletal muscle cells exceeds its oxidation, which leads to the accumulation of fatty acid derivatives, such as diacylglycerol (DAG), which can then activate a number of different serine kinases that negatively regulate insulin action. Thus, DAG is a potent allosteric activator of protein kinase Cθ (PKCθ), which is the most abundant PKC isoform in skeletal muscle (Griffin et al., 1999; Cortright et al., 2000; Itani et al., 2000). This PKC isoform inhibits the action of insulin by phosphorylating certain serine residues on insulin receptor substrate 1 (IRS1), including Ser[307] in the rodent IRS-1 protein (reviewed in ref. (Gual et al., 2005)). This phosphorylation impairs insulin-receptor signaling through several distinct mechanisms (Hotamisligil et al., 1996). PKCθ also impairs insulin sensitivity by activating another serine kinase, IκB kinase β (IKKβ) (Perseghin et al., 2003). In addition to phosphorylating IRS-1 in Ser[307], IKKβ phosphorylates IκB. Thus, it activates the pro-inflammatory transcription factor NF-κB, which has been linked to fatty acid-induced impairment of insulin action in skeletal muscle in rodents (Kim et al., 2001; Yuan et al., 2001). Once activated, NF-κB regulates the expression of multiple inflammatory mediators, including IL-6. This cytokine correlates strongly with insulin resistance and type 2 diabetes (Pickup et al., 1997; Kern et al., 2001; Pradhan et al., 2001) and its plasma levels are 2-3 times higher in patients with obesity and type 2 diabetes than in lean control subjects (Kern et al., 2001).

Accumulation of fatty acid derivatives can be attenuated by mitochondrial β-oxidation. The rate-limiting step for β-oxidation of long-chain fatty acids is their transport into mitochondria via CPT-1. The activity of this enzyme is inhibited by malonyl-CoA, the product of acetyl-CoA carboxylase, which, in turn, is inhibited by AMPK. This kinase is a metabolic sensor that detects low ATP levels and increases oxidative metabolism (Reznick & Shulman, 2006), by reducing the levels of malonyl-CoA. Interestingly, activation of fatty acid oxidation by overexpressing CPT-1 in cultured skeletal muscle cells (Sebastian et al., 2007) and in mouse skeletal muscle (Bruce et al., 2009) improves lipid-induced insulin resistance. Hence, this approach may provide a valid therapeutic strategy to prevent this pathology. Activation of PPARβ/δ by its ligands (including GW501516) enhances fatty acid catabolism in adipose tissue and skeletal muscle, thereby delaying weight gain (for a review see (Barish et al., 2006)). This increase in fatty acid oxidation in human skeletal muscle cells following PPARβ/δ activation by GW501516 is dependent on both PPARβ/δ and AMPK (Kramer et al., 2007). AMPK is activated by GW501516 by modulating the ATP:AMP ratio (Kramer et al., 2007). Despite these data, little information was available on whether the increase in fatty acid oxidation attained after PPARβ/δ activation prevented fatty acid-induced inflammation and insulin resistance in skeletal muscle cells. However, we have recently reported that the PPARβ/δ ligand GW501516 prevented palmitate-induced inflammation and insulin resistance in skeletal muscle cells (Coll et al., 2010b). Treatment with GW501516 enhanced the expression of two-well known PPARβ/δ-target genes involved in fatty acid oxidation, CPT-1 and pyruvate dehydrogenase kinase 4 (PDK-4), and increased the phosphorylation of AMPK. This prevented the reduction in fatty acid oxidation caused by palmitate exposure. In agreement with these changes, GW501516 treatment reversed the increase in DAG and PKCθ activation caused by palmitate. These effects were abolished in the presence of the CPT-1 inhibitor etomoxir, thereby implicating increased fatty acid oxidation in the changes. Consistent with these findings, PPARβ/δ activation by GW501516 blocked palmitate-induced NF-κB DNA-binding activity. Likewise, drug treatment inhibited the increase in IL-6 expression caused by palmitate in C2C12 myotubes and human skeletal muscle cells, as well as the protein secretion of this cytokine. Overall, these findings indicate that PPARβ/δ attenuates fatty acid-induced NF-κB activation and the subsequent development of insulin resistance in skeletal muscle cells by reducing DAG accumulation. Interestingly, it has been suggested that the hypotrigliceridemic effect of GW501516 in humans is dependent of the increase in CPT-1 expression observed in skeletal muscle (Riserus et al., 2008).

7. Conclusion

Reduction of LDL-C, the main target of hypolipidemic therapy, has been proved effective reducing morbidity and mortality associated to CVD. However, a high proportion of patients receiving statins, the most lipid-lowering family of drugs used, do not reach optimal LDL-C levels. In addition, even in those patients reaching the optimal LDL-C levels following statin treatment, a residual risk remains, probably due to the presence of other risk factors, including the presence of atherogic dyslipidemia (described by the presence of high triglycerides, low HDL-C levels, and the presence of small dense LDL particles), glucose metabolism alterations and additional non-lipid-related risk factors. Several studies have confirmed that PPARβ/δ plays an important role in the regulation of lipoprotein metabolism, leading to reductions in the levels of plasma triglycerides and LDL-C and increases in HDL-C in different animal models. Taken together, these effects attained following PPARβ/δ activation on lipoprotein metabolism are so promising that this nuclear receptor has been considered a therapeutic target to prevent and treat dyslipidemia. However, as with any drug designed for human therapy, a great deal of research will be needed on the efficacy and safety of PPARβ/δ activators before they reach clinical use.

8. Acknowledgments

The author's work that is summarized in this review was supported by grants from the Ministerio de Ciencia e Innovación of Spain (SAF2009-06939). CIBER de Diabetes y Enfermedades Metabólicas Asociadas (CIBERDEM) is an Instituto de Salud Carlos III project. L.S-M. and L.S. were supported by FPI grants from the Spanish Ministerio de Ciencia e Innovación. We would like to thank the University of Barcelona's Language Advisory Service for its help.

9. References

Third Report of the National Cholesterol Education Program (NCEP) Expert Panel on Detection, Evaluation, and Treatment of High Blood Cholesterol in Adults (Adult Treatment Panel III) final report. *Circulation* 2002;106:3143-421.

Adiels M, Olofsson SO, Taskinen MR, Boren J. Overproduction of very low-density lipoproteins is the hallmark of the dyslipidemia in the metabolic syndrome. *Arterioscler Thromb Vasc Biol* 2008;28:1225-36.

Akira S, Uematsu S, Takeuchi O. Pathogen recognition and innate immunity. *Cell* 2006;124:783-801.

Akiyama TE, Lambert G, Nicol CJ et al. Peroxisome proliferator-activated receptor beta/delta regulates very low density lipoprotein production and catabolism in mice on a Western diet. *J Biol Chem* 2004;279:20874-81.

Auwerx J, Baulieu E, Beato M et al. A unified nomenclature system for the nuclear receptor superfamily. *Cell* 1999;97:161-63.

Bansal S, Buring JE, Rifai N, Mora S, Sacks FM, Ridker PM. Fasting compared with nonfasting triglycerides and risk of cardiovascular events in women. *JAMA* 2007;298:309-16.

Barak Y, Liao D, He W et al. Effects of peroxisome proliferator-activated receptor delta on placentation, adiposity, and colorectal cancer. *Proc Natl Acad Sci U S A* 2002;99:303-8.

Barish GD, Narkar VA, Evans RM. PPAR delta: a dagger in the heart of the metabolic syndrome. *J Clin Invest* 2006;116:590-597.

Barroso E, Rodriguez-Calvo R, Serrano-Marco L et al. The PPAR{beta}/{delta} Activator GW501516 Prevents the Down-Regulation of AMPK Caused by a High-Fat Diet in Liver and Amplifies the PGC-1{alpha}-Lipin 1-PPAR{alpha} Pathway Leading to Increased Fatty Acid Oxidation. *Endocrinology* 2011;152:1848-59.

Barter P, Gotto AM, LaRosa JC et al. HDL cholesterol, very low levels of LDL cholesterol, and cardiovascular events. *N Engl J Med* 2007;357:1301-10.

Berger J, Leibowitz MD, Doebber TW et al. Novel peroxisome proliferator-activated receptor (PPAR) gamma and PPARdelta ligands produce distinct biological effects. *J Biol Chem* 1999;274:6718-25.

Boden G. Role of fatty acids in the pathogenesis of insulin resistance and NIDDM. *Diabetes* 1997;46:3-10.

Boden G, Jadali F, White J et al. Effects of fat on insulin-stimulated carbohydrate metabolism in normal men. *J Clin Invest* 1991;88:960-966.

Bou KM, Sundaram M, Zhang HY et al. The level and compartmentalization of phosphatidate phosphatase-1 (lipin-1) control the assembly and secretion of hepatic VLDL. *J Lipid Res* 2009;50:47-58.

Braissant O, Foufelle F, Scotto C, Dauca M, Wahli W. Differential expression of peroxisome proliferator-activated receptors (PPARs): tissue distribution of PPAR-alpha, -beta, and -gamma in the adult rat. *Endocrinology* 1996;137:354-66.

Bruce CR, Hoy AJ, Turner N et al. Overexpression of carnitine palmitoyltransferase-1 in skeletal muscle is sufficient to enhance fatty acid oxidation and improve high-fat diet-induced insulin resistance. *Diabetes* 2009;58:550-558.

Cani PD, Amar J, Iglesias MA et al. Metabolic endotoxemia initiates obesity and insulin resistance. *Diabetes* 2007;56:1761-72.

Canto C, Gerhart-Hines Z, Feige JN et al. AMPK regulates energy expenditure by modulating NAD+ metabolism and SIRT1 activity. *Nature* 2009;458:1056-60.

Castelli WP. Epidemiology of triglycerides: a view from Framingham. *Am J Cardiol* 1992;70:3H-9H.

Cederberg H, Saukkonen T, Laakso M et al. Postchallenge glucose, A1C, and fasting glucose as predictors of type 2 diabetes and cardiovascular disease: a 10-year prospective cohort study. *Diabetes Care* 2010;33:2077-83.

Chakravarthy MV, Lodhi IJ, Yin L et al. Identification of a physiologically relevant endogenous ligand for PPARalpha in liver. *Cell* 2009;138:476-88.

Chakravarthy MV, Pan Z, Zhu Y et al. "New" hepatic fat activates PPARalpha to maintain glucose, lipid, and cholesterol homeostasis. *Cell Metab* 2005;1:309-22.

Chan DC, Watts GF. Dyslipidaemia in the metabolic syndrome and type 2 diabetes: pathogenesis, priorities, pharmacotherapies. *Expert Opin Pharmacother* 2011;12:13-30.

Chawla A, Lee CH, Barak Y et al. PPARdelta is a very low-density lipoprotein sensor in macrophages. *Proc Natl Acad Sci U S A* 2003;100:1268-73.

Chen Z, Gropler MC, Norris J, Lawrence JC, Jr., Harris TE, Finck BN. Alterations in hepatic metabolism in fld mice reveal a role for lipin 1 in regulating VLDL-triacylglyceride secretion. *Arterioscler Thromb Vasc Biol* 2008;28:1738-44.

Chung S, Lapoint K, Martinez K, Kennedy A, Boysen SM, McIntosh MK. Preadipocytes mediate lipopolysaccharide-induced inflammation and insulin resistance in primary cultures of newly differentiated human adipocytes. *Endocrinology* 2006;147:5340-5351.

Coll T, Barroso E, Alvarez-Guardia D et al. The Role of Peroxisome Proliferator-Activated Receptor beta/delta on the Inflammatory Basis of Metabolic Disease. *PPAR Res* 2010a;2010.

Coll T, Alvarez-Guardia D, Barroso E et al. Activation of peroxisome proliferator-activated receptor-{delta} by GW501516 prevents fatty acid-induced nuclear factor-{kappa}B activation and insulin resistance in skeletal muscle cells. *Endocrinology* 2010b;151:1560-1569.

Cortright RN, Azevedo JL, Zhou Q et al. Protein kinase C modulates insulin action in human skeletal muscle. *American Journal of Physiology-Endocrinology and Metabolism* 2000;278:E553-E562.

Daynes RA, Jones DC. Emerging roles of PPARs in inflammation and immunity. *Nat Rev Immunol* 2002;2:748-59.

deGoma EM, Leeper NJ, Heidenreich PA. Clinical significance of high-density lipoprotein cholesterol in patients with low low-density lipoprotein cholesterol. *J Am Coll Cardiol* 2008;51:49-55.

Delerive P, De Bosscher K, Vanden Berghe W, Fruchart JC, Haegeman G, Staels B. DNA binding-independent induction of I kappa B alpha gene transcription by PPAR alpha. *Molecular Endocrinology* 2002;16:1029-39.

Delerive P, De BK, Besnard S et al. Peroxisome proliferator-activated receptor alpha negatively regulates the vascular inflammatory gene response by negative cross-talk with transcription factors NF-kappaB and AP-1. *J Biol Chem* 1999;274:32048-54.

Desreumaux P, Dubuquoy L, Nutten S et al. Attenuation of colon inflammation through activators of the retinoid X receptor (RXR)/peroxisome proliferator-activated receptor gamma (PPARgamma) heterodimer. A basis for new therapeutic strategies. *J Exp Med* 2001;193:827-38.

Dreyer C, Krey G, Keller H, Givel F, Helftenbein G, Wahli W. Control of the peroxisomal beta-oxidation pathway by a novel family of nuclear hormone receptors. *Cell* 1992;68:879-87.

Du J, Guan T, Zhang H, Xia Y, Liu F, Zhang Y. Inhibitory crosstalk between ERK and AMPK in the growth and proliferation of cardiac fibroblasts. *Biochem Biophys Res Commun* 2008;368:402-7.

Eckel RH, Grundy SM, Zimmet PZ. The metabolic syndrome. *Lancet* 2005;365:1415-28.

Estall JL, Kahn M, Cooper MP et al. Sensitivity of lipid metabolism and insulin signaling to genetic alterations in hepatic peroxisome proliferator-activated receptor-gamma coactivator-1alpha expression. *Diabetes* 2009;58:1499-508.

Feige JN, Gelman L, Michalik L, Desvergne B, Wahli W. From molecular action to physiological outputs: peroxisome proliferator-activated receptors are nuclear receptors at the crossroads of key cellular functions. *Prog Lipid Res* 2006;45:120-159.

Finck BN, Gropler MC, Chen Z et al. Lipin 1 is an inducible amplifier of the hepatic PGC-1alpha/PPARalpha regulatory pathway. *Cell Metab* 2006;4:199-210.

Forman BM, Chen J, Evans RM. Hypolipidemic drugs, polyunsaturated fatty acids, and eicosanoids are ligands for peroxisome proliferator-activated receptors alpha and delta. *Proc Natl Acad Sci U S A* 1997;94:4312-17.

Fruchart JC, Sacks FM, Hermans MP et al. The Residual Risk Reduction Initiative: a call to action to reduce residual vascular risk in dyslipidaemic patient. *Diab Vasc Dis Res* 2008;5:319-35.

Gouni-Berthold I, Giannakidou E, Faust M, Berthold HK, Krone W. The peroxisome proliferator-activated receptor delta +294T/C polymorphism in relation to lipoprotein metabolism in patients with diabetes mellitus type 2 and in non-diabetic controls. *Atherosclerosis* 2005;183:336-41.

Griffin ME, Marcucci MJ, Cline GW et al. Free fatty acid-induced insulin resistance is associated with activation of protein kinase C theta and alterations in the insulin signaling cascade. *Diabetes* 1999;48:1270-1274.

Grundy SM. Atherogenic dyslipidemia: lipoprotein abnormalities and implications for therapy. *Am J Cardiol* 1995;75:45B-52B.

Grundy SM, Cleeman JI, Daniels SR et al. Diagnosis and management of the metabolic syndrome. An American Heart Association/National Heart, Lung, and Blood Institute Scientific Statement. Executive summary. *Cardiol Rev* 2005;13:322-27.

Gual P, Le Marchand-Brustel Y, Tanti JF. Positive and negative regulation of insulin signaling through IRS-1 phosphorylation. *Biochimie* 2005;87:99-109.

Gustafson B, Gogg S, Hedjazifar S, Jenndahl L, Hammarstedt A, Smith U. Inflammation and impaired adipogenesis in hypertrophic obesity in man. *Am J Physiol Endocrinol Metab* 2009.

Haber EP, Hirabara SM, Gomes AD, Curi R, Carpinelli AR, Carvalho CR. Palmitate modulates the early steps of insulin signalling pathway in pancreatic islets. *FEBS Lett* 2003;544:185-88.

Higashida K, Higuchi M, Terada S. Potential role of lipin-1 in exercise-induced mitochondrial biogenesis. *Biochem Biophys Res Commun* 2008;374:587-91.

Hirabara SM, Curi R, Maechler P. Saturated fatty acid-induced insulin resistance is associated with mitochondrial dysfunction in skeletal muscle cells. *J Cell Physiol* 2010;222:187-94.

Hirabara SM, Silveira LR, Abdulkader F, Carvalho CR, Procopio J, Curi R. Time-dependent effects of fatty acids on skeletal muscle metabolism. *J Cell Physiol* 2007;210:7-15.

Hondares E, Pineda-Torra I, Iglesias R, Staels B, Villarroya F, Giralt M. PPARdelta, but not PPARalpha, activates PGC-1alpha gene transcription in muscle. *Biochem Biophys Res Commun* 2007;354:1021-27.

Hotamisligil GS, Peraldi P, Budavari A, Ellis R, White MF, Spiegelman BM. IRS-1-mediated inhibition of insulin receptor tyrosine kinase activity in TNF-alpha- and obesity-induced insulin resistance. *Science* 1996;271:665-68.

Itani SI, Zhou Q, Pories WJ, MacDonald KG, Dohm GL. Involvement of protein kinase C in human skeletal muscle insulin resistance and obesity. *Diabetes* 2000;49:1353-58.

Jeninga EH, Schoonjans K, Auwerx J. Reversible acetylation of PGC-1: connecting energy sensors and effectors to guarantee metabolic flexibility. *Oncogene* 2010;29:4617-24.

Johnson TE, Holloway MK, Vogel R et al. Structural requirements and cell-type specificity for ligand activation of peroxisome proliferator-activated receptors. *J Steroid Biochem Mol Biol* 1997;63:1-8.

Kamei Y, Xu L, Heinzel T et al. A CBP integrator complex mediates transcriptional activation and AP-1 inhibition by nuclear receptors. *Cell* 1996;85:403-14.

Kannel WB. High-density lipoproteins: epidemiologic profile and risks of coronary artery disease. *Am J Cardiol* 1983;52:9B-12B.

Kern PA, Ranganathan S, Li C, Wood L, Ranganathan G. Adipose tissue tumor necrosis factor and interleukin-6 expression in human obesity and insulin resistance. *Am J Physiol Endocrinol Metab* 2001;280:E745-E751.

Kersten S. Peroxisome proliferator activated receptors and lipoprotein metabolism. *PPAR Res* 2008;2008:132960.

Kersten S, Desvergne B, Wahli W. Roles of PPARs in health and disease. *Nature* 2000;405:421-24.

Kim JK, Kim YJ, Fillmore JJ et al. Prevention of fat-induced insulin resistance by salicylate. *Journal of Clinical Investigation* 2001;108:437-46.

Kliewer SA, Forman BM, Blumberg B et al. Differential expression and activation of a family of murine peroxisome proliferator-activated receptors. *Proc Natl Acad Sci U S A* 1994;91:7355-59.

Kramer DK, Al-Khalili L, Guigas B, Leng Y, Garcia-Roves PM, Krook A. Role of AMP kinase and PPARdelta in the regulation of lipid and glucose metabolism in human skeletal muscle. *J Biol Chem* 2007;282:19313-20.

Krey G, Braissant O, L'Horset F et al. Fatty acids, eicosanoids, and hypolipidemic agents identified as ligands of peroxisome proliferator-activated receptors by coactivator-dependent receptor ligand assay. *Mol Endocrinol* 1997;11:779-91.

Lan F, Cacicedo JM, Ruderman N, Ido Y. SIRT1 modulation of the acetylation status, cytosolic localization, and activity of LKB1. Possible role in AMP-activated protein kinase activation. *J Biol Chem* 2008;283:27628-35.

Lee CH, Olson P, Hevener A et al. PPARdelta regulates glucose metabolism and insulin sensitivity. *Proc Natl Acad Sci U S A* 2006a;103:3444-49.

Lee WJ, Kim M, Park HS et al. AMPK activation increases fatty acid oxidation in skeletal muscle by activating PPARalpha and PGC-1. *Biochem Biophys Res Commun* 2006b;340:291-95.

Leibowitz MD, Fievet C, Hennuyer N et al. Activation of PPARdelta alters lipid metabolism in db/db mice. *FEBS Lett* 2000;473:333-36.

Lewis GF. Fatty acid regulation of very low density lipoprotein production. *Curr Opin Lipidol* 1997;8:146-53.

Li M, Pascual G, Glass CK. Peroxisome proliferator-activated receptor gamma-dependent repression of the inducible nitric oxide synthase gene. *Mol Cell Biol* 2000;20:4699-707.

Lorenzo C, Wagenknecht LE, Hanley AJ, Rewers MJ, Karter AJ, Haffner SM. A1C between 5.7 and 6.4% as a marker for identifying pre-diabetes, insulin sensitivity and secretion, and cardiovascular risk factors: the Insulin Resistance Atherosclerosis Study (IRAS). *Diabetes Care* 2010;33:2104-9.

Mathieu P, Lemieux I, Despres JP. Obesity, inflammation, and cardiovascular risk. *Clin Pharmacol Ther* 2010;87:407-16.

Mathieu P, Pibarot P, Despres JP. Metabolic syndrome: the danger signal in atherosclerosis. *Vasc Health Risk Manag* 2006;2:285-302.

Miller M, Cannon CP, Murphy SA, Qin J, Ray KK, Braunwald E. Impact of triglyceride levels beyond low-density lipoprotein cholesterol after acute coronary syndrome in the PROVE IT-TIMI 22 trial. *J Am Coll Cardiol* 2008;51:724-30.

Nguyen MT, Favelyukis S, Nguyen AK et al. A subpopulation of macrophages infiltrates hypertrophic adipose tissue and is activated by free fatty acids via Toll-like receptors 2 and 4 and JNK-dependent pathways. *J Biol Chem* 2007;282:35279-92.

Okazaki M, Iwasaki Y, Nishiyama M et al. PPARbeta/delta regulates the human SIRT1 gene transcription via Sp1. *Endocr J* 2010;57:403-13.

Oliver WR, Jr., Shenk JL, Snaith MR et al. A selective peroxisome proliferator-activated receptor delta agonist promotes reverse cholesterol transport. *Proc Natl Acad Sci U S A* 2001;98:5306-11.

Perseghin G, Petersen K, Shulman GI. Cellular mechanism of insulin resistance: potential links with inflammation. *Int J Obes Relat Metab Disord* 2003;27 Suppl 3:S6-11.

Peters JM, Lee SS, Li W et al. Growth, adipose, brain, and skin alterations resulting from targeted disruption of the mouse peroxisome proliferator-activated receptor beta(delta). *Mol Cell Biol* 2000;20:5119-28.

Pickup JC, Mattock MB, Chusney GD, Burt D. NIDDM as a disease of the innate immune system: association of acute-phase reactants and interleukin-6 with metabolic syndrome X. *Diabetologia* 1997;40:1286-92.

Pradhan AD, Manson JE, Rifai N, Buring JE, Ridker PM. C-reactive protein, interleukin 6, and risk of developing type 2 diabetes mellitus. *JAMA* 2001;286:327-34.

Reznick RM, Shulman GI. The role of AMP-activated protein kinase in mitochondrial biogenesis. *J Physiol* 2006;574:33-39.

Riserus U, Sprecher D, Johnson T et al. Activation of peroxisome proliferator-activated receptor (PPAR)delta promotes reversal of multiple metabolic abnormalities, reduces oxidative stress, and increases fatty acid oxidation in moderately obese men. *Diabetes* 2008;57:332-39.

Robitaille J, Gaudet D, Perusse L, Vohl MC. Features of the metabolic syndrome are modulated by an interaction between the peroxisome proliferator-activated receptor-delta -87T>C polymorphism and dietary fat in French-Canadians. *Int J Obes (Lond)* 2007;31:411-17.

Roden M, Perseghin G, Petersen KF et al. The roles of insulin and glucagon in the regulation of hepatic glycogen synthesis and turnover in humans. *J Clin Invest* 1996;97:642-48.

Rodriguez-Calvo R, Serrano L, Coll T et al. Activation of peroxisome proliferator-activated receptor beta/delta inhibits lipopolysaccharide-induced cytokine production in adipocytes by lowering nuclear factor-kappaB activity via extracellular signal-related kinase 1/2. *Diabetes* 2008;57:2149-57.

Rosenson RS, Otvos JD, Freedman DS. Relations of lipoprotein subclass levels and low-density lipoprotein size to progression of coronary artery disease in the Pravastatin Limitation of Atherosclerosis in the Coronary Arteries (PLAC-I) trial. *Am J Cardiol* 2002;90:89-94.

Ruderman NB, Xu XJ, Nelson L et al. AMPK and SIRT1: a long-standing partnership? *Am J Physiol Endocrinol Metab* 2010;298:E751-E760.

Sanderson LM, Boekschoten MV, Desvergne B, Muller M, Kersten S. Transcriptional profiling reveals divergent roles of PPARalpha and PPARbeta/delta in regulation of gene expression in mouse liver. *Physiol Genomics* 2010;41:42-52.

Schrauwen P, Schrauwen-Hinderling V, Hoeks J, Hesselink MK. Mitochondrial dysfunction and lipotoxicity. *Biochim Biophys Acta* 2010;1801:266-71.

Sebastian D, Herrero L, Serra D, Asins G, Hegardt FG. CPT I overexpression protects L6E9 muscle cells from fatty acid-induced insulin resistance. *Am J Physiol Endocrinol Metab* 2007;292:E677-E686.

Serrano-Marco L, Rodriguez-Calvo R, El K, I et al. Activation of Peroxisome Proliferator-Activated Receptor-{beta}/-{delta} (PPAR-{beta}/-{delta}) Ameliorates Insulin Signaling and Reduces SOCS3 Levels by Inhibiting STAT3 in Interleukin-6-Stimulated Adipocytes. *Diabetes* 2011;60:1990-1999.

Shaw N, Elholm M, Noy N. Retinoic acid is a high affinity selective ligand for the peroxisome proliferator-activated receptor beta/delta. *J Biol Chem* 2003;278:41589-92.

Shepherd J, Barter P, Carmena R et al. Effect of lowering LDL cholesterol substantially below currently recommended levels in patients with coronary heart disease and diabetes: the Treating to New Targets (TNT) study. *Diabetes Care* 2006;29:1220-1226.

Shepherd J, Betteridge J, Van GL. Nicotinic acid in the management of dyslipidaemia associated with diabetes and metabolic syndrome: a position paper developed by a European Consensus Panel. *Curr Med Res Opin* 2005;21:665-82.

Shi H, Kokoeva MV, Inouye K, Tzameli I, Yin H, Flier JS. TLR4 links innate immunity and fatty acid-induced insulin resistance. *J Clin Invest* 2006;116:3015-25.

Shoelson SE, Lee J, Goldfine AB. Inflammation and insulin resistance. *J Clin Invest* 2006;116:1793-801.

Silveira LR, Fiamoncini J, Hirabara SM et al. Updating the effects of fatty acids on skeletal muscle. *J Cell Physiol* 2008;217:1-12.

Skogsberg J, Kannisto K, Cassel TN, Hamsten A, Eriksson P, Ehrenborg E. Evidence that peroxisome proliferator-activated receptor delta influences cholesterol metabolism in men. *Arterioscler Thromb Vasc Biol* 2003;23:637-43.

Sugden MC, Caton PW, Holness MJ. PPAR control: it's SIRTainly as easy as PGC. *J Endocrinol* 2010;204:93-104.

Sznaidman ML, Haffner CD, Maloney PR et al. Novel selective small molecule agonists for peroxisome proliferator-activated receptor delta (PPARdelta)--synthesis and biological activity. *Bioorg Med Chem Lett* 2003;13:1517-21.

Takada I, Yu RT, Xu HE et al. Alteration of a single amino acid in peroxisome proliferator-activated receptor-alpha (PPAR alpha) generates a PPAR delta phenotype. *Mol Endocrinol* 2000;14:733-40.

Tan NS, Michalik L, Noy N et al. Critical roles of PPAR beta/delta in keratinocyte response to inflammation. *Genes Dev* 2001;15:3263-77.

Tanaka T, Yamamoto J, Iwasaki S et al. Activation of peroxisome proliferator-activated receptor delta induces fatty acid beta-oxidation in skeletal muscle and attenuates metabolic syndrome. *Proc Natl Acad Sci U S A* 2003;100:15924-29.

Taskinen MR. Diabetic dyslipidaemia: from basic research to clinical practice. *Diabetologia* 2003;46:733-49.

Turner RC, Millns H, Neil HA et al. Risk factors for coronary artery disease in non-insulin dependent diabetes mellitus: United Kingdom Prospective Diabetes Study (UKPDS: 23). *BMJ* 1998;316:823-28.

van d, V, Kruit JK, Havinga R et al. Reduced cholesterol absorption upon PPARdelta activation coincides with decreased intestinal expression of NPC1L1. *J Lipid Res* 2005;46:526-34.

Wallace JM, Schwarz M, Coward P et al. Effects of peroxisome proliferator-activated receptor alpha/delta agonists on HDL-cholesterol in vervet monkeys. *J Lipid Res* 2005;46:1009-16.

Wang YX, Zhang CL, Yu RT et al. Regulation of muscle fiber type and running endurance by PPARdelta. *PLoS Biol* 2004;2:e294.

Wellen KE, Hotamisligil GS. Inflammation, stress, and diabetes. *J Clin Invest* 2005;115:1111-19.

Xu HE, Lambert MH, Montana VG et al. Molecular recognition of fatty acids by peroxisome proliferator-activated receptors. *Mol Cell* 1999;3:397-403.

Yu K, Bayona W, Kallen CB et al. Differential activation of peroxisome proliferator-activated receptors by eicosanoids. *J Biol Chem* 1995;270:23975-83.

Yuan MS, Konstantopoulos N, Lee JS et al. Reversal of obesity- and diet-induced insulin resistance with salicylates or targeted disruption of IKK beta. *Science* 2001;293:1673-77.

Zamir I, Zhang J, Lazar MA. Stoichiometric and steric principles governing repression by nuclear hormone receptors. *Genes Dev* 1997;11:835-46.

Zenimaru Y, Takahashi S, Takahashi M et al. Glucose deprivation accelerates VLDL receptor-mediated TG-rich lipoprotein uptake by AMPK activation in skeletal muscle cells. *Biochem Biophys Res Commun* 2008;368:716-22.

Zhang BB, Zhou G, Li C. AMPK: an emerging drug target for diabetes and the metabolic syndrome. *Cell Metab* 2009;9:407-16.

Zhang Y, Castellani LW, Sinal CJ, Gonzalez FJ, Edwards PA. Peroxisome proliferator-activated receptor-gamma coactivator 1alpha (PGC-1alpha) regulates triglyceride metabolism by activation of the nuclear receptor FXR. *Genes Dev* 2004;18:157-69.

Zheng Y, Zhang W, Pendleton E et al. Improved insulin sensitivity by calorie restriction is associated with reduction of ERK and p70S6K activities in the liver of obese Zucker rats. *J Endocrinol* 2009;203:337-47.

12

Liver Glucokinase and Lipid Metabolism

Anna Vidal-Alabró, Andrés Méndez-Lucas, Jana Semakova,
Alícia G. Gómez-Valadés and Jose C. Perales
Department of Physiological Sciences II,
University of Barcelona, Barcelona,
Spain

1. Introduction

Control of energy metabolism is crucial for optimal functioning of organs and tissues. Amongst all nutrients, glucose is the principal energy source for most cells and, therefore, minimum blood glucose levels must be guaranteed. Alterations in glycaemia can lead to hyperglycaemic states (producing protein glycosylation and toxicity in glucose-sensitive cells) or hypoglycaemic states (that can affect brain function), both harmful. Therefore, mechanisms must exist to keep glycaemia in a narrow physiological range (4-8 mM) independently of the nutritional state. To achieve control of blood glucose levels, our body has a complex, interorgan signaling system using nutrients (glucose, lipids, amino acids), hormones (insulin, glucagon, ghrelin, etc.) and the autonomic nervous system. In response to these signals, organs and tissues (mainly intestine, endocrine pancreas, liver, skeletal muscle, adipose tissue, brain and adrenal glands) adapt their function to energetic requirements.

The liver plays a pivotal role in the maintenance of glucose homeostasis by continuously adapting its metabolism to energetic needs. In the fed state, when blood glucose levels are high and there is insulin, liver takes-up part glucose to replenish glycogen stores. Besides, when glucose stores are full, the liver has the capacity to synthesize lipids *de novo* from glucose for-long term energy storage. Lipids are packaged in very low-density lipoprotein (VLDL) particles and then transported to the adipose tissue. Conversely during starvation, when glycaemia falls and glucagon increases, the liver produces glucose to maintain circulating glucose levels by breaking down glycogen stores or by synthesizing glucose de novo through gluconeogenesis. Gluconeogenesis, as an energy-consuming pathway, is linked to β-oxidation of fatty acids (fuel supplier pathway).

From this introduction on the regulation of glucose homeostasis, one can appreciate the close relation that exists between carbohydrate metabolism and lipid metabolism in the liver. Therefore, alterations in hepatic carbohydrate metabolic pathways may directly affect hepatic and/or blood lipid levels. Particularly, this chapter will focus on evaluating the incidence of glucokinase (GK) –the first enzyme of the glycolytic pathway in the liver- on lipidemia and on hepatic lipid content. But first, an introductory overview of the physiology behind the first-pass metabolism of dietary glucose in the liver will be presented.

2. Liver glucose metabolism

After a meal rich in carbohydrates, high levels of glucose reach the liver via portal vein. Glucose enters passively the hepatocyte through GLUT-2, a facilitated glucose transporter, and then is rapidly phosphorylated by GK at the sixth carbon to obtain glucose-6-phosphate which cannot escape the cell. From a functional perspective, it is important to recognize that both GLUT2 and glucokinase are expressed in cell types in which glucose metabolism has to vary accordingly to extracellular glucose concentration (glucose sensors). The high Km for glucose of both proteins, and the absence of product inhibition by glucose-6-phosphate, ensure that glucose uptake and phosphorylation in these cells are proportional to extracellular glucose concentration throughout the physiological range of glycaemia

The product of GK reaction, glucose-6-phosphate, is the gateway to the major pathways of glucose utilization: glycogen synthesis, glycolysis, oxidation of glucose and pentose phosphate pathway. It should be noted that hepatic glycolysis provides pyruvate principally for lipid synthesis rather than for oxidation. As glucose is the main substrate for fatty acid synthesis, hepatic glycolytic enzymes can be considered an extension of the lipogenic pathway. Glucose, insulin and parasympathetic nervous system orchestrate these glucose metabolic pathways in the fed state, with the aim of maintaining normal levels of blood sugar.

2.1 Glycogen synthesis

Two enzymes, glycogen synthase and glycogen phosphorylase, control glycogen levels. Both enzymes are regulated by phosphorylation and allosteric modulators. Specifically in the fed state, insulin activates glycogen synthase (limiting enzyme for glycogen synthesis) by promoting its dephosphorylation and, at the same time inhibits glycogen phosphorylase (important for glycogen breakdown). Meanwhile, glucose-6-phosphate binding to glycogen synthase favours its dephosphorylation, promoting glycogen synthase activity (Bollen, 1998; Agius, 2008). As a result, glucose coming from bloodstream fills hepatic glycogen stores.

2.2 Lipogenesis *de novo*

Hepatic lipogenesis is induced upon ingestion of excess carbohydrates to convert extra carbohydrates to triglyceride for long-time energy storage. Once inside the hepatocyte, glucose enters glycolytic pathway and provides pyruvate, which enters mitochondrion where it is converted into acetyl-CoA by pyruvate dehydrogenase. On the other side, in the cytoplasm glucose is also oxidized through the pentose phosphate pathway and NADPH is obtained. Acetyl-CoA will serve for fatty acid and also cholesterol synthesis. The initial steps for fatty acid synthesis are the transfer of acetyl-CoA from mitochondria to the cytoplasm and its conversion into malonyl-CoA under the action of the enzyme acetyl-CoA carboxylase. Importantly, malonyl-CoA is a regulatory molecule because it inhibits carnitine palmitoyltransferase-1, a rate limiting enzyme in β-oxidation of fatty acids. Therefore, increasing malonyl-CoA favours lipogenesis. Malonyl-CoA is elongated using NADPH under the action of the enzyme fatty acid synthase. Once obtained, fatty acids can be esterified with glycerol to form diglyceride and triglyceride. Most of the triglyceride is produced for export to the adipose tissue, but in order to be secreted, it must be packaged in very low-density lipoprotein (VLDL) particles together with cholesterol, phospholipids and apolipoprotein B (Figure 1).

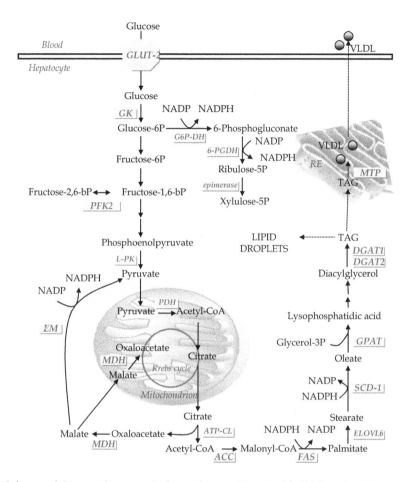

Fig. 1. Scheme of de novo lipogenesis from glucose. Once inside the hepatocyte, glucose is metabolized on one hand through glycolysis to pyruvate (GK means glucokinase; PFK-2, 6, phosphofructo-2-kinase/fructose-2,6-bisphosphatase; L-PK, liver-pyruvate kinase). On the other hand, glucose is oxidized through pentose phosphate pathway to obtain NADPH (G6P-DH means glucose-6-phosphate dehydrogenase; 6-PGDH, 6-phosphogluconate dehydrogenase). Pyruvate enters the mitochondrion to obtain citrate (PDH means, pyruvate dehydrogenase; MDH, malate dehydrogenase and EM, malic enzyme). De novo synthesis of fatty acids starts with citrate (ATP-CL means ATP citrate lyase; ACC, acetyl-CoA carboxylase) and after suffering elongation and desaturation reactions (ELOVL6 means elongase that catalyzes the conversion of palmitate to stearate; SCD-1, stearoyl-coenzyme A desaturase), fatty acids are converted to triglyceride (TAG) (GPAT means glycerol-3-phosphate acyltransferase; DGAT, diacylglycerol acyltransferase). Triglyceride can be stored in the liver but are mostly packaged into VLDL (very low-density lipoprotein) and secreted to bloodstream (MTP means microsomal triglyceride transfer protein). Original artwork.

In mammals, hepatic lipogenesis is controlled by several transcription factors, mainly SREBP-1c (sterol regulatory element binding protein 1c) and ChREBP (carbohydrate-responsive element-binding protein), but also by PPAR-γ (peroxisome proliferator-activated receptor gamma), LXR-α (liver X receptor alpha) and XBP1, all of them regulated by nutritional and hormonal conditions.

SREBP-1c plays a major role in the induction of lipogenic genes by insulin. SREBP-1c is a member of the bZIP transcription factor family that was originally identified as a mediator of sterol signaling (Wang, 1994), and is produced as a precursor form that reside in the endoplasmic reticulum in an inactive state. On one hand insulin stimulates SREBP-1c gene transcription, and on the other hand, induces the maturation of SREBP-1c precursor (Shimomura, 1998). Mature SREBP-1c moves to nucleus and activates transcription of several lipogenic genes with SRE (sterol regulatory elements) sequences in their promoters, for instance fatty acid synthase (FAS), stearoyl-Coenzyme A desaturase 1 (SCD-1), etc. (Figure 2) (Foretz, 1999; Ferre, 2010).

Glucose regulates genes of glycolytic and lipogenic pathways by activating ChREBP (Iizuka, 2008). ChREBP is a transcription factor that binds to ChoRE sequences present in the promoter of ACC (acetyl Coenzyme-A carboxylase), fatty acid synthase (FAS), stearoyl-Coenzyme A desaturase 1 (SCD-1), L-pyruvate kinase (L-PK), etc. (Uyeda, 2006). Under basal conditions, ChREBP is phosphorylated at Ser196 and remains in the cytosol. When glycaemia increase, glucose enters the hepatocyte and is metabolized. Therefore there is an increase in some glucose metabolites such as xylulose-5P, which promotes ChREBP dephosphorylation (Kabashima, 2003). Then, ChREBP rapidly moves to the nucleus and will activate transcription of its target genes (Figure 2).

SREBP-1c and ChREBP are also transcriptionally activated by liver X receptor apha (LXR-α), which could be a glucose sensor although it is controversial (Mitro, 2007; Denechaud, 2008). LXR-α is classically activated by oxysterols and it is important for the transcription of some lipogenic genes, a part form SREBP-1c and ChREBP, since their promoters contain LXRE (LXR response element) sequences (Chen, 2004; Cha, 2007).

XBP1, a transcription factor best known as a key regulator of the unfolded protein response (UPR), has been surprisingly associated with *de novo* fatty acid synthesis in the liver. It seems to be induced by diet carbohydrates and its deletion in mice causes hypocholesterolemia and hypotriglyceridemia, attributed to diminished hepatic lipid production (Lee, 2008). But, there are still some questions about its function to answer: what is its binding site in the promoter regions of these genes? Does it act alone or in partnership with other known transcription factors such as SREBP, ChREBP and LXR?

In summary, hepatic lipogenesis is regulated by several transcription factors that may probably work synergistically (Figure 2). With this complex system, carbons from glucose can be directed to fatty acid synthesis only when there is substrate availability and glycogen depots have been replenished. Altered fatty acid synthesis in the liver can lead to changes in lipid secretion, and consequently to dyslipidemia (Ginsberg, 2006).

2.3 Inhibition of hepatic glucose production

During fasting, liver produces glucose that enters bloodstream in order to maintain glycaemia, ensuring fuel supply for brain and red blood cells. But after a meal, when diet glucose arrives, hepatocytes must switch glucose production to glucose uptake. Insulin and high glucose levels coordinate the inhibition of glycogenolysis and gluconeogenesis (glucose producing pathways).

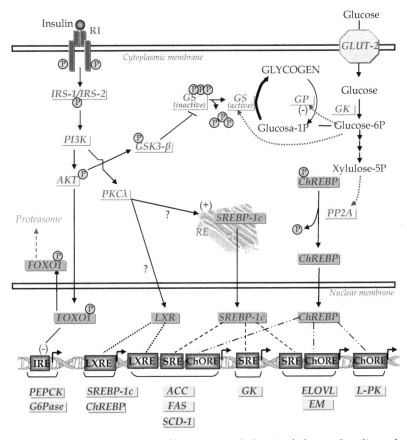

Fig. 2. Main regulatory mechanisms of hepatic metabolism in fed state. Insulin and glucose direct gene transcription to switch from glucose producing pathways to glucose uptake and storage. Briefly, insulin signaling promotes the phosphorylation of FOXO1 that results in its nuclear exclusion and proteasome degradation; consequently, transcription of gluconeogenic genes is inhibited. Besides, insulin stimulates transcription of lipogenic genes through SREBP-1c activation and probably through LXR-α, as well. Finally, insulin signaling causes activation of glycogen synthase function. Glucose also controls allostericaly glycogen synthesis and promote transcription of lipogenic genes via activation of ChREBP. IR means insulin receptor, IRS, insulin receptor substrate; PI3K, phosphoinositide 3-kinse; AKT, Ser/Thr protein kinase; GSK3-β, glycogen synthase kinase 3.beta; FOXO1, forkhead box O1; PCK, protein kinase C; LXR, liver X receptor; SREBP-1c, sterol regulatory element binding protein 1c; ChREBP, carbohydrate response element binding protein; GS, glycogen synthase; GP, glycogen phosphorylase; GK, glucokinase; PP2A, protein phosphatase 2A); IRE, insulin response element; LXRE liver X receptor response element; SRE, sterol regulatory elements; ChORE, carbohydrate-response elements; PEPCK-C, cytosolic phosphoenolpyruvate carboxykinase; G6Pase, glucose-6-phosphatase; ACC, Acyl-CoA carboxylase; FAS, fatty acid synthase; SCD-1, stearoyl-CoA desaturase 1; ELOVL , EM, malic enzyme and L-PK, liver-pyruvate kinase. Original artwork.

Insulin directly inhibits the transcription of gluconeogenic genes by promoting the phosphorylation of FOXO1 (forkhead box O), a transcription factor necessary for the induction of gluconeogenesis in conjunction with PGC-1α (PPAR-gamma coactivator 1-alpha) (Puigserver, 2003). In addition, SREBP-1c promotes the inhibition of some gluconeogenic genes. Insulin also represses glycogenolysis by phosphorylating glycogen synthase (Bollen, 1998). On the other hand, insulin regulates hepatic glucose production indirectly: a) it suppresses lipolysis in adipose tissue causing a reduction in glycerol (gluconeogenic substrate) availability; b) it inhibits glucagon secretion in the pancreas; and c) it activates hypothalamic pathways important for glucose homeostasis.

Synergistically with insulin, glucose inhibits glycogenolysis allosterically (Bollen, 1998). Glucose inhibition on gluconeogenesis is mediated by glucose metabolites, specifically fructose-2,6-bisphosphate (Wu, 2001) and xylulose-5-phosphate (Massillon, 1998).

3. Glucokinase regulates the fate of glucose carbons in the liver

In order to enter the lipogenic pathway, glucose must be metabolized. The first and rate-limiting step is the phosphorylation of glucose at the 6th carbon to obtain glucose-6-phosphate. This reaction is catalyzed by glucokinase (GK; EC 2.7.1.1), a member of the hexokinase family. However, GK differs from other hexokinases in its particular kinetic properties: affinity for glucose that is within the physiological plasma concentration range ($S_{0.5}$ for glucose of 8 mM), positive cooperativity for glucose although it is a monomeric enzyme, and lack of inhibition by glucose-6-phosphate (Table 1).

	HEXOKINASES 1-3	GLUCOKINASE
Molecular weight	100 KDa	50 KDa
Substrates	Hexoses	Glucose
$S_{0.5}$ for glucose	< 0.5 mM	8 mM
Kinetic	Hyperbolic	Sigmoidal
Product inhibition	Yes	No

Table 1. Hexokinase family kinetic properties

As a result of its kinetic characteristics, intracellular glucose phosphorylation rate inside the hepatocyte correlates with glycaemia. Hence, GK can be considered an intracellular glucose sensor. Consequently, apart from hepatocytes, GK is expressed in glucosensitive cells of the pancreas, hypothalamus, anterior pituitary gland, and entero-endocrine K and L cells of the gut (Schuit, 2001; Zelent, 2006; Vieira, 2007; Iynedjian, 2009), all of them crucial in the control of the whole-body glucose homeostasis.

Liver contains 99.9% of the body GK. Therefore, is not surprising that this enzyme influences intermediary metabolism and energy storage. GK reaction controls the flux of glucose through several metabolic pathways: glycolysis, glucose oxidization, glycogenesis, triglyceride synthesis, phospholipids and cholesterol synthesis, glycogenolysis and gluconeogenesis. For that reason, GK is an enzyme highly regulated in the liver, both at the transcriptional and the post-transcriptional level.

3.1 Regulation of GK activity in the liver

Gck gene has two distinct promoters and one of them directs gene transcription specifically in the liver (Postic, 1995). Hepatic GK expression responds to nutritional changes; it is activated by insulin and inhibited by glucagon. Insulin induction of Gck gene expression is through the PI$_3$-kinase/Akt signaling. However, no IRE (insulin response element) has been described in Gck promoter, and it is not clear which transcription factor mediates insulin-directed Gck expression. SREBP-1c is a candidate to mediate insulin-directed expression of Gck, although controversial results exist (Foretz, 1999; Gregory, 2006). Probably, SREBP-1c is not essential for rapid induction of GK transcription, but it can have a role for long-term expression. Other candidates to mediate insulin-dependent expression of Gck gene are the complex HIF-α/HNF-4/p300 (Roth, 2004), and ERR-α -estrogen-related receptor alpha-(Zhu, 2010).

GK can be modulated by covalent modifications such as nitrosylation and phosphorylation. However, the physiological importance of these modifications is still not determined. More importantly, protein interaction affects GK activity and even intracellular distribution. It has been described that GK in the liver can interact with GKRP (glucokinase regulatory protein), BAD (Bcl-xL/Bcl-2-Associated Death Promoter), PFK-2 (6-phosphofructo-2-kinase/fructose-2,6-bisphosphatase), GKAP (glucokinase-associated protein), etc. (Massa, 2010). From all GK protein partners, GKRP is the best studied and has high physiological relevance in the liver.

3.1.1 Post-transcriptional regulation by GKRP

GKRP regulation of GK affects both the activity and subcellular localization of the enzyme. GKRP is a competitive inhibitor with respect to glucose. Van Shaftingen *et al* proposed a mechanistic model (Van Shaftingen, 2004); GKRP exists in two conformations, one with low affinity for GK and the other with high affinity. Fructose-1-phosphate and fructose-6-phosphate bind to the same binding site in the GKRP protein. When fructose-1-phosphate is bound to GKRP, GKRP adopts a conformation with low affinity for GK, and on the contrary, when the binding of fructose-6-phosphate to GKRP favours its interaction with GK.

But, Kamata *et al* also described that GK can exist in different conformations with different affinity for glucose (Kamata, 2004); in the absence of glucose, the enzyme exists in a super-open conformation thermodynamically stable and with low affinity for substrate. When glucose binds to it, there is a conformational change to an open form and next to a closed conformation that binds ATP. Then the catalytic cycle completes, after reaction products are released, GK can relax to an open or to a super-open conformation, depending on glucose concentrations (considering that the open conformation has higher affinity for glucose). GK conformation is important for GKRP protein interaction, as it can only take place when GK is in the super-open conformation (Anderka, 2008). From these conformational models of GKRP and GK, one can extrapolate the exquisite influence of carbohydrate concentration in regulating GKRP/GK binding and, consequently, GK phosphorylating activity.

GKRP also plays a fundamental role in importing GK to the nucleus, as it can be deduced from animals null for GKRP that present GK permanently in the cytosol (Farrelly, 1999). At low glucose concentrations, GKRP binds to GK and the formation of GKRP/GK complex results in entry and sequestration of both proteins in the nucleus of hepatocytes. However, it is still not resolved how GK is translocated to the nucleus. On the other hand, in metabolic states with high glucose concentrations, accompanied or not by high fructose levels, and sufficient ATP, there is the dissociation of the GKRP/GK complex. GK has a nuclear export signal sequence. Therefore, once dissociated from the complex, GK can be exported to the cytoplasm (Shiota, 1999). Insulin also favours the dissociation of the complex.

The physiological function of GKRP consists of inhibiting GK activity by sequestering it to the nucleus. GKRP binding also serves to stabilize GK protein and protect it from degradation. Thus, thanks to GKRP a big reservoir of GK exists in the nucleus of the hepatocyte at low glucose concentration. After a meal, this reservoir of GK can be rapidly mobilized (translocation is complete within 30 minutes) to the cytosol in order to promote glucose uptake and storage in the liver. This regulation process is much more fast and efficient than the synthesis de novo of GK promoted by insulin. Conversely, when glucose uptake has finished, GK returns to the nucleus in order to save energy because, on one hand, this translocation avoids the futile cycle between glucose and glucose-6-phosphate, and on the other hand, it ends the glucose signal generated by GK activity that activate transcription of glycolytic and lipogenic genes (Figure 3). The consequence of GK translocation to the nucleus in the post-absorptive state is the induction of glycogenolysis and gluconeogenesis.

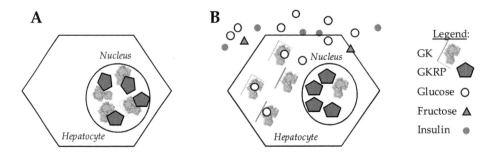

Fig. 3. Subcellular localization of GK regulated by GKRP. (A) During fasting, GK is sequestered in the nucleus where it remains bound to GKRP and inactive. After a meal, nutritional signals (i.e. insulin, glucose and fructose) induce the dissociation of the GK/GKRP complex and free GK translocates to the cytosol. Original artwork.

To summarize, thanks to its kinetic properties and its subtle regulation, GK enables the liver to adapt its metabolism for glucose uptake or glucose production as required, and consequently to regulate energy homeostasis.

3.2 GK modulation in the liver: impact on carbohydrate and lipid metabolism

Numerous natural mutations in GK gene have been associated to disease (Gloyn, 2003 & Osbak, 2009), reinforcing the concept that it is a crucial enzyme in the control of whole-body glucose homeostasis. Mutations that cause decrease or loss of GK activity are associated to maturity onset diabetes of the young-2 (MODY-2) or to permanent neonatal diabetes mellitus (PNDM). In diabetes, as a result of impairment in insulin secretion, the capacity of the liver to uptake glucose is diminished. On the other hand, activating mutations of GK cause persistent hyperinsulinemic hypoglycemia in infancy (PHHI). The phenotype of all these pathologies is mainly dominated by GK function in the pancreatic β-cell, where it regulates glucose-dependent insulin secretion. As insulin controls hepatic GK transcription and influences GKRP regulation, it is difficult to elucidate which are the specific consequences of these mutations on hepatic GK independently of insulin.

Some animal models have been developed to study the specific role of liver GK on metabolism.

3.2.1 Genetic suppression of hepatic GK

A liver specific GK knock-out was obtained using the LoxP-Cre system (Postic, 1999). Transgenic mice showed mild hyperglycemia and hyperinsulinemia in basal conditions, without changes in hepatic glycogen, plasma non-esterified fatty acids, triglycerides or β-hydroxybutyrate. In hyperglycaemic clamp studies, reduced hepatic glucose uptake and glycogen levels were observed in KO animals; however, results on lipid profile were not provided.

3.2.2 Genetic overexpression of GK in the liver

Several liver GK gain-of-function studies, both using transgenic animals and by means of adenovirus gene transfer, have been performed in healthy animals and models of diabetes such as streptozotocin induced type I and type II induced by ingestion of high fat/high carbohydrate diet. Due to heterogeneity, these studies will be examined according to the animal model and analysis conditions.

a. Overexpression of GK in the liver of fed, healthy animals is summarized in Table 2 (Ferre, 1996a, 1996b, 2003; O'Doherty, 1999; Scott, 2003).

Study variables	Ferre 1996a, 1996b Ferre 2003		O'Doherty 1999; Scott 2003	
Animal model	Mus musculus Transgenic PEPCK-C promoter		Rattus norvegicus Adenoviral gene transfer CMV promoter	
GK activity over control	x 2		x 3	x 6.4
Age at analysis	2 months	12 months	5 days post-injection (Rats 200-250 g)	
Glycaemia	decrease	-	no change	Decrease
Blood lactate	-	-	increase	Increase
Blood triglycerides	~ increase	-	~ increase	Increase
NEFA	~ increase	-	no change	increase
Insulin	decrease	increase	no change	decrease
Hepatic glucose-6-P	increase	~ increase	-	-
Hepatic glycogen	increase	decrease	no change	no change
Hepatic triglycerides	no change	increase	-	-
Modulation of enzymes and transcription factors	↑ L-PK ↓PEPCK-C, GLUT-2, TAT	-	↑ L-PK, ACC1, FAS, G6Pase. No change in PEPCK-K	-

Table 2. Hepatic GK overexpression studies in healthy fed animals. Comments: decrease, increase and no change are referred to control group. "~" means no statistically significant; "-", no determined; "CMV", cytomegalovirus; "PEPCK-C", cytosolic phosphoenolpyruvate carboxykinase; "L-PK", liver pyruvate kinase; "TAT", tyrosine aminotransferase; "ACC1", Acetyl-Coenzyme A carboxylase 1; "FAS", fatty acid synthase; and "G6Pase", glucose-6 phosphatase.

In these models, enhancing hepatic glucose uptake by GK overexpression results in a direct reduction of glycaemia. As a consequence of lower blood glucose levels, pancreatic β-cell secretes less insulin. Therefore, a decrease in insulinemia is a secondary effect of increasing hepatic GK activity. But, O'Doherty et al demonstrate that the influence of GK activity on blood glucose and insulin levels could be dose-dependent, as it occurs only with high doses of their transgene. In the hepatocyte, glucose-6-phosphate derived from GK activity is directed to glycogen synthesis and, consequently, hepatic glycogen levels are increased in the study by Ferre et al. However, glycogen content is not modified by GK overexpression in the study of O'Doherty et al, maybe for intrinsic limitations. In both animal models, increasing GK activity results in glucose signaling that activates transcription of glycolytic and lipogenic genes. Lipogenic proteins together with high availability of citrate and ATP (derived from augmented glucose metabolism) lead to enhanced *de novo* lipogenesis in the liver, and consequently, higher secretion of VLDL to bloodstream that could explain the observed increase in blood triglycerides. Augmented blood fatty acids might be explained by insulin levels; low levels of this hormone result in low inhibition of lipolysis in the adipose tissue, and consequently fatty acids raise in the bloodstream. Importantly, Ferre et al show that long-term GK overexpression drives to hyperinsulinemia and hepatic steatosis.

b. Studies of GK overexpression in the liver of fasted, healthy mice are listed in Table 3 (Hariharan, 1997; O'Doherty, 1999; Desai, 2001; Ferre, 2003 & Scott, 2003)

Study variables	Hariharan 1997	Desai 2001	Ferre 2003	O'Doherty 1999 Scott 2003
Animal model	M. musculus Transgenic	M. musculus Adenovirus	M. musculus Transgenic	R. norvegicus Adenovirus
Promoter	apoA1-SV40	RSV	PEPCK-C	CMV
GK activity over control	x5	x1.5	x2	x2.1 or x3
Age at analysis	5 weeks	3 weeks post-injection	12 months	4-5 days post-injection
Glycaemia	Decrease	no change	-	no change
Blood lactate	Decrease	no change	-	~ decrease
Blood triglycerides	no change	no change	increase	increase
NEFA	~ increase	no change	-	no change
Insulin	Decrease	decrease	increase	no change
Hepatic glucose-6-P	-	-	~ increase	-
Hepatic glycogen	-	-	no change	increase
Hepatic triglycerides	-	-	increase	-
Modulation of enzymes and transcription factors	-	-	-	↑ L-PK, ACC1 No change: PEPCK-C, PFK-2

Table 3. Hepatic GK overexpression studies in healthy fasted animals. Comments: decrease, increase and no change are referred to control group. "~" means no statistically significant; "-", no determined; "CMV", cytomegalovirus; "RSV", rose sarcoma virus; "apoA1-SV40", apolipoprotein A1 enhancer and simian vacuolating virus 40 promoter; "PEPCK-C", cytosolic phosphoenolpyruvate carboxykinase; "L-PK", liver pyruvate kinase; "ACC1", Acetyl-Coenzyme A carboxylase 1; "PFK-2", 6-phosphofructo-2-kinase/fructose-2,6-bisphosphatase.

In fast state, the influence of hepatic GK overexpression on glycaemia is not clear. Hariharan et al showed a decrease in glycaemia, accompanied by a decrease in insulinemia that could explain a reduction of glycolysis in skeletal muscle, causing the observed decline in serum lactate. Low insulin levels can also explain the increment of blood fatty acids. Interestingly, 20-weeks old mice were smaller than controls and presented reduced body mass index. On the contrary, long-term analysis of transgenic mice developed by Ferre et al showed that increasing GK activity in the liver lead to hepatic steatosis, hyperglycemia, hyperinsulinemia, obesity and insulin resistance. On the other hand, adenoviral gene transfer models for hepatic GK overexpression in fasting revealed induction of lipogenesis and consequently a tendency to increase blood triglycerides, without affecting glycaemia.

c. Studies on hepatic GK overexpression in the context of type 1 diabetes mellitus: This is an autoimmune disease with specific destruction of insulin-producing β-cells in the pancreas, and results in loss of insulin production. As insulin stimulates the transcription of Gck gene in the liver, type 1 diabetic subjects do not have GK protein in their livers and consequently hepatic glucose metabolism is impaired. Gene therapy has been tested to restore liver glucose uptake capacity by increasing hepatic GK protein (Ferre, 1996a; Morral, 2002, 2007). In type 1 diabetic liver, all models present a similar phenotype. When restoring glucose signaling in diabetic hepatocytes via GK, glucose catabolic pathways are induced and, on the contrary, hepatic glucose production is inhibited. Consequently there is a reduction of diabetic hyperglycemia accompanied by incremented hepatic glycogen depots and de novo lipogenesis. Decreasing blood glucose levels forces muscle and adipose tissue to use fatty acids as energetic substrates, and in consequence, serum fatty acids are decreased in type 1 diabetic mice expressing GK in the liver. Lower blood fatty acids, together with increased glucose metabolism in the liver, inhibit hepatic β-oxidation of fatty acids. Therefore, these models suggest that hepatic overexpression of GK in type 1 diabetes leads to normoglycaemia thanks to increments in hepatic glucose uptake and fatty acid oxidation in peripheral tissues.

d. Finally, hepatic GK overexpression in the context of type 2 diabetes: type 2 diabetes is a complex metabolic disorder caused by two physiologic defects: insulin resistance in combination with insulin secretion deficiency. Type 2 diabetes is characterized by glucose metabolism alterations such as failure of insulin to inhibit hepatic gluconeogenesis and impaired skeletal muscle glucose uptake. However, lipid metabolism is also altered. This is often reflected by increased circulating free fatty acids and triglycerides together with increased fat accumulation in non-adipose tissues. Thus, changes in the equilibrium between glucose and fatty acid metabolism in liver and muscle could be responsible for glucose homeostasis alterations. Obesity, hyperinsulinemia, in combination with hyperglycemia, inhibits fatty acid oxidation in many tissues. As a result, lipogenesis is favored over fatty acid oxidation leading to an increase in fat accumulation and a decrease in energy expenditure. A hypothetical strategy for type 2 diabetes therapy is increasing glucokinase activity, with the aim of enhancing glucose uptake in the liver that could contribute to gluconeogenesis inhibition with consequent restoration of glycaemia. If glycaemia is restored, plasma insulin levels could be secondarily lowered and it could be able to elevate energy expenditure and reduce obesity.

However, liver GK activity is increased in mild type 2 diabetes, but diminished in morbid obese diabetic patients. Animal diabetic models linked to obesity, show that GK deficiency in the liver occurs only in the case of obesity, and in severe or long-term forms of the disease. Although hepatic GK expression is different depending on disease stage, some strategies based on increasing GK activity in the liver have been tested in some models of high fat diet induced type 2 diabetes (Desai, 2001 & Ferre, 2003) , in obesity models (Wu, 2005 & Torres, 2009) and in transgenic mice with hepatic insulin resistance (Okamoto, 2007). All these studies have in common that the increase in hepatic GK activity produces glycaemia normalization. Hepatic GK, through glycolysis and glycogenesis activation, increases blood glucose clearance while it inhibits hepatic glucose production. On the other hand, liver GK activity results in increased malonyl-CoA, a lipogenic substrate and inhibitor of β-oxidation. It is difficult to draw clear conclusions when evaluating consequences of liver GK overexpression on lipid metabolism in type 2 diabetic models. Wu et al report an expected increase in hepatic and serum triglycerides, together with higher serum fatty acids. However, Wu et al report that, although hepatic fatty acid β-oxidation was decreased, muscle increased fatty acid oxidation as a consequence of lower glycaemia and insulinemia. Conversely, Desai et al showed no changes in hepatic and serum lipid levels. Otherwise, Torres et al & Okamoto et al obtained an increase in serum triglycerides with no changes in fatty acid levels. The most striking model is presented by Ferre et al: under high fat diet, liver GK-transgenic mice became insulin resistant faster than controls and showed hepatic steatosis. It contrasts with results obtained in GK gene locus transgenic mice (Shiota, 2001). Besides exhibiting a reduction of the blood glucose concentration, mice with a greater than normal amount of GK also exhibited a dramatic resistance to the development of hyperglycemia and hyperinsulinemia normally brought on by consumption of a high fat diet.

Taken together, all these models have convincingly demonstrated that increasing GK protein in the liver leads to a direct reduction of glycaemia, but sometimes it can be accompanied with the risk of serious alterations in lipid metabolism deriving in hepatic steatosis and/or overt dyslipidemia. This aspect is essential when considering the possibility of using GK overexpression in the liver for diabetes therapy. At this point, it would be important to find out which are the causes of the different phenotypes observed in those animal models of hepatic GK overexpression previously described. There are several possible reasons:

a.   Species-specific results: one possibility is that GK overexpression in mouse liver may be more effective stimulating glucose disposal than the same degree of expression in a larger animal such as rat.

b.   Side-effects of gene transfer technology: when using adenoviral gene transfer, adenoviruses involve *per se* hepatic metabolic changes. When using transgenic, germ-line manipulated animals overexpress GK throughout life, including intrauterine life, possibly resulting in compensatory changes in insulin secretion, insulin action, or in other metabolic variables that do not occur with acute manipulation of GK via adenovirus technology.

c.   Promoter that directs transgene expression can affect two important variables. On one hand, taking into account the metabolic hepatic zonation concept (Jungermann, 1995), the promoter determines which set of hepatocytes express the transgene. It is well known that physiological GK expression predominates in the perivenous area of the liver (Moorman, 1991; Jungerman, 1995 & Jungerman, 2000). However, most studies of hepatic GK gain of function did not use perivenous promoters. For instance, Ferre et al used a PEPCK promoter that directs the transgene to the periportal area of the liver, specialized in gluconeogenesis. In contrast, RSV or CMV promoters are ubiquitous promoters that transfect both perivenous and periportal hepatocytes. On the other hand, promoter directs the regulation of transgene expression by nutrients and hormones. For instance, GK under the PEPCK promoter is expressed under glucagon signaling and is inhibited by glucose and insulin. Therefore, hepatic GK transgenic mice described by Ferre et al express GK at the periportal area of the liver during fasting, and not in fed state.

d.   Transgene dose: Desai et al and O'Doherty et al described different metabolic impact of hepatic GK overexpression depending on the dose of transgene that they used.

In our laboratory we aimed to re-examine the conclusions of these studies and the differentiated effects that GK activity could have on the metabolism, clearly differentiated, of periportal and perivenous hepatocytes. To evaluate the issue, we have developed a hydrodynamic gene transfer technique that served us to pursuit GK overexpression studies exclusively in perivenous liver (Liu, 1999; Zhang, 1999; Gomez-Valades, 2006; Budker, 2006 & Suda, 2007). With the injection of a plasmid for green fluorescent protein (GFP) and immunohistochemistry for PEPCK (periportal marker), we could visualize that hydrodynamic injection generate two separate populations of hepatocytes: green hepatocytes that expressed GFP and red hepatocytes showing PEPCK-C staining (Figure 4). We could conclude that in our conditions the hydrodynamic gene transfer technique delivered the transgene only in the hepatocytes surrounding the central vein of the liver acinus.

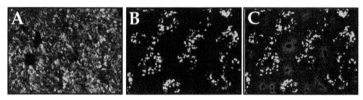

Fig. 4. Visualization of liver transfection achieved with adenoviral and hydrodynamic gene transfer techniques. (A) Healthy mice were injected with 5.5 ·10⁹ IU of an adenovirus that codified for the green fluorescent protein (GFP). Green fluorescence was observed in liver sections (200X), demonstrating a homogeneous presence of the transgene all over the liver acinus. (B) A plasmid for GFP was hydrodynamically injected to healthy mice and, as it can see appreciated in liver sections, resulted in non-homogenous green fluorescence signal. (C) Slices from hydrodynamically-injected mice were immunostained for PEPCK-C (red signal), a periportal marker.

Our results represent the first attempt to overexpress pGK in perivenous hepatocytes. The first approach was the hydrodynamic injection of a plasmid with the Gck gene to healthy mice (Vidal-Alabró; publication pending). Forty-eight hours post-injection, increased GK in perivenous hepatocytes had clear effects on glucose homeostasis (Figure 5A). There was a reduction of glycaemia and insulinemia in the fed state, probably as a direct consequence of increased hepatic glucose uptake. Therefore perivenous GK gain of function reproduced results of periportal GK (Ferre, 1996), and liver-homogeneous GK overexpression (O'Doherty, 1999; Desai, 2001 & Scott, 2003). However, 16 hours-fasted mice did not show differences in blood glucose and insulin levels (data not shown), as Desai et al and O'Doherty et al had obtained with adenoviral GK transfer. Fifty days post-injection, perivenous GK overexpressing-mice presented blood glucose levels similar to control animals but accompanied by hyperinsulinism (Figure 5B). Long-term augmented GK activity in perivenous liver resulted in hepatic insulin resistance, since mice presented a phenotype very similar to liver-specific insulin receptor knock-out mice named LIRKO (Michael, 2000). Briefly, hyperinsulinism was probably due to reduced hepatic insulin clearance. Since peripheral tissues were still insulin-sensitive, hyperinsulinism inhibited lipolysis and induced lipogenesis in adipose tissue. Adipose tissue function together with reduced hepatic lipogenesis *de novo* could explain the observed decrease in circulating triglycerides and free fatty acids. Although having increased GK activity in the liver, neither glycogen synthesis nor glycolysis was stimulated in those mice. Besides, gluconeogenesis was not inhibited in fed state. Therefore, considering the bibliography, our perivenous model resembled transgenic mice that expressed GK transgene under PEPCK-C promoter at periportal hepatocytes (Ferre, 2003). However, periportal GK overexpressing model showed whole-body insulin resistance linked to obesity and hepatic steatosis. It must be considered that their analysis was in 12 months old mice. If the study was extended to 12 months, we would be able to tell if hepatic insulin resistance observed in our mice model leads to general insulin resistance or, on the contrary, confirm its resemblance to LIRKO animals.

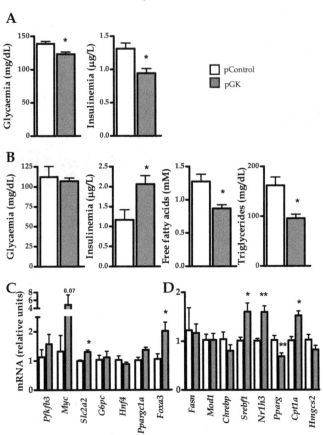

Fig. 5. Analysis of GK-overexpressing healthy mice. (A) Shows glycaemia and insulinemia, 48 hours post-injection of the plasmid that contained the GK gene. Columns represent media ± standard error. (B) 50 days post-injection results on serum nutrients (glucose, free fatty acids and triglycerides) together with insulin levels are represented. (C) After 50 days post-injection, expression of glycolytic and gluconeogenic genes from liver were analyzed by Real-Time PCR. Calculations were done following $\Delta\Delta$Ct algorithm (Applied Biosystems), using β-microglobulin gene expression as a housekeeping gene. (D) The same for lipogenic and lipolysis genes. * $p<0.05$ and ** $p<0.01$ vs control, determined by t-Student.

In the context of type 1 diabetes induced with streptozotocin, perivenous liver GK gain of function restored hepatic glucose uptake and reduced gluconeogenesis. Therefore, typical increases in hepatic glucose depots (glycogen, triglyceride) occurred and resulted in a reduction of diabetic glycaemia, albeit small. But, perivenous GK expressing mice showed a significant increase in triglyceride and free fatty acid serum concentration, and hepatic lipids (Figure 6) (Vidal-Alabró; publication pending). Therefore our work in type 1 diabetes model reproduces those of periportal GK overexpression (Ferre, 1996a) and those of liver homogeneous GK overexpression (Morral, 2002, 2007) in terms of glycaemia. However, our results on lipid metabolism are more deleterious, probably because perivenous hepatocytes have higher lipogenic potential than periportal hepatocytes (Jungermann, 1995).

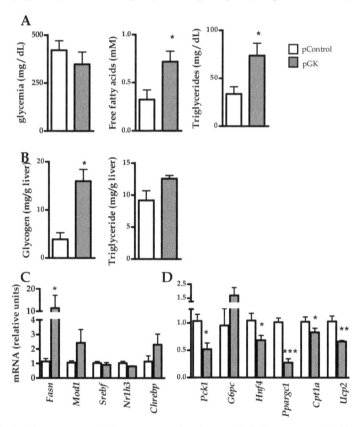

Fig. 6. Analysis of perivenous GK overexpression in type 1 diabetic mice. (A) Shows glycaemia, serum triglycerides and free fatty acids, 48 hours post-injection of the plasmid that contained the GK gene. Columns represent media ± standard error. (B) Hepatic glucose storage was evaluated by measuring glycogen and triglyceride levels. (C) Expression of lipogenic genes in the liver was analyzed by Real-Time PCR. Calculations were done following $\Delta\Delta$Ct algorithm (Applied Biosystems), using β-microglobulin gene expression as a housekeeping gene. (D) The same for gluconeogenic and lipolysis genes. * $p<0.05$, **$p< 0.01$ and *** $p<0.001$ vs control, determined by t-Student.

All in all, our review of the literature together with our own results on the subject will convey that pGK-overexpression in the liver, independent of zonation, will result in changes in glycaemia but with the risk of non-desirable lipid alterations and insulin resistance. However, several undetermined factors influence the results obtained in GK overexpression studies, reinforcing the concept that hepatic GK is a key regulator of whole-body homeostasis, so that little changes in its activity and/or in its regulation affect glucose and lipid metabolism.

4. GKRP modulates the impact of GK activity on glucose and lipid homeostasis

GKRP is the best-known regulator of the hepatic GK at the post-transcriptional level. Therefore, impairments in GKRP should affect GK and consequently glucose metabolism, since GK plays a central role in glucose homeostasis. Nevertheless, mutations in the GKRP gene (Gckr) that caused disease or alterations in glucose metabolism have never been described until now. Recently, several whole-genome analysis have associated polymorphisms in the Gckr gene with fast hypoglycemia and increased serum triglyceride in humans, even though these subjects have reduced risk to type 2 diabetes (Køster, 2005; Sparsø, 2007; Vaxillaire, 2008; Orho-Melander, 2008 & Beer, 2009). The mechanism underlying this phenotype seems to be a reduction in GK inhibition by the variant regulatory protein (Beer, 2009). But, before exploring this issue it should be convenient to consider some aspects of GKRP biology.

Although GKRP research has been focused in the liver, there are evidences that the GKRP protein is also present in hypothalamic neurons (Schuit, 2001; Alvarez, 2002 & Roncero, 2009). GK/GKRP system in the hypothalamus could play a role in glucose-sensing important for the regulation of energy homeostasis by balancing energy intake, expenditure and storage. On the other hand, there is some controversy in the literature as to whether GKRP also regulates GK in pancreatic β-cells. The vast majority of studies state that GKRP is not expressed in rodent β-cells. However, it has been demonstrated that human islets express GKRP at very low levels (Beer, 2009). This issue should be revisited because of the recent publication of several genome-wide association studies that associate GK, GCKR, G6PC2, MTNR1B with type 2 diabetes risk linked to β-cell function (Reiling, 2009 & Bonetti, 2011). Whether, β-cell GK function is affected directly by a hypothetic pancreatic GKRP, or indirectly by liver GKRP impaired activity, still needs clarification. Another question that remains to be resolved is whether GKRP is also expressed and functional in other GK expressing cells, for instance, in the gut and in the pituitary gland.

Consequently, when considering studies of genome-wide association, mutant GKRP protein might affect GK activity in the brain, in the liver and perhaps in the β-cell. Therefore it is difficult to explain the phenotype only taking into account the hepatic GK/GKRP system. The same occurs with the characterization of GKRP-deficient mice (Farrelly, 2002 & Grimsby, 2000). GKRP knock-out mice models, whether heterozygous or homozygous, had normal weight. Interestingly focusing in liver analysis, those mice displayed reduced production of hepatic GK protein while having the same levels of GK mRNA than control animals, and GK protein was localized exclusively in the cytoplasm. That showed the importance of hepatic GKRP in stabilizing and protecting the intracellular GK pool. These animal models exhibited impaired postprandial glycemic control, with lower hepatic glycogen content and lack of inhibition of PEPCK-C gene expression, albeit with no noteworthy loss in insulin secretion or changes in fasting blood glucose concentrations. Moreover, when challenged with a high-sucrose/high-fat diet the knock-out and normal mice gained body weight at a similar rate but the knock-out mice were hyperglycaemic and hyperinsulinemic. Importantly, no changes in plasma triglycerides and non-esterified fatty acids were observed in basal conditions as well as with a high-sucrose/high-fat diet. In summary, absence of GKRP results in decreased hepatic GK protein content, affecting glucose metabolism without disturbing lipid parameters.

On the other hand, GKRP gain of function in the liver has also been assessed. In vitro studies with HepG2 cells simultaneously transduced with an adenoviral vector expressing GKRP and another adenoviral vector for GK had significantly elevated GK protein and activity levels compared with cells transduced with the GK adenovirus alone (Slosberg, 2001). These data suggest that GKRP serves to stabilize and protect a pool of GK protein (i.e., extend half-life), and is consistent with data obtained in GKRP knock-out studies. But in vivo studies revealed a more complicated situation. Adenoviral-mediated hepatic overproduction of GKRP in mice with high-fat diet-induced diabetes resulted in 23% decrease in GK enzymatic activity. Although reduction of GK activity is commonly associated to diabetes, hepatic GKRP-expressing mice had improved fasting and glucose-induced glycaemia with a concomitant increase in insulin sensitivity and TAG levels, and a decrease in leptin levels. A possible explanation for discrepancies between in vivo and in vitro results on GK levels when overexpressing GKRP is that GK expression in vivo is influenced by insulin and other physiological regulators. To understand how decreased GK activity improved type 2 diabetes phenotype in this model, a possibility is that GK activity may be applied in a more efficient manner toward metabolizing blood glucose. The subcellular compartmentalization by scaffolding proteins of enzymes or signaling proteins into clusters is often used as a means of increasing system efficiencies.

Coming back to genome-wide studies that associate Gckr with fast hypoglycemia and high triglycerides, Beer et al reported that P446L-GKRP has reduced regulation by physiological concentrations of fructose-6-phosphate, resulting indirectly in increased GK activity (Beer, 2009). They predicted that this increased GK activity in the liver enhanced glycolytic flux, promoting hepatic glucose metabolism and elevating concentrations of malonyl-CoA, a substrate for *de novo* lipogenesis, providing a mutational mechanism for the reported association of this variant with raised triglycerides and lower glucose levels. However, their predictions are conflictive with in vivo studies by Slosberg et al (Slosberg, 2001), since GKRP gain of function reduced hepatic GK activity and also resulted in a decrease of blood glucose levels accompanied by an increase of blood triglycerides. Therefore, any other undetermined factor/s must exist to really understand the complex physiology of the GK/GKRP system. Another possibility is that brain P446L-GKRP and β-cell P446L-GKRP (if existent) may exert determinant influences on phenotype.

Another study that may bring light to this issue, relates to defects in glucokinase translocation identified in Zucker diabetic fatty (ZDF) (Fujimoto, 2004 & Shin, 2007). Although having normal GK protein content, GK was predominantly localized in the nucleus regardless of plasma glucose and insulin levels. Nevertheless, sorbitol restored GK translocation. Clearly, there must be two distinct mechanisms bringing about the dissociation of GK from GKRP. How they are related and what differentiate them are questions currently under investigation. Since this defect was discovered in early stage of diabetes, it could cause of the progression to diabetes seen in the adult ZDF rat. Consistently, a MODY-2 mutation in the Gck gene has been reported to increase the physical interaction of GK and GKRP (García-Herrero, 2007). But, again these data are in conflict with other studies that reported some new GK mutations causing MODY-2 that reduced GK inhibition by GKRP (Veiga-da-Cunha, 1996; Gloyn, 2005 & Sagen, 2006). Once more, it is difficult to draw conclusions, but the importance of proper GK/GKRP function on metabolism and disease is reinforced, as subtle changes in its activity and/or regulation lead to contrary phenotypes.

Several naturally occurring activating mutations have been described that are localized at the same region where synthetic GK activators bind (Kamata, 2004; Heredia, 2006 & Matschinsky, 2009). Both activating mutations and synthetic activators stabilize the open conformation of the GK protein, resulting in higher affinity for glucose and a reduction of the interaction between GK and GKRP, since the super-open conformation of the enzyme (inactive) is not possible. In humans, activation of GK by naturally occurring mutations is associated to persistent hyperinsulinemic hypoglycemia of the infancy (PHHI), syndrome with a heterogeneous phenotype even in the same family but generally with a normal lipid profile. On the other hand, GK activation through administration of GK activation drugs has been tested for their potential in the therapy of type 2 diabetes, considering principally their capacity to increase glucose-stimulated insulin release at the β-cell (Grimsby, 2003; Brocklehurst, 2004; Efanov, 2005; Leighton, 2005; Coope, 2006 & Matschinsky, 2009). Whole-body effects of glucokinase activator drugs demonstrated a dose-dependent reduction of glycaemia, associated with increased insulin secretion in the pancreas and net glucose uptake in the liver. Besides, the administration of a GK activator prevented the development of diabetes in a diet-induced obesity animal model (Grimsby, 2003). Surprisingly, most in vivo studies with GK activators drugs do not show the lipid profile (Grimsby, 2003; Brocklehurst, 2004; Efanov, 2005; Leighton, 2005 & Coope, 2006), except one where treatment of ob/ob mice with GK activator PSN-GK1 did not produce any significant change blood lipids (Fyfe, 2007).

With all this puzzling background, we intended to study the expression of an activated mutant form of GK with the aim to decipher the metabolic consequences in the liver of having a GK not regulated by GKRP, with theoretical antidiabetic properties. Particularly we proposed the overexpression of glucokinase A456V (identified in patients of persistent hyperinsulinemic hypoglycemia of the infant), with a $S_{0.5}$ for glucose of 3 mM instead of 8 mM for the wild-type enzyme (Christesen, 2002), and without GKRP regulation (Heredia, 2006). We postulated that GK-A456V overexpression (also as a model for the liver-specific consequences of activating drugs on GK) could increase glucose uptake compared with the wild-type enzyme at equal levels of expression, whilst the metabolic fate of glucose might be different from that of wild-type GK due to its different capacity of interaction with other regulating proteins (GKRP and maybe PFK-2).

By means of hydrodynamic gene transfer of an expression plasmid for GK-A456V in healthy mice, we have been able to demonstrate that the perivenous overexpression of GK-A456V results in a sustained improvement in blood glucose, insulinemia and glucose tolerance, in the absence of dyslipidemia or hepatic lipidosis nor long-term insulin resistance (Vidal-Alabró; publication pending). Importantly, GK-A456V protein levels were similar to GK-control group, suggesting GK-A456V stability although not being directly regulated by GKRP. Its mechanism of action could be explained by its lower $S_{0.5}$ for glucose, so that glucose uptake is stimulated in later phases after ingestion (post absorptive phase) and during early fasting. It is tempting to speculate that glucose taken-up in perivenous liver, both in postprandial and post-absorptive periods, could be directed towards the glycolytic and oxidative metabolism and not through the pentose phosphate pathway that would favor lipid biosynthesis. This hypothesis is reinforced by results published by Wu et al (Wu, 2005) in which adenovirus expression of wild-type GK in the liver activate the pentose phosphate pathway, in marked contrast to the overexpression of the kinase domain from PFK-2 that stimulates flux through the glycolytic pathway. Surprisingly, GK-A456V transfected animals showed a marked increase in glucose-6-phosphatase. GK overexpression in perivenous hepatocytes does not significantly affect Glc6Pase expression, suggesting that zonation is an important experimental variable not sufficiently addressed to date in the field.

Transfecting GK-A456V in type 1 diabetic mice induced with streptozotocin, also caused an important reduction of diabetic hyperglycemia without dyslipidemia, in contrast with GK overexpression. Again, an induction of glucose-6-phosphatase transcription was observed in the liver GK-A456V -expressing animals (Figure 7) (Vidal-Alabró; publication pending).

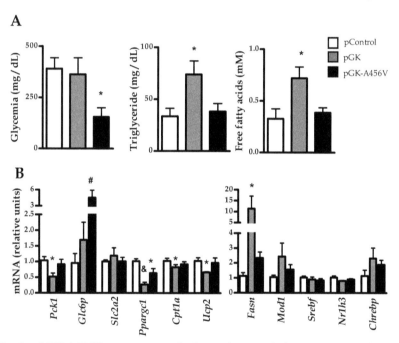

Fig. 7. Study of GK-A456V expression in the liver of type 1 diabetic mice. (A) Shows glycaemia, serum triglyceride and free fatty acid levels, 48 h post-injection of the plasmid for the GK-A456V gene. Columns represent media ± standard error. (B) Expression of gluconeogenic and lipolysis genes from liver was analyzed by Real-Time PCR. Calculations were done following $\Delta\Delta Ct$ algorithm (Applied Biosystems), using β-microglobulin gene expression as a housekeeping gene. (C) The same for lipogenic genes. * $p<0.05$, # $p<0.05$ vs control and pGK, and & $p<0.001$ vs control and $p<0.05$ vs pGK-A456V, as determined by One-way ANOVA.

Our results lead us to consider the physiology of glucose-6-phosphatase in the context of glucose and lipid metabolism. Glucose-6-phosphatase dephosphorylates glucose-6-phosphate in the endoplasmic reticulum to obtain glucose, as the last step in the gluconeogenic pathway. Its transcription is regulated by insulin, so that it is repressed in fed state and induced during fasting. However, glucose induces transcription of this enzyme although the physiological significance of this induction is still not resolved (Nordlie, 2010). Finally glucose-6-phosphatase deficiency causes severe hyperlipidemia and hepatic steatosis (Bandsma, 2002, 2008), therefore giving rise that this enzyme may also participate or influence the GK/GKRP system in the regulation of hepatic glucose fate. To support this hypothesis, Reiling and colleagues described combined effects of single-nucleotide polymorphisms in GK, GKRP and glucose-6-phosphatase on fasting plasma glucose and type 2 diabetes (Reiling, 2009). Therefore, it is a field that needs further exploration.

5. Conclusion

Subtle changes in GK activity or in GKRP function have consequences in glucose and lipid metabolism. However, further studies must be done to completely understand the mechanism underlying GK/GKRP biology. Our results on increasing GK protein in the liver of both healthy and insulin-deficient mice (lacking endogenous GK) resulted in dyslipidemia. On the other hand, our analysis of the metabolic consequences of GK-GKRP deregulation by overexpressing a GK activating mutant (GKA456V) in the liver of both healthy and type 1 diabetic mice demonstrates an impact on glycaemia in the absence of dyslipidemia or hepatic lipid deposition. These data provide novel insights into the capacity of the complex GK-GKRP to influence the fate of metabolized glucose in the liver, providing a framework for further research on GK activating drugs in the liver.

We conclude that GKRP regulation impairment and GK-A456V altered kinetics greatly influence liver metabolism, in line with results in humans carrying a mutant GKRP (Køster, 2005; Sparsø, 2007; Vaxillaire, 2008 & Orho-Melander, 2008). Besides, it suggests that activating GK exclusively in the liver could be a feasible strategy to funnel excess glucose from the diet out of circulation, widening the scope for GK synthetic activators research.

6. Acknowledgments

We thank Sandra M. Ocampo, Francesc X. Blasco and the Research Support Services from the Biology Unit of Bellvitge (University of Barcelona) for their technical assistance, and Dr. Maria Molas for invaluable assistance in reviewing the manuscript. A.V.A received a fellowship from DURSI (Generalitat de Catalunya), A.M.L. received a fellowship from F.P.I. (Ministerio de Educación y Ciencia, Spain). This study was supported by a grant from the Ministerio de Educación y Ciencia (BFU2006-02802 and BFU2009-07506).

7. References

Agius, L. (2008). Glucokinase and molecular aspects of liver glycogen metabolism. *The Biochemical Journal*, Vol.414, No.1, (August 2008), pp. 1-18, ISSN 0264-6021

Alvarez, E., Roncero, I, Chowen, J.A., Vázquez, P. & Blázquez, E. (2002). Evidence that glucokinase regulatory protein is expressed and interacts with glucokinase in rat brain. *Journal of neurochemistry*, Vol. 80, No. 1, (January 2002), pp. 45-53, ISSN 0022-3042

Anderka, O., Boyken, J., Aschenbach, U., Batzer, A., Boscheinen, O. & Schmoll, D. (2008). Biophysical characterization of the interaction between hepatic glucokinase and its regulatory protein. *The Journal of Biological Chemistry*, Vol.283, No. 46, (November 2008), pp. 31333-31340, ISSN 0021-9258

Beer, N.L., Tribble, N.D., McCulloch, L.J., Roos, C., Johnson, P.R., Orho-Melander, M. & Gloyn, A.L. (2009). The P446L variant in GCKR associated with fasting plasma glucose and triglyceride levels exerts its effect through increased glucokinase activity in liver. *Human Molecular Genetics*, Vol 18, No. 21, (November 2009), pp. 4081-4088, ISSN 0964-6906

Bollen, J., Keppens, S. & Stalmans, W. (1998). Specific features of glycogen metabolism in the liver. *The Biochemical Journal*, Vol.336, No.1, (November 1998), pp. 19-31, ISSN 0264-6021

Bonetti, S., Trombetta, M., Boselli, M.L., Turrini, F., Malerba, G., Trabetti, E., Pignatti, P.F., Bonora, E. & Bonadonna, R.C. (2011). Variants of GCKR affect both β-cell and kidney function in patients with newly diagnosed type 2 diabetes: the Verona newly diagnosed type 2 diabetes study 2. *Diabetes care*, Vol. 34, No. 5, (May 2011), pp 1205-1210, ISSN 0149-5992

Brocklehurst, K. J., Payne, V.A., Davies, R.A., Carroll, D., Vertigan, H.L., Wightman, H.J., Aiston, S., Waddell, I.D., Leighton, B., Coghlan, M.P. & Agius, L. (2004). Stimulation of hepatocyte glycose metabolism by a novel small molecule glucokinase activators. *Diabetes*, Vol. 53, No. 3, (March 2004), pp. 535-541, ISSN 0012-1797

Budker, V.G., Subbotin, V.M., Budker, T., Sebestyén, M.G., Zhang, G. & Wolff, J.A. (2006). Mechanism of plasmid delivery by hydrodynamic tail vein injection. II. Morphological studies. *The journal of gene medicine,* Vol. 8, N. 7, (July 2006), pp. 874-888, ISSN 1099-498X

Cha, J.Y. & Repa, J.J. (2007). The liver X receptor (LXR) and hepatic lipogenesis. The carbohydrate-response element-binding protein is a target gene of LXR. *The Biochemical Journal*, Vol.282, No. 1, (January 2007), pp. 743-751, ISSN 0264-6021

Chen, G., Liang, G., Ou, J., Goldstein, J. L. & Brown, M.S. (2004). Central role for liver X receptor in insulin-mediated activation of Srebp-1c transcription and stimulation of fatty acid synthesis in liver. *Proceedings of the National Academy of Sciences,* Vol. 101, No. 31, (August 2004), pp. 11245-11250, ISSN 0027-8424

Christesen, H.B., Jacobsen, B.B., Odili, S., Buettger, C., Cuesta-Munoz, A., Hansen, T., Brusgaard, K., Massa, O., Magnuson, M.A., Shiota, C., Matschinsky, F.M & Barbetti, F. (2002). The second activating glucokinase mutation (A456V): implications for glucose homeostasis and diabetes therapy. *Diabetes,* Vol. 51, No. 4, (April 2002), pp. 1240-1246, ISSN 0012-1797

Coope, G.J., Atkinson, A.M., Allot, C., McKerrecher, D., Johnstone, C., Pike, K.G., Holme, P.C., Vertigan, H., Gill, D., Coghlan, M.P. & Leighton, B. (2006). Predictive blood glucose lowering efficacy by glucokinase activators in high fat fed female Zucher rats. *British Journal of pharmacology*, Vol. 149, No. 3, (October 2006), pp. 328-335, ISSN 0007-1188

Denechaud, P.D., Bossard, P., Lobaccaro, J.A., Millatt, L., Staels, B., Girard, J. & Postic, C. (2008). ChREBP, but not LXRs, is required for the induction of glucose-regulated genes in mouse liver. *The Journal of Clinical Investigation,* Vol. 118, No. 3, (March 2008), pp. 956-964, ISSN 0021-9738

Desai, U.J., Slosberg, E.D., Boettcher, B.R., Caplan, S.L., Fanelli, B., Stephan, Z., Gunther, V.J, Kaleko, M. & Connelly, S. (2001). Phenotypic correction of diabetic mice by adenovirus-mediated glucokinase expression. *Diabetes*, Vol. 50, No. 10, (October 2001), pp. 2287-2295, ISBN 0012-1797

Efanov, A.M., Barrett, D.G., Brenner, M.B., Briggs, S.L., Delaunois, A., Durbin, J.D., Giese, U., Guo, H., Radloff, M., Gil, G.S., Sewing, S., Wang, Y., Weixhert, A., Zaliani, A. & Gromada, J. (2005). A novel glucokinase activator modulates pancreatic islet and hepatocyte function. *Endocrinology*, Vol. 146, No. 9, (September 2005), pp. 3696-3701, ISSN 0013-7227

Farrely, D., (1999). Mice mutant for glucokinase regulatory protein exhibit decreased liver glucokinase: a sequestration mechanism in metabolic regulation. *Proceedings of the National Academy of Sciences*, Vol. 96, No. 25, (December 1999), pp. 14511-14516, ISSN 0027-8424

Ferre, P. & Foufelle, F. (2010). Hepatic steatosis: a role for *de novo* lipogenesis and the transcription factor SREBP-1c. *Diabetes, Obesity and Metabolism*, Vol.12, (October 2010), pp. 83-92, ISSN 1462-8902

Ferre, T., Pujol, A., Riu, E., Bosch, F. & Valera, A. (1996a). Correction of diabetic alterations by glucokinase. *Proceedings of the National Academy of Sciences*, Vol. 93, No. 14, (July 1996), pp. 7225-7230, ISSN 0027-8424

Ferre, T., Riu, E., Bosch, F.& Valera, A. (1996b). Evidence from transgenic mice that glucokinase is rate limiting for glucose utilization in the liver. *The FASEB Journal*, Vol. 10, No. 10, (August 1996), pp. 1213-1218, ISSN 0892-6638

Ferre, T., Riu, E., Franckhauser, S., Agudo, J & Bosch, F. (2003). Long-term overexpression of glucokinase in the liver of transgenic mice leads to insulin resistance. *Diabetologia*, Vol. 46, No. 12, (December, 2003), pp. 1662-1668, ISSN 0012-186X

Foretz, M., Guichard, C., Ferre, P. & Foufelle, F. (1999). Sterol regulatory element binding protein-1c is a major mediator of insulin action on the hepatic expression of glucokinase and lipogenesis-related genes. *Proceedings of the National Academy of Sciences*, Vol. 96, No. 22, (October 1999), pp. 12737-12742, ISSN 0027-8424

Fujimoto, Y., Donahue, E. D. & Shiota, M. (2004). Defect in glucokinase translocation in Zucher diabetic fatty rats. *American Journal of Physiology. Endocrinology and Metabolism*, Vol. 287, No. 3, (September 2004), pp. E414-E423, ISSN 0193-1849

Fyfe, M.C., White, J.R., Taylor, A., Chatfield, R., Wargent, E., Printz, R.L., Suplice, T., McCormack, J.G., Procter, M.J., Teynet, C., Widdowson, P.S. & Wong-Kai-In, P. (2007). Glucokinase activator PSN-GK1 displays enhanced antihyperglycaemic and insulinotropic actions. *Diabetologia*, Vol. 50, No. 6, (June 2007) pp. 1277-1287, ISSN 0012-186X

García-Herrero, C.M., Galán, M., Vincent, O., Flández, B., Gargallo, M., Delgado-Alvarez, E., Blázquez, E. & Navas, M.A. (2007). Functional analysis of human glucokinase gene mutations causing MODY2: exploring the regulatory mechanisms of glucokinase activity. *Diabetologia*, Vol. 50, No. 2, (February 2007), pp. 325-333, ISSN 0012-186X

Gavrilova, O., Haluzik, M., Matsuse, K., Custon, J.J., Johnson, L., Dietz, K.R., Nicol, C.J., Vinson, C., Gonzalez, F.J. & Reitman, M.L. (2003). Liver peroxisome proliferator-activated receptor gamma contributes to hepatic steatosis, triglyceride clearance, and regulation of body fat mass. *The Journal of Biological Chemistry*, Vol.278, No. 36, (September 2003), pp. 34268-34276, ISSN 0021-9258.

Ginsberg, H.N., Zhang,Y., Hernandez-Ono, A. (2006). Metabolic Syndrome: Focus on Dyslipidemia. *Obesity*, Vol.14, Suppl.1, (February 2006), pp. 41S-49S, ISSN 1930-7381.

Gloyn, A.L. (2003). Glucokinase (GCK) mutations in hyper- and hypoglycemia: maturity-onset diabetes of the young, permanent neonatal diabetes, and hyperinsulinemia of infancy. *Human mutation*, Vol. 22, No. 5, (November 2003), pp. 353-362, ISSN 1059-7794

Gloyn, A.L., Odili, S., Zelent, D., Buettger, C., Castleden, H.A., Steele, A. M., Stride, A., Shiota, C., Magnuson, M.A., Lorini, R., d'Annunzio, G., Stanley, C.A., Kwagh, J., van Schaftingen E., Veiga-da-Cunha, M., Barbetti, F., Dunten, P., Han, Y., Grimsby, J., Taub, R., Ellard, S., Hattersley, A. T.& Matschinsky, F.M. (2005). Insights into the structure and regulation of glucokinase from a novel mutation (V62M), which causes maturity-onset diabetes of the young. *The Journal of Biological Chemistry*, Vol. 280, No. 14, (April 2005), pp 14105-14113, ISSN 0021-9258

Gómez-Valadés, A. G., Vidal-Alabro, A., Molas, M., Boada, J., Bermúdez, J., Bartrons, R. & Perales, J.C. (2006). Overcoming diabetes-induced hyperglycemia through inhibition of hepatic phosphoenolpyruvate carboxykinase (GTP) with RNAi. *Molecular Therapy*, Vol. 13, No. 2; (February 2006), pp. 401-410, ISSN 1525-0016

Gregori, C., Guillet-Deniau, I., Girard, J., Decaux, J.F. & Pichard, A.L. (2006). Insulin regulation of glucokinase gene expression: evidence against a role for sterol regulatory element binding protein 1 in primary hepatocytes. *FEBS Letters*, Vol. 580, No. 2, (January 2006), pp. 410-414, ISSN 0014-5793

Grimsby, J., Coffey, J.W., Dvorozniak, M.T., Magram, J., Li, G., Matschinsky, F.M., Shiota, C., Kaur, S., Magnuson, M.A. & Grippo, J.F. (2000). Characterization of glucokinase regulatory protein-deficient mice. *The Journal of biological chemistry*, Vol. 275, No. 11, (March 2000), pp. 7826-7831, ISSN 0021-9258

Grimsby, J., Sarabu, R., Corbett, W.L., Haynes, N.E., Bizzarro, F.T., Coffey, J.W., Guertin, K.R., Hilliard, D.W., Kester, R.F., Mahaney, P.E., Marcus, L., Qi, L., Spence, C.L., Tengi, J., Magnuson, M.A., Chu, C.A., Dvorozniak, M.T., Matschinsky, F.M. & Grippo, J.F. (2003). Allosteric activators of glucokinase: potential role in diabetes therapy. *Science*, Vol. 301, No. 5631, (July 2003), pp. 370-373, ISSN 0036-8075

Hariharan, N., Farrelly, D., Hagan, D., Hillyer, D., Arbeeny, C., Sabrah, T., Treloar, A., Brown, K., Kalinowski, S. & Mookhtiar, K. (1997). Expression of human hepatic glucokinase in transgenic mice liver results in decreased glucose levels and reduced body weight. *Diabetes*, Vol. 46, No. 1, (January 1997), pp. 11-16, ISSN 0012-1797

Heredia, V.V., Carlson, T.J, Garcia, E. & Sun, S. (2006). Biochemical basis of glucokinase activation and the regulation by glucokinase regulatory protein in naturally occurring mutations. *The Journal of biolobical chemistry*, Vol. 281, No. 52, (December 2006), pp. 40201-40207, ISSN 0021-9258

Iizuka, K. & Horikawa, Y. (2008). ChREBP: A Glucose-activated Transcription Factor Involved in the Development of Metabolic Syndrome. *Endocrine Journal*. Vol. 55, No. 4, (August 2008), pp. 617-624, ISSN 0918-8959

Iynedjian, P.B., (2009). Molecular physiology of mammalian glucokinase. *Cellular and Molecular Life Sciences*, Vol. 66, No. 1, (January 2009), pp. 27-42, ISSN 1420-682X

Jungermann, K., (1995). Zonation of metabolism and gene expression in liver. *Histochemistry and cell biology*, Vol. 103, No. 2,(February 1995), pp. 81-91, ISSN 0948-6143

Jungermann, K. & Kietzmann, T. (2000). Oxygen: modulator of metabolic zonation and disease of the liver. *Hepatology*, Vol. 31, No. 2, (February 2000), pp. 255-260, ISSN 0270-9139

Kabashima, T., Kawaguchi, T., Wadzinski, B.E. & Uyeda, K. (2003). Xylulose-5-phosphate mediates glucose-induced lipogenesis by xylulose-5-phosphate-activated protein phosphatase in rat liver. *Proceedings of the National Academy of Sciences*, Vol. 100, No. 9, (April, 2003), pp. 5107-5112, ISSN 0027-8424

Kamata, K., Mitsuya, M., Nishimura, T., Eiki, J. & Nagata, Y. (2004). Structural basis for allosteric regulation of the monomeric allosteric enzyme human glucokinase. *Structure*, Vol. 12, No. 3, (March 2004), pp. 429-438, ISSN 0969-2126

Køster, B., Fenger, M., Poulsen, P., Vaag, A. & Bentzen, J. (2005). Novel polymorphisms in the GCKR gene and their influence on glucose and insulin levels in a Danish twin population. *Diabetic medicine: a journal of the British Diabetic Association*, Vol. 22; No. 12 (December 2005), ISSN 0742-3071

Lee, A., Scappa, E.F., Cohen, D.E. & Glimcher, L.H. (2008) Regulation of Hepatic Lipogenesis by the Transcription Factor XBP1. *Science*, Vol. 320, No. 5882, (June 2008), pp. 1492-1496, ISSN 0036-8075

Leighton, B., Atkinson, A. & Coghlan, M.P., (2005). Small molecule glucokinase activators as novel anti-diabetic agents. *Biochemical Society transactions*, Vol. 33, No. Pt 2, (April 2005), pp. 371-374, ISSN 0300-5127

Liu, F., Song, Y. & Liu, D. (1999). Hydrodynamics-based transfection in animals by systemic administration of plasmid DNA. *Gene Therapy*, Vol. 6, No. 7, (July 1999), pp. 1258-1266, ISSN 0969-7128

Massa, M.L., Gagliardino, J.J. & Francini, F. (2011). Liver glucokinase: an overview on the regulatory mechanisms of its activity. *IUBMB Life*, Vol. 63, No. 1, (January 2011), pp. 1-6, ISSN 1521-6543

Massillon, D., Chen, W., Barzilai, N., Prus-Wertheimer, D., Hawkins, M., Liu, R., Taub, R. & Rossetti, L. (1998). Carbon flux via the pentose phosphate pathway regulates the hepatic expression of the glucose-6-phosphatase and phosphoenolpyruvate carbokykinase genes in conscious rats. *The Journal of Biological Chemistry*, Vol.273, No. 1, (January 1998), pp. 228-234, ISSN 0021-9258.

Matschinsky, F.M. Assessing the potential of glucokinase activators in diabetes therapy. *Nature reviews. Drug discovery*, Vol 8, No. 5, (May 2009), pp. 399-416, ISSN 1474-1776

Michael, M.D., Kulkarni, R.N., Postic, C., Previs, S.F., Shulman, G.I., Magnuson, M.A. & Kahn, C.R. (2000). Loss of insulin signaling in hepatocytes leads to severe insulin resistance and progressive hepatic dysfunction. *Molecular Cell*, Vol. 6, No. 1, (July 2000), pp. 87-97, ISSN 1097-2765

Mitro, N., Mak, P.A., Vargas, L., Godio, C., Hampton, E., Molteni, V., Kreusch, A. & Saez, E. (2007). The nuclear receptor LXR is a glucose sensor. *Nature*, Vol. 445, (January 2007), pp. 219-223, ISSN 0028-0836

Moorman, A.F., de Boer, P.A., Charles, R. & Lamers, W.H. (1991). Pericentral expression pattern of glucokinase mRNA in the rat liver lobulus. *FEBS letters*, Vol. 287, No. 1-2, (August 1991), pp. 47-52, ISSN 0014-5793

Morral, N., McEvoy, R., Dong, H., Meseck, M., Altomonte, J., Thung, S. & Woo, S.L. (2002). Adenovirus-mediated expression of glucokinase in the liver as an adjuvant treatment for type 1 diabetes. *Human gene therapy*, Vol. 13; No. 13, (September 2002), pp. 1561-1570, ISSN 1043-0342

Morral, N., Edenberg, H.J., Witting, S.R., Altomonte, J., Chu, T. & Brown, M. (2007). Effects of glucose metabolism on the regulation of genes of fatty acid synthesis and triglyceride secretion in the liver. *Journal of lipid research*, Vol. 48, No. 7, (July 2007), pp. 1499-1510, ISSN 0022-2275

Nordlie, R.C. & Foster, J.D. (2010). A retrospective review of the roles of multifunctional glucose-6-phosphatase in blood glucose homeostasis: Genesis of the tuning/retuning hypothesis. *Life sciences*, Vol. 87, No. 11-12, (September 2010), pp. 339-349, ISSN 0024-3205

O'Doherty, R.M., Lehman, D.L., Télémaque-Potts, S. & Newgard, C.B. (1999). Metabolic impact of glucokinase overexpression in liver: lowering of blood glucose in fed rats is accompanied by hyperlipidemia. *Diabetes*, Vol. 48, No. 10, (October, 1999), pp. 2022-2027, ISSN 0012-1797

Okamoto, Y., Ogawa, W., Nishizawa, A., Inoue, H., Teshigawara, K., Kinoshita, S., Matsuki, Y., Watanabe, E., Hiramatsu, R., Sakaue, H., Noda, T. & Kasuga, M. (2007). Restoration of glucokinase expression in the liver normalizes postprandial glucose disposal in mice with hepatic deficiency of PDK1. *Diabetes*, Vol. 56, No. 4, (April 2007), pp. 1000-1009, ISSN 0012-1797

Orho-Melander, M., Melander, O., Guiducci, C., Perez-Martinez, P., Corella, D., Roos, C., Tewhey, R., Rieder, M.J., Hall, J., Abecasis, G., Tai, E.S., Welch, C., Arnett, D.K., Lyssenko, V., Lindholm, E., Saxena, R., de Bakker, P.I., Burtt, N., Voight, B.F., Hirschhorn, J.N., Tucker, K.L., Hedner, T., Tuomi, T., Isomaa, B., Eriksson, K.F., Taskinen, M.R., Wahlstrand, B., Hughes, T.E., Parnell, L.D., Lai, C.Q., Berglund, G., Peltonen, L., Vartiainen, E., Jousilahti, P., Havulinna, A.S., Salomaa, V., Nilsson, P., Groop, L., Altshuler, D., Ordovas, J.M. & Kathiresan, S. (2008). Common missense variant in the glucokinase regulatory protein gene is associated with increased plasma triglyceride and C-reactive protein but lower fasting glucose concentrations. *Diabetes*, Vol. 57, No. 11, (November 2008), pp. 3112-3121, ISSN 0012-1797

Osbak, K.K., Colclough, K., Saint-Martin, C., Beer, N.L., Bellanné-Chantelot, C., Ellard, S. & Gloyn, A.L. (2009). Update on mutations in glucokinase (GCK), which cause maturity-onset diabetes of the young, permanent neonatal diabetes, and hyperinsulinemic hypoglycemia. *Human mutation*, Vol. 30, No. 11, (November, 2009), pp. 1512-1526, ISSN 1059-7794

Postic, C., Niswender, K.D., Decaux, J.F., Parsa, R., Shelton, K.D., Gouhot, B., Pettepher, C.C., Granner, D.K., Girard, J. & Magnuson, M.A. (1995). *Genomics*, Vol. 29, No. 3, (October 1995), pp. 740-750, ISSN 0888-7543

Postic, C., Shiota, M., Niswender, K.D., Jetton, T.L., Chen, Y., Moates, J.M., Shelton, K.D., Lindner, J., Cherrington, A.D. & Magnuson, M.A. (1999) Dual roles for glucokinase in glucose homeostasis as determined by liver and pancreatic beta cell-specific gene knock-outs using Cre recombinase. *The Journal of Biological Chemistry*, Vol.274, No. 1, (January 1999), pp. 305-315, ISSN 0021-9258.

Puigserver, P., (2003). Insulin-regulated hepatic gluconeogenesis through FOXO1-PGC-1alpha interaction. *Nature,* Vol. 423, (May 2003), pp. 550-555, ISSN 0028-0836

Reiling, E., van't Riet, E., Groenewould, M.J., Welschen, L.M., van Hove, E.C., Nijpels, G., Maassen, J.A., Dekker, J.M. & 't Hart, L.M. (2009). Combined effects of single-nucleotide polymorphisms in GCK, GCKR, G6PC2 and MTNR1B on fasting plasma glucose and type 2 diabetes risk. *Diabetologia,* Vol. 52, No. 9, (September 2009) pp. 1866-1870, ISSN 0012-186X

Roncero, I., Sanz, C., Alvarez, E., Vázquez, P., Barrio, P.A. & Blázquez, E. (2009). Glucokinase and glucokinase regulatory proteins are functionally coexpressed before birth in the rat brain. *Journal of Neuroendocrinology,* Vol. 21; No. 12, (December 2009), pp. 973-981, ISSN 0953-8194

Roth, U., Curth, K., Unterman, T.G., & Kietzmann, T. (2004). The transcription factors HIF-1 and HNF-4 and the coactivator p300 are involved in insulin-regulated glucokinase gene expression via the phosphatidylinositol 3-kinase/ protein Kinase B pathway. *The Journal of Biological Chemistry,* Vol.279, No. 4, (January 2004), pp. 2623-2631, ISSN 0021-9258.

Sagen, J.V., Odili, S., Bjørkhaug, L., Zelent, D., Buettger, C., Kwagh, J., Stanley, C., Dahl-Jørgensen, K., de Beaufort, C., Bell, G.I., Han, Y., Grimsby, J., Taub, R., Molven, A., Søvik, O., Njølstad, P.R. & Matschinsky, F.M. (2006). From clinicogenetic studies of maturity-onset diabetes of the young to unravelling complex mechanisms of glucokinase regulation. *Diabetes,* Vol. 55, No. 6, (June 2006), pp. 1713-1722, ISSN 0012-1797

Schuit, F.S., Huypens, P., Heimberg, H. & Pipeleers, D.G. (2001). Glucose Sensing in Pancreatic β-Cells. A Model for the Study of Other Glucose-Regulated Cells in Gut, Pancreas, and Hypothalamus. *Diabetes,* Vol. 50, No. 1, (January 2001), pp. 1-11, ISSN 0012-1797

Scott, D.K., Collier, J.J., Doan, T.T., Bunnell, A.S., Daniels, M.C., Eckert, D.T. & O'Doherty, R.M. *Molecular and cellular biochemistry,*Vol. 254, No. 1-2, (December 2003), pp. 327-337, ISSN 0300-8177

Shimomura, I., Shimano, H., Korn, B.S., Bashmakow, Y., & Horton, J.D. (1998). Nuclear sterol regulatory element-binding proteins activate genes responsible for the entire program o unsaturated fatty acid biosynthesis in transgenic mouse liver. *The Journal of Biological Chemistry,* Vol.273, No. 52, (December 1998), pp. 35299-35306, ISSN 0021-9258.

Shin, J.S., Torres, T.P., Catlin, R.L., Donahue, E.P. & Shiota, M. (2007). A defect in glucose-induced dissociation of glucokinase from the regulatory protein in Zucker diabetic fatty rats in the early stage of diabetes. *American Journal of Phisiology. Regulatory, integrative and comparative physiology.* Vol. 292, No. 4, (April 2007), pp. R1381-R1390, ISSN 0363-6119

Shiota, C., Coffey, J., Grimbsy, J., Grippo, J.F. & Magnuson, M.A. (1999). Nuclear import of hepatic glucokinase depends upon glucokinase regulatory protein, whereas export is due to a nuclear export signal sequence in glucokinase. *The Journal of Biological Chemistry,* Vol. 274, No. 52, (December 1999), pp. 37125-37130, ISSN 0021-9258.

Shiota, M., Postic, C., Fujimoto, Y., Jetton, T.L., Dixon, K., Pan, D., Grimsby, J., Grippo, J.F., Magnuson, M.A. & Cherrington, A.D. (2001). Glucokinase gene locus transgenic mice are resistant to the development of obesity-induced type 2 diabetes. *Diabetes*, Vol. 50, No. 3, (March 2001), pp. 622-629, ISSN 0012-1797

Slosberg, E.D., Desai, U.J., Fanelli, B., St. Denny, I., Connelly, S., Kaleko, M., Boettcher, B.R. & Caplan, S.L. (2001). Treatment of type 2 diabetes by adenoviral-mediated overexpression of the glucokinase regulatory protein. *Diabetes*, Vol. 50, No. 8, (August 2001), pp. 1813-1820, ISSN 0012-1797

Sparsø, T., Andersen, G., Nielsen, T., Burgdorf, K.S., Gjesing, A.P., Nielsen, A.L., Albrechtsen, A., Rasmussen, S.S., Jørgensen, T., Borch-Johnsen, K., Sandbæk, A., Lauritzen, T., Madsbad, S., Hansen, T. & Pedersen, O. (2008). The GCKR rs780094 polymorphism is associated with elevated fasting serum triacylglycerol, reduced fasting and OGTT-related insulinaemia, and reduced risk of type 2 diabetes. *Diabetologia*, Vol. 51, No. 1, (January 2008), pp. 70-75, ISSN 0012-186X

Suda, T., Gao, X., Stolz, D.B. & Liu, D. (2007). Structural impact of hydrodynamic injection on mouse liver. *Gene Therapy*, Vol. 14, No. 2, (January 2007), pp. 129-137, ISSN 0969-7128

Torres, T.P., Catlin, R.L., Chan, R., Fujimoto, Y., Sasaki, N., Printz, R.L., Newgard, C.B. & Shiota, M. (2009). Restoration of hepatic glucokinase expression corrects hepatic glucose flux and normalizes plasma glucose in zucker diabetic fatty rats. *Diabetes*, Vol. 58, No. 1, (January 2009), pp. 78-86, ISSN 0012-1797

Uyeda, K. & Repa, J.J. (2006). Carbohydrate response element binding protein, ChREBP, a transcription factor coupling hepatic glucose utilization and lipid synthesis. *Cell Metabolism*, Vol. 4, No. 2, (August 2006), pp. 107-110, ISSN 1550-4131

Van Shaftingen, E. & Veiga da Cunha, M. (2004). Discovery and role of glucokinase regulatory protein, In: *Glucokinase and Glycemic Disease: From Basics to Novel Therapeutics*, Matschinsky, F.M., Magnuson, M.A. (eds), pp. 193-207, Karger, ISBN 3-8055-7744-3, Basel (Switzerland)

Vaxillaire, M., Cavalcanti-Proença, C., Dechaume, A., Tichet, J., Marre, M., Balkau, B. & Froguel, P., for the DESIR Study Group (2008). The common P446L polymorphism in GCKR inversely modulates fasting glucose and triglyceride levels and reduces type 2 diabetes risk in the DESIR prospective general French population. *Diabetes*, Vol. 57, No. 8, (August 2008), pp. 2253-2257, ISSN 0012-1797

Veiga-da-Cunha, M., Xu, L.Z., Lee, Y.H., Marotta, D., Pilkis, S.J. & Van Schaftingen, E. (1996). Effect of mutations on the sensitivity of human beta-cell glucokinase to liver regulatory protein. *Diabetologia*, Vol. 39, No. 10, (October 1996), pp. 1173-1179, ISSN 0012-186X

Vieira, E., Salehi, A & Gylfe, E. (2007). Glucose inhibits glucagon secretion by a direct effect on mouse pancreatic alpha cells. *Diabetologia*, Vol. 50. No. 2, (February 2007), pp. 370-379, ISSN 0012-186X

Wang, X., Sato, R., Brown, MS., Hua, X. & Goldstein, JL. (1994). SREBP-1, a membrane-bound transcription factor released by sterol-regulated proteolysis. *Cell*, Vol. 77, No.1, (April 1994), pp. 53-62, ISSN 0092-8674.

Wu, C., Okar, D.A., Newgard, C.B. & Lange, A.J. (2001) Overexpression of 6-phosphofructo-2-kinase/fructose-2,6-bisphosphatase in mouse liver lowers blood glucose by suppressing hepatic glucose production. *The Journal of Clinical Investigation*, Vol. 107, No. 1, (January 2001), pp. 91-98, ISSN 0021-9738

Wu, C., Kang, J.E., Peng, L.J., Li, H., Khan, S.A., Hillard, C.J., Okar, D.A. & Lange, A.J. (2005) Enhancing hepatic glycolysis reduces obesity: differential effects on lipogenesis depend on site of glycolytic modulation. *Cell Metabolism*, Vol. 2, No. 2, (August 2005), pp. 131-140, ISSN 1550-4131

Zelent, D., Golson, M.L., Koeberlein, B., Quintens, R., van Lommel, L., Buettger, C., Weik-Collins, H., Taub, R., Grimsby, J., Schuit, F., Kaestner, K.H. & Matschinsky, F.M. (2006). A Glucose Sensor Role for Glucokinase in Anterior Pituitary Cells. *Diabetes*, Vol. 55, (July 2006), pp. 1923-1929, ISSN 0012-1797

Zhang, G., Budker, V. & Wolff, J.A. (1999). High levels of foreign gene expression in hepatocytes after tail vein injections of naked plasmid DNA. *Human Gene Therapy*, Vol. 10, No. 10, (July 1999), pp. 1735-1737, ISSN 1043-0342

Zhu, L.L., Liu, Y., Cui, A.F., Shao, D., Liang, J.C., Liu, X.J., Chen, Y., Gupta, N., Fang, F.D., & Chang, Y.S. (2010). PGC-1alpha coactivates estrogen-related receptor-alpha to induce the expression of glucokinase. *American Journal of Physiology. Endocrinology and metabolism*. Vol 298. No. 6, (June 2010), pp.E1210-8, ISSN 0193-1849

Permissions

The contributors of this book come from diverse backgrounds, making this book a truly international effort. This book will bring forth new frontiers with its revolutionizing research information and detailed analysis of the nascent developments around the world.

We would like to thank Prof. Roya Kelishadi, for lending her expertise to make the book truly unique. She has played a crucial role in the development of this book. Without her invaluable contribution this book wouldn't have been possible. She has made vital efforts to compile up to date information on the varied aspects of this subject to make this book a valuable addition to the collection of many professionals and students.

This book was conceptualized with the vision of imparting up-to-date information and advanced data in this field. To ensure the same, a matchless editorial board was set up. Every individual on the board went through rigorous rounds of assessment to prove their worth. After which they invested a large part of their time researching and compiling the most relevant data for our readers. Conferences and sessions were held from time to time between the editorial board and the contributing authors to present the data in the most comprehensible form. The editorial team has worked tirelessly to provide valuable and valid information to help people across the globe.

Every chapter published in this book has been scrutinized by our experts. Their significance has been extensively debated. The topics covered herein carry significant findings which will fuel the growth of the discipline. They may even be implemented as practical applications or may be referred to as a beginning point for another development. Chapters in this book were first published by InTech; hereby published with permission under the Creative Commons Attribution License or equivalent.

The editorial board has been involved in producing this book since its inception. They have spent rigorous hours researching and exploring the diverse topics which have resulted in the successful publishing of this book. They have passed on their knowledge of decades through this book. To expedite this challenging task, the publisher supported the team at every step. A small team of assistant editors was also appointed to further simplify the editing procedure and attain best results for the readers.

Our editorial team has been hand-picked from every corner of the world. Their multi-ethnicity adds dynamic inputs to the discussions which result in innovative outcomes. These outcomes are then further discussed with the researchers and contributors who give their valuable feedback and opinion regarding the same. The feedback is then collaborated with the researches and they are edited in a comprehensive manner to aid the understanding of the subject.

Apart from the editorial board, the designing team has also invested a significant amount of their time in understanding the subject and creating the most relevant covers. They scrutinized every image to scout for the most suitable representation of the subject and create an appropriate cover for the book.

The publishing team has been involved in this book since its early stages. They were actively engaged in every process, be it collecting the data, connecting with the contributors or procuring relevant information. The team has been an ardent support to the editorial, designing and production team. Their endless efforts to recruit the best for this project, has resulted in the accomplishment of this book. They are a veteran in the field of academics and their pool of knowledge is as vast as their experience in printing. Their expertise and guidance has proved useful at every step. Their uncompromising quality standards have made this book an exceptional effort. Their encouragement from time to time has been an inspiration for everyone.

The publisher and the editorial board hope that this book will prove to be a valuable piece of knowledge for researchers, students, practitioners and scholars across the globe.

List of Contributors

Annamaria Fulghesu and Roberta Magnini
Department of Obstetrics and Gynecology, University of Cagliari, Cagliari, Italy

Maryam Shalileh
Islamic Azad University of Hamedan Branch, Iran

Lei Zhang and Qing Qiao
Hjelt Institute, University of Helsinki, Helsinki, Finland

Lei Zhang and Yanhu Dong
Qingdao Endocrine & Diabetes Hospital, Qingdao, China
Weifang Medical University, Weifang, China

Lei Zhang and Qing Qiao
National Institute for Health and Welfare, Helsinki, Finland

Hasniza Zaman Huri
Department of Pharmacy, Faculty of Medicine, University of Malaya, Kuala Lumpur, Malaysia

Nora L. Nock and Aiswarya L.P. Chandran Pillai
Case Western Reserve University, USA

Roya Kelishadi
Faculty of Medicine & Child Health Promotion Research Center, Isfahan University of Medical Sciences, Isfahan, Iran

Parinaz Poursafa
Environment Research Center, Isfahan University of Medical Sciences, Isfahan, Iran

Hiroshi Koriyama, Hironori Nakagami, Tomohiro Katsuya and Ryuichi Morishita
Osaka University, Japan

Jozef Ukropec and Barbara Ukropcova
Institute of Experimental Endocrinology Slovak Academy of Sciences, Slovakia

Barbara Ukropcova
Institute of Pathological Physiology, Faculty of Medicine Comenius University, Slovakia

Patricia Aspichueta, Nerea Bartolomé, Xabier Buqué, María José Martínez, Begoña Ochoa and Yolanda Chico
Department of Physiology, Faculty of Medicine, University of the Basque Country, Spain

Vassilis Zannis, Andreas Kateifides, Panagiotis Fotakis and Eleni Zanni
Molecular Genetics, Boston University School of Medicine Boston, MA, USA

Vassilis Zannis, Andreas Kateifides, Panagiotis Fotakis and Dimitris Kardassis
University of Crete Medical School, Greece, Greece

Emma Barroso, Lucía Serrano-Marco, Laia Salvadó, Xavier Palomer and Manuel Vázquez-Carrera
Department of Pharmacology and Therapeutic Chemistry, Spanish Biomedical Research Centre in Diabetes and Associated Metabolic, Disorders(CIBERDEM)-Instituto de SaludCarlos III and IBUB, (Biomedicine Institute of the University of Barcelona), Faculty of Pharmacy, University of Barcelona, Barcelona, Spain

Anna Vidal-Alabró, Andrés Méndez-Lucas, Jana Semakova, Alícia G. Gómez-Valadés and Jose C. Perales
Department of Physiological Sciences II, University of Barcelona, Barcelona, Spain